Enhancing the Quality of Life of People with Intellectual Disabilities

Social Indicators Research Series

Volume 41

This new series aims to provide a public forum for single treatises and collections of papers on social indicators research that are too long to be published in our journal Social Indicators Research. Like the journal, the book series deals with statistical assessments of the quality of life from a broad perspective. It welcomes the research on a wide variety of substantive areas, including health, crime, housing, education, family life, leisure activities, transportation, mobility, economics, work, religion and environmental issues. These areas of research will focus on the impact of key issues such as health on the overall quality of life and vice versa. An international review board, consisting of Ruut Veenhoven, Joachim Vogel, Ed Diener, Torbjorn Moum, Mirjam A.G. Sprangers and Wolfgang Glatzer, will ensure the high quality of the series as a whole.

For futher volumes:
http://www.springer.com/series/6548

Ralph Kober
Editor

Enhancing the Quality of Life of People with Intellectual Disabilities

From Theory to Practice

Springer

Editor
Associate Prof. Ralph Kober
Department of Accounting and Finance
Monash University
Caulfield East
VIC 3145
Australia
ralph.kober@monash.edu

ISSN 1387-6570
ISBN 978-90-481-9649-4 e-ISBN 978-90-481-9650-0
DOI 10.1007/978-90-481-9650-0
Springer Dordrecht Heidelberg London New York

Library of Congress Control Number: 2010933253

Printed on acid-free paper

Springer is part of Springer Science+Business Media (www.springer.com)

Foreword

This book brings together contributions from leading international experts in the area of quality of life research for people with intellectual disabilities. Though not the only book focusing on quality of life (QOL) for people with intellectual disabilities, this is the first in the Social Indicators Research Series. However, that alone does not justify the publication of another book. What is unique about this book is its breadth of coverage, both in terms of its coverage of multiple areas relating to QOL research for people with intellectual disabilities and also its international scope. There are chapters on individual QOL for people with disabilities, as well as the emerging areas of QOL of children with intellectual disabilities and family quality of life (FQOL). In regards to the international scope of the book, the chapters include research relating to 17 countries of various cultural backgrounds; these being Australia, Bangladesh, Canada, China, Hong Kong, Korea, Macedonia, Mongolia, The Netherlands, Nigeria, Poland, Slovenia, Spain, Taiwan, Thailand, the UK, and the United States.

The 22 chapters included in this book have been categorized into five main areas. Parts I and II provide a comprehensive overview of the general field of QOL research for individuals with intellectual disabilities; the chapters in Part I (Chapters 1 to 5) deal with issues relating to the measurement and use of QOL and Part II (Chapters 6 and 7) follows with two literature reviews. Part III (Chapters 8–11) focuses on international perspectives relating to individual QOL and comprises four chapters that deal with QOL applications, policies, and practices across four countries (China, The Netherlands, Nigeria, Poland). Part IV (Chapters 12–14) continues the theme of individual QOL, focusing specifically on issues pertaining to the QOL of children with intellectual disabilities. Part V (Chapters 15–20) diverges from individual QOL to the emerging area of FQOL for families that have a child with an intellectual disability. This part contains chapters that provide a broad overview of the area of FQOL, as well as chapters that focus on FQOL across different countries (Australia, Canada, Korea, Slovenia, Spain, and Taiwan) and on specific groups (e.g., older-aged families with adult children with intellectual disabilities). The book concludes with Part VI (Chapters 21 and 22) which provides a description of two programs specifically focused on enhancing QOL for people with intellectual disabilities.

As mentioned in the preceding paragraph, Part I contains chapters that relate to the measurement and use of QOL. In Chapter 1 Robert Schalock discusses both the measurement of QOL-related personal outcomes and their three primary uses. The author commences by discussing a QOL conceptual and measurement model comprising of eight domains. In relation to this model the author also suggests several guidelines to ensure that the measurement of QOL-related personal outcomes is conceptually and psychometrically sound. The author concludes the chapter by discussing the use of QOL as: (i) a framework for service delivery; (ii) a basis for evidenced-based practices; and (iii) a catalyst to implement quality improvement programs. Chapter 2, written by Robert Schalock, Kenneth Keith, Miguel Verdugo, and Laura Gómez, extends the discussion on the measurement and use of QOL from Chapter 1 to focus on QOL model development and use in the field of intellectual disabilities. The chapter has four main parts in which the authors: (i) describe the formulation and validation of their model; (ii) describe the operationalization of their model; (iii) suggest criteria to evaluate any empirically derived model; and (iv) report on applications of their model.

Chapters 3 and 4 refine the discussion on model development by focusing specifically on the development of instruments to measure the quality of life (subjective well-being) of people with intellectual disabilities. In Chapter 3 Robert Cummins, Anna Lau, Gareth Davey, and Jane McGillivray present the Personal Wellbeing Index – Intellectual Disability (PWI-ID), a parallel version of the regular PWI used for general population samples. The PWI-ID scale is described with an emphasis on formal administrative procedures, and some illustrative results are presented. The authors conclude that the PWI-ID represents a psychometrically valid instrument to measure subjective well-being for people with intellectual disabilities. In Chapter 4 Miguel Verdugo, Laura Gómez, Benito Aria, and Robert Schalock describe the QOL Integral Scale; a QOL questionnaire that assess both objective and subjective QOL for people with intellectual disabilities. The QOL Integral Scale is demonstrated to be psychometrically reliable and valid, leading the authors to conclude that the scale is a suitable basis for the developing person-centered plans and quality improvement strategies in organizations.

Having described the development of instruments to assess the quality of life (subjective well-being) of people with intellectual disabilities in Chapters 3 and 4, Chapter 5, by Ralph Kober and Ian Eggleton, extends the discussion on the use of quality of life by arguing that agencies that assist people with intellectual disabilities can use QOL as one potential measure of performance. This is demonstrated with reference to research conducted on the effect of different methods of employment on the QOL for people with intellectual disabilities.

Part II (Chapters 6 and 7) provides two literature reviews relating to quality of life for people with intellectual disabilities. Chapter 6, by Gordon Lyons, presents a comprehensive review of the literature on QOL for people with intellectual disabilities. The author provides the reader with an understanding of this field of study so as to better engage with the other chapters of this book. The author commences by outlining the evolution of informative conceptual and theoretical perspectives and terms, followed by a summary of relevant research. Chapter 7, by Ralph Kober continues with a review of the literature on QOL, but narrows its focus by specifically evaluating studies on employment. The author provides a review of the literature on the effect of employment on the QOL of people with intellectual disabilities, and whether QOL differs based on method of employment.

Part III (Chapters 8–11) expands the focus on QOL for people with intellectual disabilities to consider applications, policies, and practices across countries of differing cultural backgrounds. In Chapter 8 Alice Schippers explores recent policy development and practice changes in relation to QOL for people with intellectual disabilities in The Netherlands and the European Union. Chapter 9, by Wojciech Otrebski, follows with an examination of differences of perceptions between users and their parents in relation to their assessment of importance and use of QOL domains in Poland. The author finds significant differences in the perception of the QOL domains between service users and their parents and that importance and use of the QOL domains and their indicators is related to demographic variables. In Chapter 10 Mian Wang provides an overview of QOL research (including FQOL which is discussed in Part V) in China, and discusses a number of important issues regarding applications of QOL and FQOL for addressing the challenges that China's special education faces. The etic (universal) and emic (culture-bound) properties of FQOL are also discussed within the Chinese context. Chapter 11, by Patrick Edewor, Oluremi Abimbola, and Olujide Adekeye, concludes this part on international perspectives by examining intellectual disability and begging in the Nigerian context. The authors consider the interface between intellectual disability and begging with a view to understanding the socio-cultural conditions that precipitate begging by people with intellectual disabilities in Nigeria. They conclude by recommending policy implementation strategies in the area of education targeted at both the person with the intellectual disability and their parents.

Part IV (Chapters 12–14) focuses specifically on the issue of QOL of children with intellectual disabilities. The part commences with Chapter 12, by Gordon Lyons and Michele Cassebohm, which explores issues associated with understanding, assessing, and improving QOL for children with profound intellectual and multiple disabilities. The authors present grounded theories regarding: (i) the nature of QOL for children with profound intellectual and multiple disabilities; and (ii) how other people can best come to know these children. The authors believe that QOL can be discerned for children with profound intellectual and multiple disabilities, that these children often experience a reasonable QOL, and that their QOL can be improved. In Chapter 13 Joanne Shearer the author presents the results of an inquiry into the lives of children with a disability who attend inclusive schools. A personal account of the children's experiences at school, home, and in the community is provided by the children and their parents through interviews. The QOL of these children appears rich, and the author discusses circumstances that enhance their lives.

Chapter 14, by Eric Emerson, concludes the part on QOL for children with intellectual disabilities with the author challenging the reader to reflect on the reliance on psychological indicators of well-being in measuring QOL. The author commences with a discussion on the two dominant approaches to conceptualizing and measuring the QOL of children with disabilities (social indicators of living conditions compared with psychological indicators of well-being). Through the presentation of international examples, the author highlights that the two approaches lead to substantially different conclusions with regard to the extent and nature of disadvantage experienced by children with disabilities.

While the first four parts of the book focused primarily on the QOL of individuals with intellectual disabilities, Part V (Chapters 15–20) focuses on the emerging area of FQOL. FQOL is the study of the QOL of the entire family unit taken as a whole, as opposed to the separate QOL of each individual that comprises the family unit. In Chapter 15, Nina Zuna, Jean Ann Summers, Ann Turnbull, Xiaoyi Hu and S. Xu present a unified theory of FQOL for families of children with intellectual disabilities. The authors depict FQOL as an interactive process in which individual family member demographics, characteristics, and beliefs interact with family-unit dynamics and characteristics within the context of individual-level and family-level supports, services, and practices. This interactive inner framework of the model is further impacted by federal, state, and local systems, policies, and programs. The chapter concludes with a working theoretical model of FQOL, which serves as a guide for researchers to generate multiple testable theoretical statements.

Chapter 16, by Nancy Jokinen and Roy Brown, continues the discussion of FQOL presented in Chapter 15, but focuses specifically on the issue of FQOL in relation to older-aged families with adult children with intellectual disabilities. The authors describe the impact of an aging population on countries' abilities to provide effective services to older-aged families with adult children with intellectual disabilities. The authors highlight research, policy, and practice implications and conclude with recommendations for future research and practice.

In Chapter 17 Fiona Rillotta, Neil Kirby, and Joanne Shearer describe and compare two FQOL questionnaires (the Beach Center FQOL Scale and the International FQOL Survey). The authors highlight the fact that both surveys make use of similar FQOL domains, but that some differences exist throughout the scales. The authors demonstrate that, while both surveys resulted in relatively comprehensive FQOL data, some components relevant to FQOL were included in one survey but not the other. The authors' evaluation of these respective instruments supports the importance of administering both FQOL scales through a mixed-methods interview. The authors conclude by providing suggestions on how the FQOL measures might be improved to better identify the factors that contribute toward a life of quality for these families.

In keeping with the international nature of this book, the remaining chapters in Part III (Chapters 18–20) focus on FQOL across countries of different cultural backgrounds (Australia, Canada, Korea, Spain, Slovenia, and Taiwan). In Chapter 18 Climent Giné, Marta Gràcia, Rosa Vilaseca, and Anna Balcells present their research-in-progress which aims to identify what Spanish families with children with intellectual disability understand by QOL. Based on this, the authors have begun developing an FQOL scale that will provide information on the support required to ensure that families receive the necessary resources to enhance their FQOL. The work presented in the chapter is still in its development stage, with the authors presenting their general approach and the results of their pilot study.

Chapter 19, by Majda Schmidt and Ralph Kober, provides data in relation FQOL in Slovenia with the authors also describing the care and support systems for children with intellectual disabilities and their families in Slovenia. The authors highlight the low FQOL scores for Slovene families with a child with an intellectual disability relative to international averages and that FQOL is correlated to financial well-being.

While Chapters 18 and 19 looked at FQOL in relation to single countries, Chapter 20, by Roy Brown, Keumja Hong, Joanne Shearer, Mian Wang, and Shin-yi Wang, concludes Part V by presenting a comprehensive comparison of FQOL across various countries (Australia, Canada, Korea, and Taiwan), as well as across different forms of intellectual disability (autism and down syndrome). The authors illustrate how different variables and factors play an important role in our understanding of FQOL. The results presented in the chapter suggest that both internal aspects of family life, including the nature of a child's disability, and external factors (e.g., community and the types of support available for the family) are highly relevant. The data presented by the authors stress family variability and therefore raise questions concerning the flexibility of support and intervention. The authors suggest changes to improve policy and practice for supporting families, while at the same time positively influencing the adaptation of the child with an intellectual disability, and as such enhancing overall FQOL.

The final part of the book, Part VI (Chapters 21 and 22), relates specifically to enhancing QOL for people with intellectual disabilities. In Chapter 21, Rhonda Faragher argues that numeracy (quantitative literacy) is a key factor in the enhancement of an individual's QOL, especially those with intellectual disabilities. Given the potential contribution that numeracy can have on QOL, the author believes there is a need for numeracy development to be approached systematically, as opposed to being left to occur by chance. The chapter presents a method of enhancing numeracy, and as such QOL, and the process is explored through a case example. Chapter 22, by Cathy Terrill and James Gardner, concludes the part on enhancing QOL by presenting an account of an organization that closed its sheltered workshops. Instead people with intellectual disabilities were offered a variety of alternative opportunities within community settings. The authors describe the resultant increase in QOL and building of social capital. The chapter concludes with guidelines for disability agencies to enhance QOL and build social capital.

Preface

The origins of this book can be traced back to the seventh annual conference of the International Society for Quality of Life Studies (ISQOLS) Conference (Grahamstown, South Africa, 17–20 July 2006) when I was approached by Springer to edit a book as part of the Social Indicators Research Series relating specifically to people with disabilities. Given the breadth and depth of research on quality of life relating to people with disabilities, it quickly became apparent that there would be insufficient space in one book to cover all disability types, and as such the decision was made to limit the focus of this book to intellectual disabilities with future books potentially looking at quality of life in relation to people with other disabilities.

Contributors to this book come mainly from members of the Quality of Life Special Interest Research Group (SIRG) of the International Association for the Scientific Study of Intellectual Disability (IASSID). ISQOLS and the IASSID Quality of Life SIRG have established a cooperative relationship with the two most recent ISQOLS conferences (San Diego, USA, 6–9 December 2007 and Florence, Italy, 19–23 July 2009) having a considerable number of presentations relating to quality of life for people with disabilities, with many of the contributors to this book presenting papers.

Caulfiled East, VIC, Australia — Ralph Kober

Acknowledgements

My sincere thanks to Bob Cummins for suggesting my name to Springer for this project. Without Bob's suggestion I would not have been involved in editing this book. To Esther Otten and Miranda Dijksman from Springer, my thanks for your helpfulness and also your patience in seeing this project to fruition. I also wish to express my gratefulness to all the people who contributed chapters for their willingness and enthusiasm to participate in this project. It goes without saying that without your contributions there would be no book. Let us hope that this book will live up to its title and contribute to the enhancement of quality of life of people with intellectual disabilities.

In addition to the people directly involved with this book, I also feel it appropriate to acknowledge several others without whom this book would not have seen the light of day. To my wife, thank you for your love and support which ensured that I completed this book. To my parents, thank you for your love and encouragement. To Ian Eggleton, my thanks for introducing me into this area and your continued support. Finally, and definitely by no means least, I wish to express my gratitude to Ivan Brown, Roy Brown, Bob Cummins, Trevor Parmenter, and Bob Schalock for all their support and guidance over the years. For someone like me, who entered this field of research without a background in psychology, your welcome and help have been invaluable.

Contents

Contributors

Oluremi H. Abimbola Department of Sociology, Covenant University, Ota, Ogun State, Nigeria, remhez@yahoo.com

Olujide A. Adekeye Department of Human Resource Development, Covenant University, Ota, Ogun State, Nigeria, jikeye@yahoo.com

Benito Arias Institute on Community Integration, University of Valladolid, Valladolid, Spain, barias@psi.uva.es

Anna Balcells Ramon Llull University, Barcelona, Spain, AnnaBB0@blanquerna.url.edu

Roy I. Brown University of Calgary, Calgary, AB, Canada; Flinders University, Adelaide, SA, Australia, roybrown@telus.net

Michele Cassebohm The University of Newcastle, chell55@bigpond.net.au

Robert A. Cummins School of Psychology, Deakin University, Geelong, VIC, Australia, cummins@deakin.edu.au

Gareth Davey Department of Psychology, University of Chester, Chester, UK, g.davey@chester.ac.uk

Patrick A. Edewor Department of Sociology, Covenant University, Ota, Ogun State, Nigeria, edeworpat@yahoo.com

Ian R.C. Eggleton School of Accounting and Commercial Law, Victoria University of Wellington, Wellington, New Zealand, Ian.Eggleton@vuw.ac.nz

Eric Emerson Centre for Disability Research, Lancaster University, Lancaster, UK; Australian Family and Disability Studies Research Collaboration, University of Sydney, Sydney, Australia, eric.emerson@lancaster.ac.uk

Rhonda M. Faragher Australian Catholic University (Canberra), P.O. Box 256, Dickson, ACT 2602, Australia, Rhonda.Faragher@acu.edu.au

James Gardner President and CEO, CQL, jfgardner@thecouncil.org

Climent Giné Ramon Llull University, Barcelona, Spain, climentgg@blanquerna.url.edu

Laura E. Gómez School of Psychology-University of Salamanca, Institute on Community Integration, University of Salamanca, Salamanca, Spain, laura_e80@msn.com

Marta Gràcia Barcelona University, Barcelona, Spain, mgraciag@ub.edu

Keumja Hong Graduate School, Tokyo University of Social Welfare, Tokyo, Japan, hongjapan@msn.com

Xiaoyi Hu Beach Center on Disability, University of Kansas, Lawrence, KS 66045, USA, huxiaoyi@ku.edu

Nancy S. Jokinen School of Social Work, University of Northern British Columbia, Prince George, BC, Canada, jokinnen@unbc.ca

Kenneth D. Keith Department of Psychology, University of San Diego, San Diego, CA, USA, kkeith@andeigo.edu

Neil Kirby School of Psychology, The University of Adelaide, Adelaide, SA, Australia

Ralph Kober Department of Accounting and Finance, Monash University, Caulfield East, VIC 3145, Australia, ralph.kober@monash.edu

Anna L.D. Lau Department of Rehabilitation Sciences, Hong Kong Polytechnic University, Kowloon, Hong Kong, rsalau@inet.polyu.edu.hk

Gordon Lyons The University of Newcastle, gordon.lyons@newcastle.edu.au

Jane McGillivray School of Psychology, Deakin University, Geelong, VIC, Australia, mcgill@deakin.edu.au

Wojciech Otrębski Department of Rehabilitative Psychology, Institute of Psychology, John Paul II Catholic University of Lublin, Lublin, Poland, Otrebski@kul.pl

Fiona Rillotta School of Psychology, The University of Adelaide, Adelaide, SA, Australia, fiona.rillotta@adelaide.edu.au

Robert L. Schalock Hastings College, Hastings, NE, USA, rschalock@ultraplix.com

Alice Schippers Disability Studies in the Netherlands, Utrecht, The Netherlands; Policy and Quality Affairs, Amsterdam, The Netherlands, alice.schippers@tiscali.nl

Majda Schmidt Faculty of Education, University of Maribor, Maribor, Slovenia, majda.schmidt@uni-mb.si

Joanne Shearer Flinders University, Adelaide, South Australia, Australia, joanneshearer@aapt.net.au

Jean Ann Summers Beach Center on Disability, University of Kansas, Lawrence, KS 66045, USA, jsummers@ku.edu

Cathy Ficker Terrill President and CEO, Ray Graham Association for People with Disabilities, Downers Grove, Illinois, USA, cathyfickerterrill@yahoo.com

Ann P. Turnbull Beach Center on Disability, University of Kansas, Lawrence, KS 66045, USA, turnbull@ku.edu

Miguel Á. Verdugo School of Psychology-University of Salamanca, Institute on Community Integration, University of Salamanca, Salamanca, Spain, verdugo@usal.es

Rosa Vilaseca Barcelona University, Barcelona, Spain, rosavilaseca@ub.edu

Mian Wang Education Department, Gevirtz Graduate School of Education, University of California, Santa Barbara, CA 93106, USA, mwang@education.ucsb.edu

Shin-yi Wang Taiwan Association of Clinical Psychology, Taipei, Taiwan, shinyi@ualberta.ca

Sheng Xu Beach Center on Disability, University of Kansas, Lawrence, KS 66045, USA, xusheng1022@163.com

Nina Zuna Beach Center on Disability, University of Kansas, Lawrence, KS 66045, USA, nzuna@ku.edu

Introduction

This book brings together contributions from leading international experts in the area of quality of life for people with intellectual disabilities. The 22 chapters present an overview of the broader area of quality of life for people with intellectual disabilities, as well as covering specific areas such as quality of life for of children with intellectual disabilities and family quality of life for families with children with an intellectual disability. The book also has a truly international flavor with authors coming from 5 continents and the presentation of research relating to 17 countries of various cultural backgrounds.

Throughout the book the focus is on enhancing the quality of life of people with intellectual disabilities, and numerous chapters provide suggestions and recommendations for both practice and policy.

Written for: Given both the theoretical and practice perspectives offered by the various chapters and also the books broad coverage, this book is will be of value to researchers and postgraduate students interested in quality of life research relating to people with intellectual disabilities, as well as to professionals and policy makers working in the area of intellectual disabilities.

Keywords: Family quality of life, Intellectual disabilities, Quality of life

Part I
Measurement and Use of Quality of Life

Chapter 1
The Measurement and Use of Quality of Life-Related Personal Outcomes

Robert L. Schalock

Overview

The purpose of this chapter is to present a framework for the measurement and use of quality of life-related personal outcomes for persons with intellectual and closely related developmental disabilities (ID/DD). The primary intent of the chapter is to provide a number of empirically based strategies and guidelines that if followed, will assure that the measurement of quality of life-related personal outcomes is conceptually and psychometrically sound, and that the application of the quality of life (QOL) conceptual model involves what is increasingly becoming its three primary uses: as a framework for service delivery, as a basis for evidence-based practices, and as a vehicle to implement quality improvement strategies.

The chapter should be read and understood within the context of two significant trends impacting current policies and practices regarding persons with ID/DD (Schalock, Gardner, & Bradley, 2007). First, there is a desire among stakeholders for quality services and personal outcomes, a focus on providing individualized supports within inclusive (i.e., community) environments, an emphasis on key performance indicators and evidence-based practices, and the use of best practices based on current knowledge regarding skill training, assistive technology, environmental modification/accommodation, natural supports, and social capital. The second trend involves the need for organizations to improve their performance and accountability through systematically collecting and analyzing QOL-related data and information, and implementing quality improvement (QI) strategies based on the analysis.

R.L. Schalock (✉)
Hastings College, Hastings, NE, USA
e-mail: rschalock@ultraplix.com

R. Kober (ed.), *Enhancing the Quality of Life of People with Intellectual Disabilities*, Social Indicators Research Series 41, DOI 10.1007/978-90-481-9650-0_1,

The Measurement of Quality of Life-Related Personal Outcomes

QOL Measurement Guidelines

A detailed review of the extensive research on QOL measurement is beyond the scope of this chapter. Reviews of that extensive literature can be found in Cummins (2004a, 2004b), Schalock (1997), Schalock et al. (2007), Schalock and Verdugo (2002), and Verdugo, Schalock, Keith, and Stancliffe (2005). Such a review suggests the following guidelines:

- Methodological pluralism (i.e., both subjective and objective data collection methods) should be used in the measurement of QOL-related personal outcomes. Subjective measures include satisfaction that while attractive are less sensitive to environmental changes and considered by many to reflect an enduring personality trait rather than a sensitive measure of intervention. There is also consensus that (a) there is a low correlation between subjective and objective QOL measures; and (b) objective measures of personal experiences and circumstances are better to use for QI purposes (Cummins, 1997; Hensel, Rose, Stenfert-Kroese, & Banks-Smith, 2002; Schalock & Felce, 2004; Schalock et al., 2007).
- Likert-type rating scales provide an efficient method for assessing quantitatively attitudes and behaviors in psychometrically sound ways (Hartley & MacLean, 2006).
- Proxies need to be used with caution and selectively (Stancliffe, 2000; Verdugo et al., 2005). Guidelines for their use will be discussed later in the chapter.
- Iconic (visual) presentation and alternative response formats should be used to facilitate both understanding and valid responding (Bonham et al., 2004; Hartley & MacLean, 2006; Heal & Sigelman, 1995).
- Consumers should be actively involved in the selection of indicator items and the collection and utilization of QOL-related data (Bonham et al., 2004; Schalock & Bonham, 2003; Schalock et al., 2007).

QOL Measurement Model

The QOL conceptual and measurement model summarized in Table 1.1 has been developed over the last decade using three sequential steps: obtaining and describing the phenomenon, concept mapping, and testing the model (Schalock & Verdugo, 2002; Wang et al., 2010). A similar process has been used to develop a family QOL measurement model (Poston et al., 2002; Summers et al., 2005). The four components of the model shown in Table 1.1 are QOL factors, domains, indicators, and indicator items.

QOL factors: higher order constructs identified on the basis of structural equation modeling employing cross-cultural data obtained from 2,800 consumers with ID/DD, parents or guardians of those consumers, and professionals providing

Table 1.1 Quality of life conceptual and measurement model

Factor	Domain	Exemplary indicators[a]
Independence	Personal development	Education status, personal skills, adaptive behavior (ADLs IADLs)
	Self-determination	Choices/decisions, autonomy, personal control, personal goals
Social participation	Interpersonal relations	Social networks, friendships, social activities, interactions, relationships
	Social inclusion	Community integration/participation, community roles, supports
	Rights	Human (respect, dignity, equality) Legal (legal access, due process)
Well-being	Emotional well-being	Safety and security, positive experiences, contentment, self-concept, lack of stress
	Physical well-being	Health and nutrition status, recreation, leisure
	Material well-being	Financial status, employment status, housing status, possessions

[a]See Table 1.2 for exemplary items to assess respective domain indicators.

services and supports to those consumers (Jenaro et al., 2005; Schalock et al., 2005; Wang et al., 2010). The three higher order constructs (independence, social participation, and well-being) shown in Table 1.1 (along with their respective QOL domains) have been confirmed for each of the three respondent groups (Wang et al., 2010).

QOL domains: The set of factors composing personal well-being. The set represents the range over which the QOL concept extends and thus defines the multi-dimensionality of a life of quality. The eight QOL domains listed in Table 1.1 were initially developed on the basis of a meta-analysis of international QOL literature and subsequently validated (in reference to both factor structure and factor stability) in a series of cross-cultural studies (Bonham et al., 2004; Jenaro et al., 2005; Schalock et al., 2005; Verdugo & Schalock, 2003; Verdugo, Gomez, Arias, & Martin, 2006).

QOL core indicators: Quality of life-related perceptions, behaviors, and conditions that give an indication of a person's well-being. *These core indicators are used to define operationally each QOL domain; their measurement results in personal outcomes*. The exemplary indicators listed in Table 1.1 are the most common indicators for each of the eight core domains based on an international review of QOL literature in the areas of education, special education, mental retardation/intellectual disability, mental/behavioral health, and aging (Schalock & Verdugo, 2002).

Indicator items: Specific items that are used to assess either the person's perceived well-being ("self report") on the item, or an objective indicator of the person's life experiences and circumstances ("direct observation") in reference to the item. Typically, two or three items are used to measure each QOL indicator. These measures provide the operational definition of QOL-related personal outcomes. Examples are shown later in Table 1.2.

Table 1.2 Exemplary items to assess QOL-domain indicators

Domain: *personal development*; *indicator*: *adaptive behavior*
Self-report: To what degree are you able to feed yourself, get up and down, toilet, and dress yourself? (Independent, with assistance, cannot)
Direct observation: ADL status: how would you rate the degree to which the person does these activities of daily living? (Generally independent, generally with assistance, cannot do on own)
Domain: *self-determination*; *indicator*: *choices*
Self-report: Are you offered choices (e.g., what to wear, what to eat, places to go)? (Yes, not sure, no)
Direct observation: To what degree is the person offered choices as to what to wear, what to eat, places to go, etc.? (Considerable, some, little, or none)
Domain: *interpersonal relations*; *indicator*: *friendships*
Self-report: Do you have friends? (Yes, not sure, no)
Direct observation: Has the person identified persons as friends and refers to them as such? (Yes, not sure, no)
Domain: *social inclusion*; *indicator*: *community participation*
Self-report: Do you take part in activities within the town where you live? (Yes, not sure, no)
Direct observation: How often is the person involved in activities within the community? (Frequently (weekly), sometimes 1–2/week, never)
Domain: *rights*; *indicator*: *dignity and respect*
Self-report: Do people around you allow privacy, ask what you think, leave you alone while bathing? (Yes, not sure, no)
Direct observation: How much respect and dignity is shown this person by staff and others? (Considerable, some, very little)
Domain: *emotional well-being*; *indicator*: *safety and security*
Self-report: Do you feel safe and secure? (Yes, not sure, no)
Direct observation: How would you rate the safety and security of the person's living and work/school environments? (Very safe, somewhat safe, not safe)
Domain: *physical well-being*; *indicator*: *health status*
Self-report: What about your health? How do you feel? (Very good, okay, not good/ill)
Direct observation: How would you evaluate the physical health of this person? (Good, fair, poor)
Domain: *material well-being*: *Indicator*: *possessions*
Self-report: Do you have personal possessions such as a radio, TV, stereo, pictures? (Yes, not sure, no)
Direct observation: How many personal possessions does the person have? (Many, some, few or none)

A Framework for Measuring QOL-Related Personal Outcomes

As an overview to this section, the reader should keep three points clearly in mind: First, *the measurement of quality indicator items results in personal outcomes*. Second, personal outcomes are defined and measured in reference to core QOL domains and indicators such as those listed in Table 1.1. Third, personal outcomes can be analyzed at the level of the individual, aggregated at the organization/program level, and complemented by other indicators such as health and safety indicators, staff turnover, and geographical/economic variables (Schalock et al., 2007).

The proposed framework for measuring personal outcomes has four components. These are that the framework: (a) is guided by conceptual principles; (b) is based on a validated QOL model; (c) reflects the etic (universal) and emic (culture-bound) properties of QOL domains and indicators; and (d) uses methodological pluralism.

Conceptual principles: Four conceptual principles guide the measurement of personal outcomes. They are that quality of life is: multi-dimensional; composed of the same domains for all people (even though the relative importance of some domains will show individual and cultural variability); influenced by personal and environmental factors and their interaction; and evaluated on the basis of both subjective and objective measures (Verdugo et al., 2005).

Validated QOL model: The measurement of personal outcomes needs to be based on a validated quality of life model whose domains have demonstrated factor structure and factor stability, and whose indicators are shown to have a significant relationship to the respective domain. Such a model was shown in Table 1.1. In addition, specific criteria should guide the selection of specific indicator items. As discussed in more detail elsewhere (e.g., Schalock et al., 2007; Walsh et al., 2010), these criteria: reflect what people want in their lives, relate to current and future policy issues, are those that the service/support provider has some control over, and can be used for reporting and quality improvement purposes.

Etic and emic properties: Cross-cultural studies (e.g., Jenaro et al., 2005; Keith & Schalock, 2000; Schalock et al., 2005; Wang et al., 2010) have demonstrated that the QOL factors and domains listed in Table 1.1 have factor stability and both etic (i.e., universal) and emic (i.e., culture-bound) properties. This same research has also shown that those indicators listed in Table 1.1 have both etic and emic properties. To reflect these two properties, efforts have been undertaken to evaluate the personal outcomes of all persons, including those with diagnoses other than ID/DD and the general population (Keith & Bonham, 2005; Schalock et al., 2007; State of Nebraska Health and Human Services, 2006). These efforts have generally employed the following six sequential steps (Verdugo & Schalock, 2007): (a) generating potential measures for each QOL core indicator listed in Table 1.1 based on the input from focus groups and published literature; (b) sorting the potential measures into groups that are consistent with both the conceptual and measurement QOL model and the values and aspirations of persons with and without disabilities; (c) developing Likert-type response formats for each potential item indicator; (d) doing initial studies to confirm reliability, domain loading, robustness, and the etic property of the selected measures; (e) selecting final items; and (f) finalizing the survey instrument, including administration and scoring instructions.

Methodological pluralism: Self-report and direct observation measures are typically employed. *Self-report measures* are based on the individual's assessment of his/her status on the respective indicator item. If the person cannot respond for themselves (either because of lack of receptive/expressive language or not completing the pre-test correctly), then proxies can be used to estimate the self-report information. However, it is clear from the literature that proxies are most effective in assessing the individual's objective circumstances and experiences—not the person's own perceptions. When proxies are used, then the following guidelines apply: (a) persons who know the individual well should be used; (b) have two persons who know the individual well respond as if they were the person and then use the average score for all subsequent purposes; (c) assessment involving proxies should be clearly identified as another person's perspective; (d) analyze separately self-report from objective measures; and (e) build the effect of proxy responses into the data analysis (Bonham et al., 2004; Schalock et al., 2007; Stancliffe, 2000; Verdugo et al., 2005).

Direct observation measures are based on the objective evaluation of the individual's personal experiences and circumstances on the respective indicator item. Respondents providing the direct observation information should follow the following four guidelines: (a) use one or more persons who know the individual well; (b) respondents should base their assessment on objective life experiences and circumstances of the person; (c) observations should be based on multiple occurrences of the experience and/or circumstances, not a single vent or experience; and (d) observation ratings should be converted into a 3–5-point Likert rating scale.

A 3–5-point Likert-type rating scale is used typically for both the self-report and direct observation measures. Likert-type rating scales are an efficient and potentially reliable method for capturing a wide range of variance in attitudes and behaviors (Hartley & MacLean, 2006). As indicated in Table 1.2, when both the self-report and direct observation evaluation of each indicator use the same item stem, the approach: is more conceptually and methodologically robust; readily permits the cross-validation and reliability determination for both measures; and provides data for those three uses of the QOL concept discussed next: as a framework for service delivery, as a basis for evidence-based practices, and as a vehicle to implement quality improvement strategies.

The Primary Uses of the QOL Conceptual Model

The concept of quality of life first emerged in the ID/DD literature in the 1980s as both a sensitizing notion as to what is important in peoples' lives, and as a social construct to guide the development of policies and practices for service recipients. Increasingly, however, it has been the author's experience that the QOL concept is increasingly being used for three primary uses: as a framework for service delivery, as a basis for evidence-based practices, and as a vehicle to implement quality improvement (QI) strategies.

Framework for Service Delivery

The importance of the QOL conceptual and measurement model summarized in Table 1.1 is that it has explanatory power and thus provides a firm foundation for not only service delivery practices, but also as a basis for the evidence-based practices and QI strategies discussed in subsequent sections of the chapter. Using the concept of QOL as a framework for service delivery involves application principles, QOL-focused program practices, and QOL-oriented program standards.

Application principles: a number of principles govern the use of the QOL conceptual model as a framework for service delivery. Chief among these are (Brown & Brown, 2005; Schalock et al., 2008a):

- QOL is multi-dimensional and has the same components for all people.
- QOL is influenced by personal and environmental factors and enhanced by self-determination, inclusion, equity, purpose in life, and a sense of belonging.
- QOL application enhances well-being within cultural contexts.
- QOL application should be evidence-based.

QOL-focused program practices: Five program practices flow logically from the QOL conceptual and measurement model and the above-referenced application principles. These are summarized in Table 1.3 (top section).

Program standards: Implementing and evaluating the effectiveness of the QOL concept as a framework for service delivery requires program standards. In quality improvement, for example, program standards are used frequently as benchmarks against which to evaluate change and progress. On the other hand, in program evaluation one of the criteria frequently used relates to fidelity to the conceptual/program model. In that regard, a number of studies have shown a positive relationship between overall [model-based] program implementation and the achievement of desired program-level outcomes (Dumas, Lynch, Laughlin, Smith, & Prinz, 2001; Kalafat, Illback, & Sanders, 2007).

Based on the author's experience, five program standards are summarized in Table 1.3 (bottom section).

Table 1.3 Quality of life-focused program practices and program standards

Program practices
- A holistic, multi-dimensional approach
- A focus on the community and organizations being bridges to the community
- The use of best practices that are empirically based strategies that reduce the discrepancy (i.e., mismatch) between people and the environments through functional skill training, the use of assistive technology devices, accessing natural supports, and environmental modification/accommodation
- The use of individualized support strategies and their alignment with core quality of life domains such as those listed in Table 1.1

Program standards
- The application of quality of life principles
- The use of quality of life-focused program practices as listed above
- The measurement of personal outcomes as a key component of evidence-based practices
- The demonstration of fidelity to the conceptual and measurement model (Table 1.1)
- The alignment of assessed support needs to quality of life domains
- The use of personal outcomes to guide organizational quality improvement

Evidence-Based Practices

The two essential ideas in evidence-based practices are first that interventions should have clear empirical support, and second that personal outcomes should be used to guide organizational change and quality improvement. A recent discussion (Veerman & Van Yperen, 2007) of four levels of evidence provides a useful framework for understanding how the QOL conceptual and measurement model summarized in Table 1.1 can serve as a basis for evidence-based practices. These four levels are: descriptive, theoretical, indicative, and causal.

- Descriptive: The essential elements of the intervention/program have been made explicit. This level of evidence is reflected in the program practices and standards summarized in Table 1.3.
- Theoretical: The intervention/program has a plausible rationale to explain why it should work. This is the essential function of an empirically based QOL conceptual model that defines operationally the concept and establishes the parameters for program planning and implementation. The theoretical rationale for why an emphasis on quality of life should work is found in the extensive international research (e.g., Brown & Brown, 2005; Cummins, 2005; Schalock et al., 2007) which suggests strongly that one's quality of life is: (a) is multi-dimensional and has the same components for all people; (b) influenced by personal and environmental factors; and (c) enhanced by self-determination, inclusion, individualized supports, and purpose in life.
- Indicative: The demonstration that the intervention/program strategies lead to the desired outcomes. This level of evidence is reflected in: (a) studies (e.g., Bonham et al., 2004; Perry & Felce, 2005) which demonstrate that personal outcomes are enhanced when QOL principles and QOL-related program practices are employed; and (b) the publishing of service provider profiles that show longitudinal changes in quality of life outcomes for all service recipients (Keith & Bonham, 2005; State of Nebraska Health and Human Services, 2006).
- Causal: The demonstration that either the outcome is caused by or related to the intervention, or that there is clear evidence showing which component of the program are predictive of the outcomes. There has been considerable work determining the significant predictors of QOL-related outcomes for persons with ID/DD. Across a number of studies (summarized in Schalock et al., 2007; Schalock et al., 2008a, b), personal characteristics (such as IQ and adaptive behavior levels), program practices (e.g., enabling choices, rights, self-determination, availability of transportation, and community inclusion), and setting characteristics (e.g., residential and employment status, setting size, and operational culture) are significant predictors of QOL outcomes.

Quality Improvement

Quality improvement (QI) refers to an organization or system's capacity to improve performance and accountability through systematically collecting and analyzing data and information, and implementing action strategies based on the analysis. Its goal is to improve the quality of life of individuals through the enhancement of policies, practices, training, and technical assistance (Schalock et al., 2007). The approach to QI presented below and on subsequent pages relies heavily on the principles underlying the learning organization (Orthner, Cook, Sabah, & Rosenfeld, 2006; Senge, 2006), program logic models (Andrews, 2004; Renger & Hurley, 2006; Schalock & Bonham, 2003), and evidence-based practices (Chorpita, 2003; Gambill, 1999; Langberg & Smith, 2006). Four QI strategies hold promise to enhance both the measurement and use of QOL-related personal outcomes and the organization and system's capacity to improve performance and accountability. These four are to: develop mental models, provide data tutorials, build learning teams, and establish benchmarks.

Develop mental models. Mental models are deeply ingrained assumptions, generalizations, and images we have to understand the world (De Walle, Van Loon, Van Hove, & Schalock, 2005; Senge, 2006). They form the vision and culture of an organization and serve as the basis for leadership, values training, service delivery, evidence-based practices, and quality improvement. Developing mental models that enhance QOL-related program policies, practices, and outcomes requires challenging those mental models that inhibit change, such as an emphasis on personal defectology, control and dependency, and organizations as mechanistic entities. These three inhibiting mental models are frequently the limiting factors to change. As stated by Senge (2006, p. 100), "to change the behavior of a system requires that one identify and change the limiting factor(s) and thereby increase one's leverage." This first QI strategy involves bringing these inhibiting mental models to the surface, challenging them, and in the process, bringing about changes within the organization's culture that:

- Incorporates an ecological perspective that focuses on the ameliorating effects of environmental factors.
- Focuses on social inclusion, self determination, personal development, community inclusion, and the provision of individualized supports.
- Reinforces thinking and doing, creativity, coordination, priority setting, and communication patterns.
- Embraces "right to left thinking" that specifies desired person-referenced outcomes and then asks, "what needs to be in place in the organization and/or the community for these outcomes to occur?"

Provide data tutorials. Three realities are found in many service provider organizations: first, staff generally do not understand data and data analysis; second, most personnel are afraid of data due to its frequent negative association with evaluation and its potential consequences regarding licensing, funding, certification, or investigation; and third, data management has frequently not been handled well in the past, and thus there has been a negative impact and expectation regarding how the organization accepts data and its use. In response to these three realities, the author has found that providing data tutorials as a QI strategy is very productive when built around the following parameters:

- Understanding statistical concepts and research/evaluation designs.
- Involving stakeholders in the formulation of research/evaluation questions, data collection, and data utilization.
- Understanding the questions being asked of the data, the alignment of those questions to the data collected and analyzed, and how well the data/data analysis answers those questions.
- An understanding of the contextual factors affecting the obtained results.
- Being provided with specific suggestions as to how the data/information can be used to enhance personal outcomes or other performance indicators.
- Stressing that the primary purpose of data collection and analysis is for QI purposes and not to evaluate the goodness (or badness) of the program or services offered.
- Emphasizing that any evaluation represents only "a point in time" and that using data for QI is a continuous process that requires a long-term commitment.

Build learning teams. As a key QI strategy, learning teams are based on the concept of synergy that is enhanced by being self-directed, maximizing equity among staff members, setting challenging new goals, and thinking outside the box about complex issues. Learning teams: foster co-mentoring in the group; utilize research literature, internal/external expertise, relevant learning models, and professional development; integrate knowledge, create potential solutions, and coordinate actions; apply potential solutions; and assess the results and share the findings (Isaacs, 1999; Lick, 2006; Spectot & Davidsen, 2006). In addition, a key function of learning teams is to take their understanding of the significant predictors of desired personal outcomes and target resources and strategies to those factors so as to enhance subsequent outcomes.

Establish benchmarks. Benchmarks have been developed and used out of a desire for organizations to achieve quality outcomes (Center for the Study of Social Policy, 1996). Although the approach used differs across application areas, the key principles underlying benchmarks are that they represent: (a) a point of reference from which measurement may be made; (b) a standard by which others may be compared; and (c) a disciplined search for best practices. The use of benchmarks as a QI strategy is exemplified in the following example from the State of Nebraska (United States) that establishes empirically based benchmarks on the basis of assessed QOL-domain scores.

Since 1998, the ARC of Nebraska in conjunction with the Nebraska Department of Health and Human Services has assessed the quality of life of service recipients with ID/DD on the eight QOL domains shown in Table 1.1. These scores are totalled to produce an index of perception of well-being (Keith & Bonham, 2005; State of Nebraska Health and Human Services, 2006). Average scores for each domain and index are reported: (a) annually for each provider agency, along with the state average for each domain; and (b) for a random sample of persons without disabilities living in the same community as the service-providing agency. Thus, there are three empirically established benchmarks: one based on the yearly trended scores for the agency, the second represented by the statewide average score per domain and total score, and the third by those living in the community without disabilities. Each empirically derived benchmark provides both a point of reference and a standard by which agencies can establish internal goals and also compare themselves with others providing similar services. The importance of the third benchmark (i.e., community-referenced) is that it, along with individual and/or aggregated consumer scores, provides an index of the discrepancy between personal QOL-related outcomes for persons with disabilities and those without disabilities. A primary purpose of QI is to reduce this discrepancy.

In summary, the successful implementation of these four QI strategies always involves leadership, and typically requires a change in the organization's culture. Basis to that cultural change is the need for organizations to redefine their roles and functions to include: being bridges to the community, developing partnerships within the community, advancing a research and evaluation mentality not a bureaucratic monitoring mentality, developing and using internal evaluation/data systems that will provide information for evidence-based practices, using strategies that focus on reducing the discrepancy between personal outcomes and community QOL indicators, and aligning supports assessment with the provision of individualized supports.

In addition, the author's experience over the last two decades is that the successful implementation of QI strategies such as those four just discussed requires obtaining a "buy-in" from multiple stakeholders. This "buy in" involves three key transitions: (a) the *movement from uncertainty to interest* requires a vision, hope, and potential answers as to how to enhance personal outcomes; (b) the *movement from interest to commitment* requires a QOL conceptual and measurement framework (such as that shown in Table 1.1), anticipated institutional support, and personal involvement in the process of change; and (c) the *movement from commitment to action* requires understanding specific strategies, seeing the value of change, and developing a sense of personal mastery to affect change.

Conclusion

The contents of this chapter are best understood within the context of current significant changes in public policy and service delivery practices for persons with ID/DD. Chief among these changes are (a) the involvement of these persons in the planning, delivery, and evaluation of person-centered services and supports; (b) the delineation of personal and organizational goals related to the core domains of a life of quality; (c) the emergence of public policy goals related to increased social inclusion, social justice, and civic participation; (d) the recognized power and potential of the community inclusion movement; (e) the changing conception of disability with its current focus on an ecological model of disability, the supports paradigm, and the importance of equity, empowerment, and social inclusion; and (f) the need for organizations and systems to demonstrate evidence-based practices, and quality improvement.

The measurement and use of QOL-related personal outcomes are an integral part of each of these changes, which explains in part the current popularity of the QOL concept as a change agent. The success of this change effort, however, will depend significantly on how well we conceptualize, measure, and use these outcomes. The suggested approach to the measurement and use of QOL-related personal outcomes in this chapter is based on two decades of research that has identified the core QOL domains and indicators to a life of quality, demonstrated the factor structure and etic and emic properties of the model's factors, domains, and indicators, and evaluated the efficacy of the proposed measurement framework.

Increasingly, the measurement and use of QOL-related personal outcomes is becoming the framework for service delivery, the basis for evidence-based practices, and the vehicle for implementing quality improvement strategies. In addition to those strategies and guidelines discussed in this chapter, two additional factors will also impact how successful the QOL-focused change will be. The first is that the organizations that will excel in the future will be the organizations that discover how to tap peoples' commitment and capacity to learn at all levels of the organization (Senge, 2006). The second factor is that as we move from the old to the new way of thinking about persons with ID/DD and doing "their business" the transition to a quality of life framework will be based less on power and force, and more on the mental models we have of persons with ID and the services and supports provided to enhance their quality of life and the achievement of personal outcomes.

References

Andrews, A. B. (2004). Start at the end: Empowerment evaluation product planning. *Evaluation and Program Planning*, *27*(3), 275–285.

Bonham, G. S., Basehart, S., Schalock, R. L., Marchand, C. B., Kirchner, N., & Rumenap, J. M. (2004). Consumer-based quality of life assessment: The Maryland Ask Me! Project. *Mental Retardation*, *42*(5), 338–355.

Brown, R. I., & Brown, I. (2005). The application of quality of life. *Journal of Intellectual Disability Research*, *49*(10), 718–727.

Center for the Study of Social Policy. (1996, August). Beyond lists. In *Moving to results-based accountability*. Washington, DC: Author.

Chorpita, B. F. (2003). The frontier of evidence-based practice. In A. E. Kazdin & J. R. Weisz (Eds.), *Evidence-based psychotherapies for children and adolescents* (pp.42–59). New York: Oxford.

Cummins, R. A. (1997). Assessing quality of life. In R. I. Brown (Ed.), *Assessing quality of life for people with disabilities: Models, research, and practice* (pp. 16–150). London: Stanley Thornes.

Cummins, R. A. (2004a). Instruments for assessing quality of life. In J. H. Hogg & A. Langa (Eds.), *Approaches to the assessment of adults with intellectual disabilities: A service providers guide*. London: Blackwell.

Cummins, R. A. (2004b). Issues in the systematic assessment of quality of life. In J. H. Hogg & A. Langa (Eds), *Approaches to the assessment of adults with intellectual disabilities: A service providers guide*. London: Blackwell.

Cummins, R. A. (2005). Moving from the quality of life concept to a theory. *Journal of Intellectual Disability Research*, *49*(10), 699–706.

De Walle, I., Van Loon, J., Van Hove, G., & Schalock, R. L. (2005). Quality of life vs. quality of care: Implications for people and programs. *Journal of Policy and Practice in Intellectual Disabilities*, *2*(3/4), 229–239.

Dumas, I. E., Lynch, A. M., Laughlin, J. E., Smith, E., & Prinz, R. J. (2001). Promoting intervention fidelity: Conceptual issues, methods, and preliminary results for the early alliance prevention trial. *American Journal of Preventive Medicine, 20*, 38–47.

Gambill, E. (1999). Evidence-based practice: An alternative to authority-based practice. *Families in Society, 80*, 341–350.

Hartley, S. L., & MacLean, W. E., Jr. (2006). A review of the reliability and validity of Likert-type scales for people with intellectual disability. *Journal of Intellectual Disability Research, 50*(part II), 813–827.

Heal, L. W., & Sigelman, C. K. (1995). Response biases in interviews of individuals with limited mental ability. *Journal of Intellectual Disability Research, 39*, 331–340.

Hensel, E., Rose, J., Stenfert-Kroese, B., & Banks-Smith, J. (2002). Subjective judgments of quality of life: A comparison study between people with intellectual disability and those without disability. *Journal of Intellectual Disability Research, 46*(2), 95–107.

Isaacs, W. (1999). *Dialogue and the art of thinking together*. New York: Currency.

Jenaro, C., Verdugo, M. A., Caballo, C., Balboni, G., Lachapele, Y., Otbrebski, W., et al. (2005). Cross-cultural study of person-centered quality of life domains and indicators: A replication. *Journal of Intellectual Disability Research, 49*(part 10), 734–739.

Kalafat, J., Illback, R. J., & Sanders, D., Jr. (2007). The relationship between implementation fidelity and educational outcomes in a school-based family support program: Development of a model for evaluating multidimensional full-service programs. *Evaluation and Program Planning, 30*(2), 136–148.

Keith, K. D., & Bonham, G. S. (2005). The use of quality of life data at the organization and systems level. *Journal of Intellectual Disability Research, 49*(part 10), 799–805.

Keith, K. D., & Schalock, R. L. (2000). *Quality of life from a cross-cultural perspective*. Washington, DC: American Association on Mental Retardation.

Langberg, J. M., & Smith, B. H. (2006). Developing evidence-based intervention for deployment into school settings: A case example highlighting key issues of efficacy and effectiveness. *Evaluation and Program Planning, 29*(4), 323–334.

Lick, D. W. (2006). A new perspective on organizational learning: Creating learning teams. *Evaluation and Program Planning, 29*(1), 88–96.

Orthner, D. K., Cook, P., Sabah, Y., & Rosenfeld, J. (2006). Organization learning: A cross-national pilot test of effectiveness in children's services. *Evaluation and Program Planning, 29*(1), 67–78.

Perry, J., & Felce, D. (2005). Factors associated with outcomes in community group homes. *American Journal on Mental Retardation, 110*, 121–135.

Poston, D., Turnbull, A., Park, J., Mannan, H., Marquis, J., & Wang, M. (2002). Family quality of life: A qualitative inquiry. *Mental Retardation, 41*, 313–328.

Renger, R., & Hurley, C. (2006). From theory to practice: Lessons learned in the application of ATM approach to developing logic models. *Evaluation and Program Planning, 29*(2), 106–119.

Schalock, R. L. (1997). *Quality of life: Vol. I: Conceptual and measurement issues*. Washington, DC: American Association on Mental Retardation.

Schalock, R. L., & Bonham, G. S. (2003). Measuring outcomes and managing for results. *Evaluation and Program Planning, 26*(3), 229–235.

Schalock, R. L., Bonham, G. S., & Verdugo, M. A. (2008a). The conceptualization and measurement of quality of life: Implications for program planning and evaluation in the field of intellectual disabilities. *Evaluation and Program Planning, 31*, 181–190.

Schalock, R. L., & Felce, D. (2004). Quality of life and subjective well-being: Conceptual and measurement issues. In E. Emerson, C. Hatton, T. Thompson, & T. R. Parmenter (Eds.), *International handbook of applied research in intellectual disabilities* (pp. 261–279). London: Wiley.

Schalock, R. L., Gardner, J. F., & Bradley, V. J. (2007). *Quality of life for persons with intellectual and other developmental disabilities: Applications across individuals, organizations, communities, and systems*. Washington, DC: American Association on Intellectual and Developmental Disabilities.

Schalock, R. L., & Verdugo, M. A. (2002). *Handbook on quality of life for human service practitioners*. Washington, DC: American Association on Mental Retardation.

Schalock, R. L., Verdugo, M. A., Bonham, G. S., Fantova, F., & Van Loon, J. S. (2008b). Enhancing personal outcomes: Organizational strategies, guidelines, and examples. *Journal of Policy and Practice in Intellectual Disabilities*, *5*, 276–285.

Schalock, R. L., Verdugo, M. A., Jenaro, W., Wang, M., Wehmeyer, M., Xu, J., et al. (2005). A cross-cultural study of quality of life indicators. *American Journal on Mental Retardation*, *110*, 298–311.

Senge, P. M. (2006). *The fifth discipline: The art and practice of the learning organization* (Rev. ed.). New York: Doubleday.

Spectot, J. M., & Davidsen, P. I. (2006). How can organizational learning be modeled and measured? *Evaluation and Program Planning*, *29*(1), 63–69.

Stancliffe, R. (2000). Proxy respondents and quality of life. *Evaluation and Program Planning*, *23*(1), 89–93.

State of Nebraska Health and Human Services. (2006). *2006 Nebraska developmental disabilities provider profiles*. Lincoln, USA: State of Nebraska Health and Human Services, Division of Developmental Disabilities.

Summers, J. A., Poston, D., Turnbull, A. P., Marquis, J., Hoffman, L., Manan, H., et al. (2005). Conceptualization and measuring family quality of life. *Journal of Intellectual Disability Research*, *49*(10), 777–783.

Veerman, J. W., & Van Yperen, T. A. (2007). Degrees of freedom and degrees of uncertainty: A developmental model for the establishment of evidence-based youth care. *Evaluation and Program Planning*, *30*(2), 212–221.

Verdugo, M. A., Gomez, L., Arias, B., & Martin, J. C. (2006). *Validation of the eight domain model of quality of life*. Presentation at the symposium on quality of life outcomes: Their empirical development, verification, and use. International Summit on Social Inclusion, Montreal, May 2–6.

Verdugo, M. A., & Schalock, R. L. (2003). *Cross-cultural Survey of QOL Indicators*. Salamanca: Institute on Community Integration-Faculty of Psychology-University of Salamanca.

Verdugo, M. A., & Schalock, R. L. (2007). *The development of quality of life indicator items*. Unpublished manuscript. Institute on Community Integration-Faculty of Psychology, University of Salamanca: Salamanca, Spain.

Verdugo, M. A., Schalock, R. L., Keith, K. D., & Stancliffe, R. (2005). Quality of life and its measurement: Important principles and guidelines. *Journal of Intellectual Disability Research*, *49*(10), 707–717.

Walsh, P. N., Emerson, E., Lobb, C., Hatton, C., Bradley, V., Schalock, R. L., & Mosley, C. (2010). Supported accommodation for people with intellectual disabilities and quality of life: An overview. *Journal of Policy and Practice in Intellectual Disabilities*, *7*, 137–142.

Wang, M., Schalock, R. L., Verdugo, M. A., & Jenaro, C. (2010). Examining the factor structure and hierarchical nature of the quality of life construct. *American Journal on Intellectual and Developmental Disabilities*, *115*, 218–233.

Chapter 2
Quality of Life Model Development and Use in the Field of Intellectual Disability

Robert L. Schalock, Kenneth D. Keith, Miguel Á. Verdugo, and Laura E. Gómez

Introduction and Overview

Models are helpful in understanding a phenomenon and identifying critical components or factors involved in its application. In program development and evaluation, for example, *logic models* provide a visual map or narrative description of how specific program components are related to a program's desired results. A logic model has many uses, including presenting a program's underlying assumptions, rationale, or theory; explaining the connections between inputs and outcomes; identifying critical factors that affect variation in program outcomes; and providing a systems approach to portraying the path toward a desired outcome. Logic model construction is an important first step in program monitoring, performance management, and evaluation (Frechtling, 2007; Kaplan & Garrett, 2005; Millar, Simeone, & Carnevale, 2001).

As distinct from a logic model, an *operational model* depicts key concepts and variables involved in understanding, operationalizing, and applying a phenomenon or, in the case of the present chapter, the quality of life (QOL) construct. An operational model allows one to operationalize a construct in regard to its definition, conceptual and measurement framework, components, and potential application. Thus, the development and evaluation of an operational model is an important first step in QOL assessment, application, and theory construction.

Although the model development and application work we describe in this chapter is based primarily on the authors' research on *individual-referenced QOL* over the last two decades, details about analogous efforts can be found elsewhere. Specifically, the interested reader can find similar model development and evaluation efforts described for (a) individual-referenced QOL (e.g., Cummins, 1996, 2005; Felce & Perry, 1995, 1996, 1997; Petry, Maes, & Vlaskamp, 2005, 2007); (b) family QOL (e.g., Summers et al., 2005; Chapter 15 by Zuna et al.); (c) health-related QOL (e.g., Byrne-Davis, Bennett, & Wilcock, 2006; Rahtz, Sirgy, & Lee,

R.L. Schalock (✉)
Hastings College, Hastings, NE, USA
e-mail: rschalock@ultraplix.com

R. Kober (ed.), *Enhancing the Quality of Life of People with Intellectual Disabilities*, Social Indicators Research Series 41, DOI 10.1007/978-90-481-9650-0_2,

2004; Taillefer, Dupuis, Roberge, & LeMay, 2003); and (d) QOL of older people (e.g., Bowling & Gabriel, 2004). Across these QOL model development and evaluation efforts, one finds reference to the need to focus on the parameters of a QOL model; understand better the relationship between domain-specific factors and external variables; develop more sophisticated models, including a better definition of the content and boundaries of the QOL concept; and validate the factor structure and hierarchical nature of the QOL construct.

This chapter has four major sections. In the first, we describe how we have approached the first step in model development: formulating and validating a QOL conceptual and measurement framework. In the second section, we describe how the model has been operationalized through its definition, components (concepts, indicators, and moderator–mediator variables), and premises. In the third section, we suggest a number of criteria that can be used to evaluate any empirically derived model. In the final section, we reference how the model has been applied in four areas important to the application of the QOL construct in the ID field. We do not suggest that the QOL operational model presented in this chapter is the only way to understand and apply the QOL construct; however, we hope it will provide an example and catalyst for discussion and further QOL model development efforts.

Formulating and Validating a QOL Conceptual and Measurement Framework

Model development involves combining sources of information including existing definitions, literature, and logical reasoning (Shoemaker, Tankard, & Lasorsa, 2004; Chapter 15 by Zuna et al.). In our case, the major source of information has come from two decades of research that has resulted in (a) identifying core QOL domains that have etic properties (Jenaro et al., 2005; Keith, Heal, & Schalock, 1996; Schalock et al., 2005); (b) developing and evaluating of domain-referenced and culturally sensitive QOL indicators used to assess QOL-related personal outcomes (van Loon, van Hove, Schalock, & Claes, 2008; Verdugo, Arias, Gómez, & Schalock, 2008a; Verdugo, Arias, Gómez, & Schalock, 2009); and (c) identifying a number of personal characteristics and environmental variables associated with QOL-related personal outcomes (Keith, 2007; Schalock & Bonham, 2003; Schalock, Gardner, & Bradley, 2007). Our approach to model development has included two steps that reflect the seminal work of Carlisle and Christensen (2006), Fawcett (1999), and Shoemaker et al. (2004): formulating the conceptual and measurement framework, and validating the conceptual and measurement framework.

Formulating the Conceptual and Measurement Framework

Observation and description. The concept of QOL became a widely used notion in national and international arenas during the 1960 and 1970s, and began to seriously influence the field of ID in the 1980s. During these three decades, observation and description concerning the QOL concept generally fit into either a social indicator/environmental perspective (e.g., Andrews & Whithey, 1976; Davis & Fine-Davis, 1991; Parmenter & Donelly, 1997) or a personal well-being/individual perspective (e.g., Brown, 1997; Cummins, 1997; Goode, 1990). Initially, this perspective incorporated personal values and satisfaction measures; gradually, however, it became apparent that the QOL concept implies some combination of subjective and objective variables and therefore researchers considered more objective indicators reflecting life events and circumstances (Cummins, 2000; Keith, 2001; Schalock, 1999).

Concept mapping. Concept mapping is a type of structural conceptualization that is useful for multiple purposes, including model development, theory construction, and program evaluation (Kane & Trochim, 2007; Rosas & Camphausen, 2007; Sutherland & Katz, 2005). Beginning in the mid to late 1980s, researchers used concept mapping to identify and define core QOL domains and their respective indicators and to develop a conceptual framework based on core domains and indicators. This work involved three activities: (a) generating ideas and listing potential domains and indicators based on input from focus groups, personal interviews, and published literature; (b) sorting the potential domains and indicators into groups that made conceptual sense and reflected both the values and aspirations of individuals with disabilities and community QOL standards; and (c) defining each domain operationally on the basis of measurable indicators (Cummins, 1997; Felce & Perry, 1997; Gardner & Carran, 2005; Hughes & Hwang, 1996; Hughes, Hwang, Kim, Eisenman, & Killian, 1995; Schalock & Keith, 1993; Schalock & Verdugo, 2002).

The net result of these activities for us was the development of the QOL conceptual and measurement framework shown in Table 2.1. In reference to this framework,

Table 2.1 Quality of life conceptual and measurement framework

Domain	Literature-based indicators
Emotional well-being	Contentment, self-concept, lack of stress
Interpersonal relations	Interactions, relationships, supports
Material well-being	Financial status, employment, housing
Personal development	Education, personal competence, performance
Physical well-being	Health and health care, activities of daily living, leisure
Self-determination	Autonomy/personal control, goals and personal values, choices
Social inclusion	Community integration and participation, community roles, social supports
Rights	Human (respect, dignity, equality) and legal (citizenship, access, due process)

The indicators listed are a synthesis of the international QOL literature in education, special education, intellectual disability/mental retardation, mental/behavioral health, and aging (Schalock & Verdugo, 2002). The three indicators listed in each domain are the three most commonly cited indicators across the five areas.

- QOL core domains represent the range over which the QOL concept extends and thus define the multidimensionality of a life of quality.
- QOL indicators are QOL-related perceptions, behaviors, and conditions that operationally define each QOL domain. Their measurement results in QOL-related personal outcomes.

Concept mapping also allowed QOL investigators to develop assessment instruments based on QOL domains and measurable indicators (see Cummins, 2004 for a review). As this work has continued, and as researchers have refined assessment instruments and strategies and made them more reliable and valid, they have laid a foundation to validate the conceptual and measurement framework.

Validating the Conceptual and Measurement Framework

A number of studies have validated the QOL conceptual and measurement framework shown in Table 2.1 by demonstrating the factor structure of the domains and determining the etic (universal) and emic (culture-bound) properties of the domains and indicators. Specifically, a series of cross-cultural studies (Jenaro et al., 2005; Schalock et al., 2005) used the *Cross-Cultural Survey of QOL Indicators* (Verdugo & Schalock, 2003) to survey three respondent groups (consumers, family/advocates, and professionals) representing four geographical groupings (Europe, Central and South America, North America, and Mainland China; 10 countries) on the *importance and use* (three-point Likert ratings) of the 24 core QOL indicators listed in Table 2.1. The total sample across the studies was 2823 (approximately equal numbers in each respondent group). Results indicated that (a) the factor structure and factor stability of the eight core QOL domains listed in Table 2.1 was confirmed; (b) there were similar domain profiles on importance and use across respondent and geographical groups, thus supporting the etic property of the QOL domains; and (c) there were significant group and geographical differences on indicator items, thus supporting the emic property of domain indicators.

Additional confirmation of the eight-domain factor structure shown in Table 2.1 is found in the recent work of Verdugo, Arias, Gómez, and Schalock (2008b, 2009, in press) and Wang, Schalock, Verdugo, and Jenaro (2010). Table 2.2 summarizes the results of this more recent causal modeling analysis that has evaluated

Table 2.2 Quality of life factors and domains

Factor	Domains
Independence	Personal development Self-determination
Social participation	Interpersonal relations Social inclusion Rights
Well-being	Emotional well-being Physical well-being Material well-being

via structural equation modeling the factor structure and hierarchical nature of the conceptual model summarized in Table 2.1. Note that in Table 2.2 the eight core domains listed in Table 2.1 are aggregated into three higher order factors: independence, social participation, and well-being.

In summary, the development and validation of a QOL conceptual and measurement framework is the first step in developing an operational QOL model. As discussed above, this three-step process involved observation and description, concept mapping, and validating the conceptual and measurement framework. The net result is that we understand better the construct's meaning and boundaries. As the first step in model development, this process also establishes the foundation for operationalizing the model's parameters. We discuss three such parameters next: an operational definition of individual-referenced quality of life, the model's components, and the model's premises.

Operationalizing the QOL Model

As noted previously, we define an operational QOL model as a way to depict key concepts and variables in understanding, operationalizing, and applying the QOL construct. Here we discuss operationalizing the QOL model, including a definition, model components, and model premises.

Definition of Individual-Referenced QOL

The grounded theory approach to model development derives directly from data, rather than a priori assumptions or untested hypotheses (Donaldson & Gooler, 2003; Taylor & Bogdan, 1998). This approach, which we used to develop the operational definition of individual-referenced quality of life that follows, incorporates three primary data sets: (a) identification and validation of core QOL domains that have etic properties (Tables 2.1 and 2.2); (b) demonstration of the cultural sensitivity of the QOL indicators used to assess each domain; and (c) identification of a number of personal and environmental variables that moderate or mediate QOL-related personal outcomes. The QOL definition

> Individual quality of life is a multidimensional phenomenon composed of core domains influenced by personal characteristics and environmental factors. These core domains are the same for all people, although they may vary individually in relative value and importance. Assessment of QOL domains is based on culturally sensitive indicators.

Model Components

Three principal components allow operationalization of a model: (a) concepts that provide a way to organize the phenomenon; (b) indicators that provide measures of the phenomenon; and (c) variables that allow explanation of factors influencing the

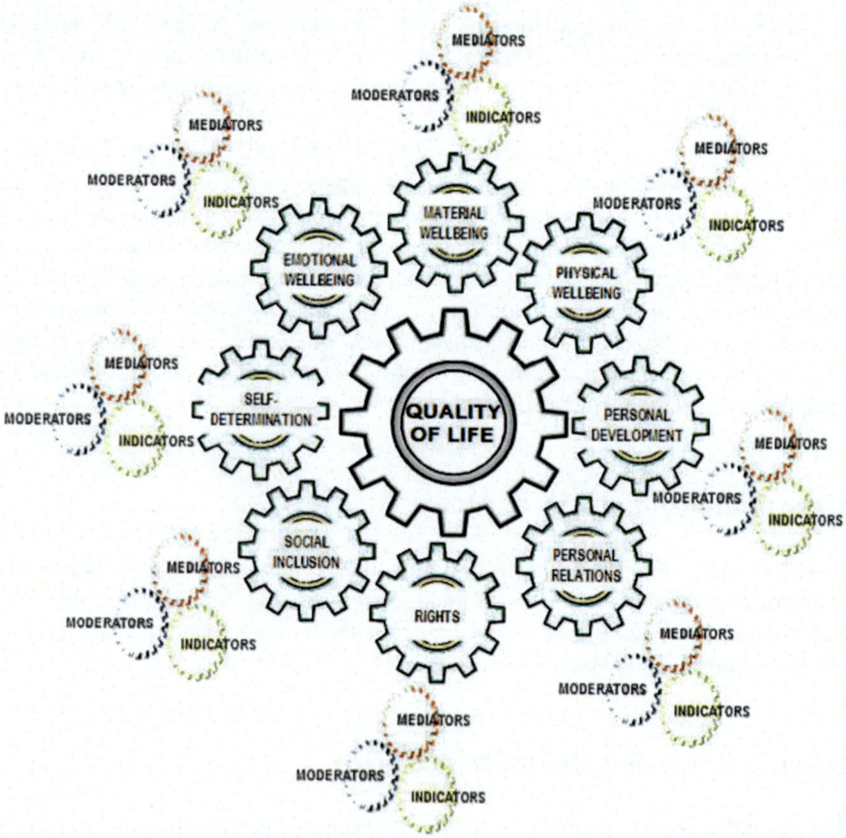

Fig. 2.1 Quality of life operational model

phenomenon. In our work to date (Fig. 2.1), *the operational model, including core QOL domains (i.e., the concept), indicators (measures), and variables (moderators and mediators), operates at the QOL domain level.*

Concepts. The QOL conceptual and measurement framework presented in Table 2.1 and the operational definition of individual-referenced QOL presented above provide the conceptual basis for an operational QOL model: QOL is multidimensional, is composed of eight core domains that are measured on the basis of personal and culturally relevant indicators, and is influenced by personal and environmental factors that act potentially as moderators or mediator. The importance of this framework and operational definition is that the QOL operational model has explanatory power and thus allows one to not only better understand essential characteristics of the QOL construct, but also better understand the role of indicators, moderator variables, and mediator variables.

Indicators. QOL indicators are quality of life-related perceptions, behaviors, and conditions that define operationally each QOL domain. *Their measurement results in personal outcomes*. For consistency and standardization purposes, indicators are selected on the basis of published research, expert panels, and stakeholder focus groups. Criteria for selecting specific indicators are that those indicator items selected: reflect what people want in their lives, are culturally sensitive, are related to current and future policy issues, are those that the individual (or service provider) has some control over, and can be used for quality improvement purposes (Verdugo, Schalock, Gomez, & Arias, 2007; Verdugo, Schalock, Keith, & Stancliffe, 2005; Walsh, Erickson, Bradley, Moseley, & Schalock, 2006).

Because there is a low correlation between subjective and objective assessments of QOL indicators (Cummins, 1997; Schalock & Felce, 2004), most current QOL assessment instruments use some combination of self-report (subjective) and directly observable (objective) indictors/measures. Both approaches *quantify the respondent's responses*, generally using a 3- to 5-point Likert scale. Such scales are easily understood and meaningful to the respondent. In the area of QOL assessment with persons with ID, Likert-type scales capture a wide range of variance in attitudes and behaviors and provide an efficient and reliable method for assessing domain-referenced indicators in psychometrically sound ways (Bonham et al., 2004; Hartley & MacLean, 2006).

The indicators used to assess a QOL domain will affect our understanding of the domain. The following three examples from four different countries reflect the emic nature of QOL indicators – even though the same criteria listed earlier were used in their selection. *Each of the three examples is referenced to the same domain*: *Personal Development*. In the first example, the six indicators used on the *Ask Me*! *Survey* are (a) "does your job and what you do make you feel important; (b) are you getting the training that will help you get a job or a better job; (c) do others give you a chance to become what you want to be; (d) are you learning things that will make you a better person; (e) do you get the information you need about sexuality; and (f) do you get the services you need?" (Bonham, Basehart, & Marchand, 2005). By comparison, the six indicators used in the *Personal Outcomes Scale* (van Loon et al., 2008), developed in Belgium and The Netherlands, uses a 3-point Likert scale to record self-report and direct observation assessments of activities and instrument activities of daily living; the learning of skills or involvement in some type of educational program; opportunities to demonstrate skills; access to information (e.g., newspaper, TV); and use of a computer, cell phone, and/or calculator. In a similar way, the *Integral Scale* (Verdugo et al., 2009), developed in Spain, uses a 4-point Likert scale to record self-report and a yes–no scale to record direct observation assessments of daily activities and involvement in educational programs and work activities. These three examples show clearly that the indicators used to assess a QOL domain will influence both our understanding of the domain and the meaning of the resultant personal outcomes.

Moderator variables. Investigators working to operationalize models typically use two classes of variables: moderators and mediators. A *moderator variable* is a qualitative (e.g., gender or race) or quantitative (e.g., IQ or SES) variable that alters the direction or strength of the relation between a predictor and an outcome (Baron & Kenny, 1986). A moderator effect is an interaction in which the effect of one variable depends on the level of the other (Frazier, Tix, & Barron, 2004; Hair, Black, Babin, Anderson, & Tatham, 2006). In reference to individual-referenced QOL outcomes research, intellectual functioning, adaptive behavior level, and level of self-determination are frequently considered moderator variables (Felce & Emerson, 2001; Gardner & Carran, 2005; Lachapelle et al., 2005; Perry & Felce, 2005; Schalock, Bonham, & Marchand, 2000; Stancliffe & Lakin, 1998; Stancliffe, Abery, & Smith, 2000; Wehmeyer & Schwartz, 1998).

Mediator variables. A *mediator* variable influences the relation between an independent variable and an outcome and exhibits indirect causation, connection, or relation (Baron & Kenny, 1986). A mediating effect is created when a third factor intervenes between the independent and outcome variable (Frazier et al., 2004; Hair et al., 2006). In the field of ID, policies, practices, services, and supports can be thought of as mediator variables. Within the individual-referenced QOL outcome research literature, residential setting, employment status, service model, organization culture and operation, and community interactions are mediator variables that affect the level of assessed personal outcomes (Bonham et al., 2004; Gardner & Carran, 2005; Perry & Felce, 2005; Tossebro, 1995; Walsh et al., 2006). An evolving literature (e.g., Cummins, 2005) suggests that at least one personal characteristic – subjective well-being homeostasis – may well serve as a mediator.

The role that moderator and mediator variables play in QOL domains and personal outcomes is not completely clear at this time. For example, Neeley-Barnes, Marcenko, and Weber (2008) reported recently that living in the community (representing a residential setting and thus a mediator variable) influenced three QOL domains: community inclusion, rights, and interpersonal relations. Analogously, particular aspects of a QOL domain may act as a mediator. For example, self-determination (a core QOL domain that includes one or more indicators related to choice, which one might consider a moderator variable) may also act as a mediator that has a causal relation to QOL-related personal outcomes (Cummins, 2005). Furthermore, in reference to logic models, mediators can act as intervening variables between inputs and outcomes (Chen, 2005; Frechtling, 2007). As research in this area continues, it is important to keep in mind that understanding the role of important moderators and mediators of personal outcomes indicates the maturity of a discipline (Aguinis, Boik, & Pierce, 2001; Hoyle & Robinson, 2003) and is also at the heart of model development and theory construction in social science (Cohen, Cohen, West, & Aiken, 2003).

Model Premises

Published literature and logical reasoning influence a model's premises. Table 2.3 summarizes the six premises that have guided this third phase of our work related to operationalizing and applying the model. These six premises not only describe key assumptions regarding the model's development but also provide the basis for evaluating and applying the model.

Table 2.3 Model premises

1. The indicators used to assess a QOL domain will affect our understanding of the domain
2. Both self-report (subjective) and direct observation (objective) measures should be obtained, because there is a low correlation between subjective and objective indicators/QOL measures (Cummins, 1997; Schalock & Felce, 2004)
3. Objective indicators of life experiences and circumstances are better than subjective measures to use for the purposes of model development and program evaluation (Cummins, 2005; Schalock & Felce, 2004; Verdugo et al., 2005)
4. Moderators and mediators are defined in reference to personal characteristics and environmental factors; can operate at any systems level (micro, meso, macro); represent a potential dynamic relationship; and can be considered as intervening variables in logic modeling that includes inputs, throughputs, outputs, and outcomes (Frazier et al., 2004; Frechtling, 2007)
5. Each QOL domain can be a moderator or mediator of any other domain and these inter-correlations are dynamic (Baron & Kenny, 1986)
6. QOL-related models are similar to a middle-range theory that consists of a limited number of concepts and propositions that are generated and tested by means of empirical research. Thus, the concepts and propositions of middle-range theories may be translated, just as with the use of a model, into variables and testable hypotheses (Fawcett, 1999)

Criteria to Evaluate an Operational Model

As the field of ID encounters more models related to constructs such as quality of life, we need to think about the criteria used to evaluate the utility and effect of models, like the one described in this chapter. In an effort to stimulate thought and discussion about relevant criteria for such models, we suggest the following questions and criteria:

1. Is the model credible? That is, is it meaningful and does it describe the phenomenon? Specific criteria would include (Hunter, 2006; Schalock & Luckasson, 2005) the following: the model is systematic (i.e., organized, sequential, logical), formal (i.e., explicit and reasoned), and transparent (i.e., apparent and clearly communicated).
2. Is the model accepted? The literature on diffusion of ideas and innovations (e.g., Rogers, 1995) has identified four key diffusion/acceptance processes: innovation; communication channels; time to involve knowledge transfer, persuasion, decision, implementation, and confirmation; and the system into which the information/idea/model is to be infused. A related series of questions include whether the model is *plausible* so that it can be followed and implemented and *practical and realistic* in taking account of the organization and system's capacities in relation to the environment (Hunter, 2006). Specific criteria include that the model is referenced in academic journals, replicated in cross-cultural studies, and used as a framework for public policy and services delivery practices.
3. Is the model testable? Criteria would include that the model generates hypotheses (e.g., of the role that moderator and mediator variables play in personal outcomes) and is modified on the basis of new information (Keith, 2001, 2007).

4. Does the use of the model change anything? Criteria would include that the model explains how program inputs, processes, and external factors potentially influence outcomes; identifies and prioritizes evaluation questions and helps align evaluation methodology to answer those questions; expands our ability to explain causality and predict results; helps to develop evidence-based practices; and facilitates capacity building for organizations and systems (Carlisle & Christensen, 2006; Corley, 2007; Rogers & Bozeman, 2001; Veerman & van Yperen, 2007).

Applying a QOL Operational Model

We have previously published application examples in four areas related to the operational QOL model presented in this chapter: (a) assessment of personal outcomes (Bonham et al., 2004; Keith, 2007; Schalock, Bonham, & Verdugo, 2008; Schalock, Verdugo, Bonham, Fantova, & van Loon, 2008; van Loon et al., 2008; Verdugo et al., 2007, 2008a, 2008b, 2009); (b) as a basis for agency reporting and provider profiles (Keith & Bonham, 2005; Keith & Ferdinand, 2000; State of Nebraska, 2008); (c) as a basis for quality improvement strategies (Bonham et al., 2005; Schalock, Verdugo, et al., 2008); and (d) as a framework for desired policy outcomes (Shogren et al., 2009) and individual support plans (van Loon, 2008). These applications are occurring at the same time that the field is discussing and evaluating the utility of logic models to both explain the connection between inputs and outcomes and identify critical factors that affect variation in quality of life-related outcomes (Isaacs, Clark, Correia, & Flannery, 2007; Schalock & Bonham, 2003; Schalock et al., 2007).

Because of this convergence, it is important to understand clearly the relationship between operational and logic models. Both have comparable developmental phases (Gugiu, Rodriguez, & Campos, 2007), provide an integrative framework for assessment and evaluation strategies (Cooksy, Gill, & Kelly, 2001), assume that information without use is information without value (Corley, 2007), and can be used as a planning and performance management tool (Kaplan & Garrett, 2005; Millar et al., 2001). Their differences lie in their intended purpose or focus. A logic model can present a program's underlying rationale, theory, and assumptions, including explaining connections between inputs and outcomes, identifying critical factors affecting variation in program outcomes, and providing a systems approach portraying the path toward a desired outcome. In distinction, an operational model operationalizes a construct, including its definition, conceptual and measurement framework, components, and potential application.

Logic and operational models intersect at the outcomes level of the logic model. The viability and strength of a logic [program] model is heavily dependent on the conceptual soundness and validity of the outcome variable(s) used, which underscores the critical need to develop QOL-related personal outcome measures based on an operational model that is formulated and validated through processes such as those discussed in this chapter. As Stancliffe and Lakin (2005) and Isaacs et al. (2007) have noted, the lack of a robust outcome measure (i.e., dependent variable) has limited both the utility of logic models in the field of IDand the generalizations that can be made about the relationship between inputs and outcomes. Furthermore, in our view, an empirically derived and validated QOL-related operational model provides the conceptual and measurement basis and framework for QOL-related theory development and QOL-related evidence-based practices.

Conclusion

Over the last three decades, we have seen significant conceptual and empirical work clarifying the concept of quality of life. Specifically, we have moved from a philosophical concept to a measurable construct, and from a measurable construct to an operational model that is supported by considerable data and serves as a basis for application and hypothesis testing. The operational QOL model presented in this chapter (a) defines QOL in terms of its empirically derived domains and measurable indicators; (b) measures QOL-related outcomes on the basis of these domain-referenced indicators; (c) operationalizes and assesses moderator and mediator variables that potentially affect variation in QOL-related personal outcomes; and (d) depicts how one or more of the model's components can be used as a basis for service delivery, program practices, and program evaluation.

Based on our experience to date, use of such a model has three implications and potential impacts. First, there should be an increased confidence (by policy makers and service delivery providers) that the QOL construct provides a valid framework for service delivery policies and program practices. Second, an operational model explains how program inputs, processes, and external factors act as moderator or mediator variables that impact QOL domain-referenced personal outcomes. Third, such a model provides an application and research framework for the emerging *trans-disciplinary approach to research and application* that involves researchers and practitioners working jointly in the production of both scientific understanding and societal application effects.

Considerable work remains to be done to evaluate this and similar operational models. This work will entail the continued exploration and identification of culturally sensitive domain-referenced indicators and the best way(s) to assess them, the identification of significant QOL domain-referenced moderator and mediator variables, and the testing of hypotheses that are based on the model. These efforts reflect the next phase in model development and theory construction in the fields of quality of life and intellectual disability.

Acknowledgment The authors are appreciative of the inputs and suggestions given by these valued colleagues at the University of Salamanca (Institute on Community Integration, School of Psychology) in Spain (Benito Arias, Maria Gómez-Vela, Pedro Jimenez Navarro, Esther Navallas, and Fabian Sainz) and Dr. Gordon Bonham (Bonham Research – Baltimore, MD).

References

Aguinis, H., Boik, R. J., & Pierce, C. A. (2001). A generalized solution for approximating the power to detect effects of categorical moderator variables using multiple regression. *Organizational Research Methods, 4*, 291–323.

Andrews, F. M., & Whithey, S. B. (1976). *Social indicators of well-being: Americans' perception of life quality*. New York: Plenum Press.

Baron, R. M., & Kenny, D. A. (1986). The moderator-mediator variable distinction in social psychological research: Conceptual, strategic, and statistical considerations. *Journal of Personality and Social Psychology, 51*, 1173–1182.

Bonham, G. S., Basehart, S., & Marchand, C. B. (2005, December). *Ask Me! FY 2006: The QOL of Marylanders with developmental disabilities receiving DDA funded supports*. Annapolis, MD: Bonham Research.

Bonham, G. S., Basehart, S., Schalock, R. L., Marchand, C. B., Kirchner, N., & Rumenap, J. M. (2004). Consumer-based quality of life assessment: The Maryland Ask Me! Project. *Mental Retardation, 42*(5), 338–355.

Bowling, A., & Gabriel, Z. (2004). An intergrational model of quality of life in older age. Results from the ESRC/MRC HSRC quality of life survey in Britain. *Social Indicators Research, 69*, 1–36.

Brown, R. I. (1997). Quality of life: The development of an idea. In R. I. Brown (Ed.), *Quality of life for people with disabilities: Models, research and practice* (2nd ed., pp. 1–10). Cheltnham: Stanley Thornes.

Byrne-Davis, L. M. T., Bennett, P. D., & Wilcock, G. K. (2006). How are quality of life ratings made? Toward a model of quality of life in people with dementia. *Quality of Life Research, 15*, 855–865.

Carlisle, P. R., & Christensen, C. M. (2006). *The cycles of theory building in management research*. Boston: School of Management-Boston University and Harvard Business School.

Chen, H. (2005). Theory-driven evaluation. In J. Mathison (Ed.), *Encyclopedia of evaluation* (pp. 415–419). Thousand Oaks, CA: Sage.

Cohen, J., Cohen, P., West, S. G., & Aiken, L. S. (2003). *Applied multiple regression/correlation analysis for the behavioral sciences* (3rd ed.). Mahwah, NJ: Erlbaum.

Cooksy, L. J., Gill, P., & Kelly, P. A. (2001). The program logic model as an integrative framework for a multimethod evaluation. *Evaluation and Program Planning, 24*(2), 119–128.

Corley, E. A. (2007). A use-and-transformation model for evaluation public R & D. *Evaluation and Program Planning, 30*(1), 21–35.

Cummins, R. A. (1996). The domains of life satisfaction: An attempt to order chaos. *Social Indicators Research, 52*, 55–72.

Cummins, R. A. (1997). Assessing quality of life. In R. I. Brown (Ed.), *Quality of life for people with disabilities: Models, research and practice* (2nd ed., pp. 116–150). Cheltenham: Stanley Thornes.

Cummins, R. A. (2000). Objective and subjective quality of life: An interactive model. *Social Indicators Research, 52*, 55–72.

Cummins, R. A. (2004). Instruments for assessing quality of life. In J. H. Hogg & A. Langa (Eds.), *Approaches to the assessment of adults with intellectual disabilities: A service providers guide* (pp. 130–152). London: Blackwell.

Cummins, R. A. (2005). Moving from the quality of life concept to a theory. *Journal of Intellectual Disability Research, 49*(10), 699–706.

Davis, E., & Fine-Davis, M. (1991). Social indicators of living conditions in Ireland with European comparisons. *Social Indicators Research, 25*(2–4), 318–353.

Donaldson, S. E., & Gooler, L. E. (2003). Theory-driven evaluation and action. *Evaluation and Program Planning, 26*(4), 355–366.

Fawcett, J. (1999). *The relationship of theory and research* (3rd ed.). Philadelphia, PA: F.A. Davis.

Felce, D., & Emerson, E. (2001). Living with support in a home in the community: Predictors of behavioural development and household and community activity. *Mental Retardation and Developmental Disabilities Research, 34*(2), 23–41.

Felce, D., & Perry, J. (1995). Quality of life: Its definition and measurement. *Research in Developmental Disabilities, 16*(1), 51–74.

Felce, D., & Perry, J. (1996). Assessment of quality of life. In R. L. Schalock (Ed.), *Quality of life: Vol. I: Conceptualization and measurement* (pp. 63–72). Washington, DC: American Association on Mental Retardation.

Felce, D., & Perry, J. (1997). Quality of life: The scope of the term and its breadth of measurement. In R. I. Brown (Ed.), *Quality of life for persons with disabilities: Models, research and practice* (2nd ed., pp. 56–71). Cheltenham: Stanley Thornes.

Frazier, P. A., Tix, A. P., & Barron, K. E. (2004). Testing moderator and mediator effects in counseling psychology research. *Journal of Counseling Psychology, 51*, 115–134.

Frechtling, J. A. (2007). *Logic modeling methods in program evaluation.* San Francisco: Jossey-Bass.

Gardner, J. F., & Carran, D. (2005). Attainment of personal outcomes by people with developmental disabilities. *Mental Retardation, 43*(3), 157–174.

Goode, D. A. (1990). Thinking about and discussing quality of life. In R. L. Schalock (Ed.), *Quality of life: Perspectives and issues* (pp. 41–57). Washington, DC: American Association on Mental Retardation.

Gugiu, P. C., Rodriguez, G., & Campos, L. (2007). Semi-structured interview protocol for constructing logic models. *Evaluation and Program Planning, 30*(4), 339–350.

Hair, J. F., Jr., Black, B., Babin, B., Anderson, R., & Tatham, R. (2006). *Multivariate data analysis* (6th ed.). Upper Saddle River, NJ: Prentice Hall.

Hartley, S. L., & MacLean, W. E., Jr. (2006). A review of the reliability and validity of Likert-type scales for people with intellectual disability. *Journal of Intellectual Disability Research, 50*(Part II), 813–827.

Hoyle, R. H., & Robinson, J. I. (2003). Mediated and moderated effects in social psychological research: Measurement, design, and analysis issues. In C. Sansone, C. Morf, & A. T. Panter (Eds.), *Handbook of methods in social psychology*. Thousand Oaks, CA: Sage.

Hughes, C., & Hwang, B. (1996). Attempts to conceptualize and measure quality of life. In R. L. Schalock (Ed.), *Quality of life: Volume I: Conceptualization and measurement* (pp. 51–61). Washington, DC: American Association on Mental Retardation.

Hughes, C., Hwang, B., Kim, J.-H., Eisenman, L. T., & Killian, D. J. (1995). Quality of life in applied research: A review and analysis of empirical measures. *American Journal on Mental Retardation, 99*(6), 623–641.

Hunter, D. E. K. (2006). Using a theory of change approach to build organizational strength, capacity, and sustainability with not-for-profit organizations in the human services sector. *Evaluation and Program Planning, 29*(2), 193–200.

Isaacs, B., Clark, C., Correia, S., & Flannery, J. (2007). The utility of logic models to plan quality of life outcomes evaluations. *Journal of Policy and Practice in Intellectual Disabilities, 4*, 177–185.

Jenaro, C., Verdugo, M. A., Caballo., C., Balboni, G., Lachapelle, Y., Otrebski, W., et al. (2005). Cross-cultural study of person-centered QOL domains and indicators: A replication. *Journal of Intellectual Disability Research, 49*(10), 734–739.

Kane, M., & Trochim, W. (2007). *A review of concept mapping for planning and evaluation.* Thousand Oaks, CA: Sage Publications.

Kaplan, S. A., & Garrett, K. E. (2005). The use of logic models by community-based initiatives. *Evaluation and Program Planning, 28*(2), 167–172.

Keith, K. D. (2001). International quality of life: Current conceptual, measurement, and implementation issues. *International Review of Research in Mental Retardation, 24*, 49–74.

Keith, K. D. (2007). Quality of life. In A. Carr, G. O'Reilly, P. N. Walsh, & J. McEvoy (Eds.), *The handbook of intellectual disability and clinical psychology practice* (pp. 143–168). London: Routledge.
Keith, K. D., & Bonham, G. S. (2005). The use of quality of life data at the organization and systems level. *Journal of Intellectual Disability Research, 49*(Part 10), 799–805.
Keith, K. D., & Ferdinand, L. R. (2000). *Project to compare quality of life of Nebraskans with developmental disabilities and citizens without disabilities*. Lincoln, NE: Governor's Planning Council on Developmental Disabilities.
Keith, K. D., Heal, L. W., & Schalock, R. L. (1996). Cross-cultural measurement of critical quality of life concepts. *Journal of Intellectual and Developmental Disability, 21*, 273–293.
Lachappelle, Y., Wehmeyer, M. L., Haelewyck, M. C., Courbois, Y., Keith, K. D., Schalock, R. L., et al. (2005). The relationship between quality of life and self-determination: An international study. *Journal of Intellectual Disability Research, 49*(10), 740–744.
Millar, A., Simeone, R. S., & Carnevale, J. T. (2001). Logic models: A systems tool for performance management. *Evaluation and Program Planning, 24*(1), 73–81.
Neeley-Barnes, S., Marcenko, M., & Weber, L. (2008). Does choice influence quality of life for people with mild intellectual disability? *Intellectual and Developmental Disabilities, 46*(1), 12–26.
Parmenter, T. R., & Donelly, M. (1997). An analysis of the dimensions of quality of life. In R. I. Brown (Ed.), *Quality of life for people with disabilities: Models, research and practice* (2nd ed., pp. 91–115). Cheltenham: Stanley Thornes.
Perry, J., & Felce, D. (2005). Factors associated with outcomes in community group homes. *American Journal on Mental Retardation, 110*, 121–135.
Petry, K., Maes, B., & Vlaskamp, C. (2005). Domains of quality of life of people with profound multiple disabilities: The perspective of parents and direct support staff. *Journal of Applied Research in Intellectual Disabilities, 18*, 35–46.
Petry, K., Maes, B., & Vlaskamp, C. (2007). Operationalizing quality of life for people with profound multiple disabilities: A Delphi study. *Journal of Intellectual Disability Research, 51*(5), 334–349.
Rahtz, D. R., Sirgy, M. J., & Lee, D.-J. (2004). Further validation and extension of the quality of life/community-health care model and measures. *Social Indicators Research, 69*, 167–198.
Rogers, E. M. (1995). *Diffusion of innovations* (4th ed.). New York: Free Press.
Rogers, J. D., & Bozeman, B. (2001). Knowledge value alliances: An alternative to the R & D project focus in evaluation. *Science Technology and Human Values, 26*(1), 23–55.
Rosas, S. R., & Camphausen, L. C. (2007). The use of concept mapping for scale development and validation in evaluation. *Evaluation and Program Planning, 30*(2), 125–135.
Schalock, R. L. (1999). Three decades of quality of life. In M. L. Wehmeyer & J. R. Patton (Eds.), *Mental retardation in the 21st century* (pp. 335–358). Austin, TX: Pro-Ed.
Schalock, R. L., & Bonham, G. S. (2003). Measuring outcomes and managing for results. *Evaluation and Program Planning, 26*(3), 229–235.
Schalock, R. L., Bonham, C. B., & Marchand, C. B. (2000). Consumer based quality of life assessment: A path model of perceived satisfaction. *Evaluation and Program Planning, 23*(1), 77–88.
Schalock, R. L., Bonham, G. S., & Verdugo, M. A. (2008). The conceptualization and measurement of quality of life: Implications for program planning and evaluation in the field of intellectual disabilities. *Evaluation and Program Planning, 31*(2), 181–190.
Schalock, R. L., & Felce, D. (2004). Quality of life and subjective well-being: Conceptual and measurement issues. In E. Emerson, C. Hatton, T. Thompson, & T. Parmenter (Eds.), *Handbook of applied research in intellectual disabilities* (pp. 261–279). New York: Wiley.
Schalock, R. L., Gardner, J. F., & Bradley, V. J. (2007). *Quality of life of persons with intellectual and other developmental disabilities: Applications across individuals, organizations, communities, and systems*. Washington, DC: American Association on Intellectual and Developmental Disabilities.

Schalock, R. L., & Keith, K. D. (1993). *Quality of life questionnaire manual*. Worthington, OH: IDS.

Schalock, R. L., & Luckasson, R. (2005). *Clinical judgment*. Washington, DC: American Association on Mental Retardation.

Schalock, R. L., & Verdugo, M. A. (2002). *Handbook on quality of life for human service practitioners*. Washington, DC: American Association on Mental Retardation.

Schalock, R. L., Verdugo, M. A., Bonham, G. S., Fantova, F., & van Loon, J. (2008). Enhancing personal outcomes: Organizational strategies, guidelines, and examples. *Journal of Policy and Practice in Intellectual Disabilities, 5*(4), 276–285.

Schalock, R. L., Verdugo, M. A., Jenaro, C., Wang, W., Wehmeyer, M., Xu, J., et al. (2005). A cross-cultural study of quality of life indicators. *American Journal on Mental Retardation, 110*, 298–311.

Shoemaker, P. J., Tankard, J. W., Jr., & Lasorsa, D. L. (2004). *How to build social science theories*. Thousand Oaks, CA: Sage Publications.

Shogren, K. A., Bradley, V. J., Gomez, S. C., Yeager, M. H., et al. (2009). Public policy and the enhancement of desired public policy outcomes for persons with intellectual disability. *Intellectual and Developmental Disabilities, 47*, 307–319.

Stancliffe, R., Abery, B., & Smith, J. (2000). Personal control and the ecology of community living settings: Beyond living-unit size and type. *American Journal on Mental Retardation, 105*, 431–454.

Stancliffe, R. J., & Lakin, C. K. (1998). Analysis of expenditures and outcomes of residential alternatives for persons with developmental disabilities. *American Journal on Mental Retardation, 102*, 552–568.

Stancliffe, R. J., & Lakin., K. C. (2005). *Costs and outcomes of community services for people with intellectual disabilities*. Baltimore, MD: Paul H. Brookes.

State of Nebraska Health and Human Services. (2008). *2008 Nebraska developmental disabilities provider profiles*. Lincoln, NE: Author (Division of Developmental Disabilities).

Summers, J. A., Poston, D. J., Turnbull, A. P., Marquis, J., Hoffman, L., Mannan, H., et al. (2005). Conceptualizing and measuring family quality of life. *Journal of Intellectual Disability Research, 49*(10), 777–783.

Sutherland, S., & Katz, S. (2005). Concept mapping methodology: A catalyst for organizational learning. *Evaluation and Program Planning, 28*(3), 257–269.

Taillefer, M.-C., Dupuis, G., Roberge, M.-A., & LeMay, S. (2003). Health-related quality of life models: Systematic review of the literature. *Social Indicators Research, 64*, 293–323.

Taylor, S. J., & Bogdan, R. (1998). *Introduction to qualitative research methods: A guidebook and resource* (3rd ed.). New York: Wiley.

Tossebro, J. (1995). Impact of size revised: Relation of number of residents to self-determination and deprivation. *American Journal on Mental Retardation, 100*, 59–67.

Van Loon, J. (2008). Aligning quality of life domains and indicators to support intensity scale data. In R. L. Schalock, J. R. Thompson, & M. J. Tasse (Eds.), *Supports intensity scale companion guide: A resource for SIS users* (pp. 80–87). Washington, DC: American Association on Intellectual and Developmental Disabilities.

Van Loon, J., van Hove, G., Schalock, R. L., & Claes, C. (2008). *Personal Outcomes Scale*. Middleburg, NL/Gent: Arduin Steichlich/Department of Special Education, University of Gent.

Veerman, J. W., & van Yperen, T. A. (2007). Degrees of freedom and degrees of certainty: A developmental model for the establishment of evidence-based youth care. *Evaluation and Program Planning, 30*(2), 136–148.

Verdugo, M. A., Arias, B., Gómez, L. E., & Schalock, R. L. (2008a). *GENCAT Scale. Formulary of the Gencat Scale. Application Manual of the Gencat Scale*. Barcelona: Department of Social action and Citizenship, Generalitat of Catalonia.

Verdugo, M. A., Arias, B., Gómez, L. E., & Schalock, R. L. (2008b). *GENCAT Scale. Final report about the development of a multidimensional scale for assessing the quality of life of human services users in Catalunya*. Barcelona: Department of Social action and Citizenship, Generalitat of Catalonia.

Verdugo, M. A., Arias, B., Gómez, L. E., & Schalock, R. L. (2009). *The integral scale*. Madrid: CEPE.

Verdugo, M. A., Arias, B., Gómez, L. E., & Schalock, R. L. (in press). Development of an objective instrument to assess quality of life in social services: Reliability and validity in Spain. *International Journal of Clinical and Health Psychology*.

Verdugo, M. A., & Schalock, R. L. (2003). *Cross-cultural survey of QOL indicators*. Salamanca: Institute on Community Integration-Faculty of Psychology-University of Salamanca.

Verdugo, M. A., Schalock, R. L., Gomez, L. E., & Arias, B. (2007). Developing multidimensional quality of life scales focusing on the context: The Gencat Scale. *Siglo Cero, 38*(4), 57–72.

Verdugo, M. A., Schalock, R. L., Keith, K. D., & Stancliffe, R. J. (2005). Quality of life and its measurement: important principles and guidelines. *Journal of Intellectual Disability Research, 49*(10), 707–717.

Walsh, P., Erickson, E., Bradley, V., Moseley, C., & Schalock, R. L. (2006). *Supported accommodation services for people with intellectual disabilities: A review of models and instruments used to measure quality of life in various settings*. Dublin: National Disability Authority.

Wang, M., Schalock, R. L., Verdugo, M. A., & Jenaro, C. (2010). Examining the factor structure and hierarchical nature of the quality of life construct. *American Journal on Intellectual and Developmental Disabilities, 115*, 218–233.

Wehmeyer, M., & Schwartz, M. (1998). The relationship between self-determination and quality of life for adults with mental retardation. *Education and Training in Mental Retardation and Developmental Disabilities, 31*(1), 3–12.

Chapter 3
Measuring Subjective Wellbeing: The Personal Wellbeing Index – Intellectual Disability

Robert A. Cummins, Anna L.D. Lau, Gareth Davey, and Jane McGillivray

Introduction

The past few decades have seen an exponential growth in quality of life (QOL) research. The results of these endeavors now form an increasingly coherent body of literature that has generated widespread interest in the wellbeing of populations and individuals. This interest is evident not just among researchers, but also in the increasing use of QOL measures as outcome indicators, and as information upon which to make policy decisions regarding the allocation of resources. However, all such applications depend critically on an understanding of the QOL construct and on the instruments used to make the necessary measurements.

Advancing a common understanding within this area has proved very challenging, not least because the field involves three disciplinary areas, and hence three different orientations to QOL measurement. These are economics, which continues to regard money as proxy for happiness (for a discussion see Ott, 2005); medicine, which regards QOL as centered on health and employs a measured construct called Health Related Quality of Life (for a critique see Cummins, Lau, & Stokes, 2004). And then there are the social sciences within which QOL is seen as an over-arching construct incorporating matters of money and health, but not restricted to these variables. It is this latter tradition that forms the basis of the following discussion.

Within the social sciences, QOL has been a topic of systematic study for over 30 years. The area was launched into scientific prominence by the publications of Andrews and Withey (1976) and Campbell, Converse, and Rodgers (1976). Both texts demonstrated the importance of clearly differentiating between the objective and the subjective dimensions of QOL. This distinction has now become the cornerstone of theory development but had to initially overcome the prejudice against subjective measurement, as being inherently unreliable.

R.A. Cummins (✉)
School of Psychology, Deakin University, Geelong, VIC, Australia
e-mail: cummins@deakin.edu.au

R. Kober (ed.), *Enhancing the Quality of Life of People with Intellectual Disabilities*, Social Indicators Research Series 41, DOI 10.1007/978-90-481-9650-0_3,

This necessary step was achieved by these two publications. They present compelling data to indicate that, not only can subjective wellbeing (SWB) be reliably measured, but that the statistical analysis of such data produced interesting results. Of particular importance, they found their measures of SWB to be remarkably stable. This was the second necessary discovery to allow for coherent theory development. It is this stability and reliability of measurement that has made SWB such an attractive new area for quantitative investigation. However, researchers in this area have also encountered some special problems in their attempt to create a systematic body of knowledge.

Two of the most difficult issues for researchers are the problems of terminology and measurement (see Diener, 2006 for a review). Terminological confusion has resulted from the lack of a single, unifying theory for SWB. Researchers approach the construct at different levels of complexity and this is reflected in the measures that they make. Then, because they create new scales to match their level of inquiry, they assume that they are measuring something different, and so coin new terms to characterize their measured variables. To sidestep this terminological complexity, for the purpose of this chapter the generic term employed to denote the mood state associated with self-perceived wellbeing will be subjective wellbeing (SWB).

The processes described above have resulted in a huge legacy of instruments. The Australian Centre on Quality of Life (ACQOL, 2008) lists many hundreds of scales that purport to measure SWB in one form or another. While such exploratory activities are, no doubt, a necessary evolutionary stage for the development of this new conceptual area, this diversity has also impeded progress in understanding SWB. These scales are of very mixed psychometric quality. Moreover, many comprise similar item content, yet with the output labeled as denoting different constructs. For example, the three core themes of perceived control, self-esteem, and optimism can be found to be represented in most of these scales. Yet, authors use items representing these basic constructs in different combinations to create scales that purport to measure something quite different. Examples are "Well-being at the school" (The Loso Well-Being Questionnaire; De Fraine, Van Landeghem, Van Damme, & Onghena, 2005) or "Self-Acceptance" (Scales of Psychological Well-Being; Ryff, 1989). While these scales may, or may not, measure something different from the basic constructs, the authors evidence no appreciation of the building blocks they are employing, and the naïve reader is lead into complexity, rather than into simplicity.

So the current state of play is that "Quality of life" is now understood to be a dual construct. It comprises an easily measured objective dimension, and a subjective dimension that is more challenging to measure and understand. Moreover, these two forms of measurement are usually, but not always, quite independent of one another. This relative independence is a crucial aspect of SWB research and demands a theoretical basis for understanding why it is so. One such model is provided by the proposition that SWB is managed by a system called SWB homeostasis (see Cummins, 2003; Cummins, Gullone, & Lau, 2002).

Homeostasis involves various mechanisms. Some of these are dispositional and include processes of adaptation, selective-attention, and cognitive-restructuring. Some of them are resources external to the person, such as money and close relationships, that can be used to shield the person from adversity. These various devices act in concert to maintain the average level of SWB at around 75% of the measurement scale maximum in Western nations (Cummins, Eckersley, Pallant, Van Vugt, & Misajon, 2003). That is, when SWB scores are standardized to a 0–100 scale (completely dissatisfied – completely satisfied) people in Australia, on average, feel 75% satisfied with their lives. However, this value differs between nations and between sub-groups mainly due to homeostatic failure. That is, the system has a limited capacity to deal with challenge and, if the level of stress exceeds the available resources, homeostasis will fail and SWB will fall below its normal range. We propose that this is the cause of depression.

This chapter concerns the measurement of SWB for people who have an intellectual disability (ID). This is a particularly challenging task. In addition to the generic difficulties of conceptualization and measurement faced by all QOL researchers, those who are concerned with measuring SWB in the context of intellectual disability face additional problems of obtaining valid and reliable self-reports. A recent review (Cummins, 2005a, 2005b) concluded that none of the measurement instruments available at that time had demonstrated adequate psychometric properties. This situation has changed marginally in the intervening years.

The special challenges associated with obtaining self-report from this population include the following:

(a) Proxy responding, which involves the provision of responses by another person (e.g., a relative, or someone who knows the person well) on behalf of the person with ID, is sometimes adopted to overcome the respondent's difficulty in meeting the cognitive demands of self-report. However, although inter-proxy concordance can be achieved, there are very serious concerns about the validity of such data, as to whether they accurately reflect the feelings of the individual concerned (Budd, Sigelman, & Sigelman, 1981; Cummins, 2002b; Perkins, 2007; Perry & Felce, 2003; Stancliffe, 1999).
(b) While a number of scales have been developed for the ID population, all of the following instruments are limited because their data cannot be norm-referenced back to the general population. These scales are the Lifestyle Satisfaction Scale (Heal & Chadsey-Rusch, 1985) and the Quality of Life Scale (Schalock & Keith, 1993), and, more recently, The Council on Quality and Leadership (2005) and the eight-domain model of quality of life (Verdugo, Gomez, & Martinez, 2007). On the other hand, most scales designed for the general population are not appropriate for use with people with an intellectual disability. As noted by Finlay & Lyons (2001), generic scales lack sensitivity to the needs of people with low cognitive capacity. It is therefore necessary to develop a scale that is suitable for administration across all sections of the population. Only by doing that can a valid and reliable comparison be made between levels of SWB in the general population and in the ID population.

These unresolved issues led to the development of the Personal Wellbeing Index (PWI). This instrument attempts to provide a valid measure of SWB for all sectors of the population through parallel versions of the scale. This development has occurred alongside the creation of a collaborative and international network of scholars who investigate the scale's performance in different cultures (International Wellbeing Group, 2006; Lau, Cummins, & McPherson, 2005).

The Development of the PWI

In response to the issues described above, the Personal Wellbeing Index (PWI) was created as a domain-based scale to serve as a universal measure of SWB. It is an improved version of an earlier scale, the Comprehensive Quality of Life Scale (ComQol). The ComQol has not only received generally favorable appraisal (Hagerty et al., 2001), but also criticism due to two features. The first is the use of importance as a weighting factor for domain satisfaction. This is now known to be a psychometrically flawed technique. The second is that the scale measures both subjective and objective life quality, but the objective scale could never be made to factor as intended. These problems have been detailed within Cummins (2002a) and will now be briefly explained. These issues continue to have relevance since a number of existing scales have the same problems.

1. The objective scale of the ComQol exhibits major problems in that, despite numerous item changes over the years, the 21 objective items do not factor into seven factors as intended, representing the seven domains. The clear implication is that the objective items do not demonstrate construct validity at the level of the domains. It may be the case that objective items simply cannot be made to conform to such psychometric requirements due to the essential independence of each variable. Certainly we are not aware of any other scale that has such a construction.
2. The subjective scale measures two variables in relation to each domain, as domain importance and domain satisfaction. Each corresponding measure of importance and satisfaction is then multiplied to yield a multiplicative composite.

This feature has considerable intuitive appeal. It seems logical to weight the satisfaction that a person experiences with any one domain by the importance they allocate to that domain. The logic of this procedure becomes more compelling when it is considered that the seven domains are measured by standard items. Thus, respondents are forced to register a satisfaction rating for each item irrespective of that domain's relevance to their life. Thus, it may be the case that someone can be "satisfied" with a domain (e.g., their material wealth), even though they do not value the domain (e.g., they have taken vows of poverty). In this case the multiplication by low importance would reduce the contribution of the domain to that person's total subjective quality of life score (obtained by summing across the domains).

Compelling though this logic seems to be, the process is flawed. The product of importance and satisfaction is a "multiplicative composite." It is, actually, an interaction term derived from the two primary variables. The difficulties and findings associated with this are as follows:

(a) It is assumed that the multiplication produces a meaningful outcome. That is, the meaning of the product can be understood in terms of each constituent variable. However, this can occur only for ratio data. Rating-scale data are quasi-interval, not ratio. The procedure is therefore statistically flawed.
(b) An additional assumption is that the psychological value of each scale choice point is equivalent between the two scales. Thus, for example, a score of 5 on a 7-point scale of importance has the same relative value as an equivalent numerical score on a scale of satisfaction. This assumption is almost certainly false. The psychometric distance between choice points is known to vary along the length of scales where the choice points are labeled (see, e.g., McHorney, Ware, Lu, & Sherbourne, 1994). Moreover, the different adjectival labels, as used for the importance and satisfaction scales, will produce different degrees of psychometric distance between adjacent scale choice points. The implication of all this is that the multiplication process is combining values with asymmetrical psychological meaning.
(c) In a similar vein, a change in an importance score from 2 to 4 should denote the same degree of perceptual shift as a corresponding score change in satisfaction. This has not been demonstrated.
(d) Data simulations demonstrate the non-linear nature of multiplicative composites derived from rating-scale data. This has been demonstrated by Trauer and Mackinnon (2001), who also argue the points made above.
(e) Because the multiplicative composite is an interaction term, its contribution to the explanation of relationships or differences can be calculated after the contribution of the main effects, importance, and satisfaction, has been calculated. Thus, for example, if the relationship between perceived health and Subjective wellbeing is to be examined, the correct procedure is to use hierarchical regression (e.g., Evans, 1991). In this procedure, Step 1 involves satisfaction, Step 2 involves importance, and Step 3 the composite (SxI). We have made this calculation on several occasions and have yet to discover any residual variance contributed by the multiplicative composite. In other words, the composite is failing to explain any additional variance beyond satisfaction and importance as separate predictive variables.

The new PWI scale was created to eliminate these problems. It deals with the problem of objective data by measuring SWB only. It also uses single questions of satisfaction without asking about importance. Both of these changes have considerably improved the conceptual structure, factorability, and psychometric properties of the scale. A detailed explanation of the changes and their justifications are provided by the International Wellbeing Group (2006).

Construction of the PWI-Adult

The PWI asks respondents to rate their satisfaction with eight life domains that collectively represent satisfaction with life as a whole. The domains are: standard of living, health, achieving in life, relationships, personal safety, community connectedness, future security, and religion/spirituality. These domains are empirically determined to represent the first-level deconstruction of satisfaction with "life as a whole." That is, each domain must contribute unique variance, as well as shared variance, to the item "How satisfied are you with your life as a whole?" Evidence for the current domain structure of the PWI has been presented by Cummins (1996), Cummins (1997), and Cummins, McCabe, Romeo, Reid and Waters (1997), International Wellbeing Group (2006), and Wills (2009).

The respondent is asked to rate their satisfaction with each domain on an 11-point end-defined scale, with anchor points of "completely dissatisfied" (0), "neutral" (5), and "completely satisfied" (10). SWB is calculated as the average of the domain scores (Cummins, 1996, 1997; International Wellbeing Group, 2006).

The PWI is designed to survey all sections of a population, as the eight domains are sufficiently broad to apply to most people. Several versions of the PWI have been developed for different groups. These include the basic scale for the general adult population (PWI-A) and modified, parallel versions for school-age children and adolescents (PWI-SC), pre-school-age children (PWI-PS), and people with an intellectual disability or other form of cognitive impairment (PWI-ID).

The scale items in each version are very similar, and the life domains they represent are common. However, the wording of some domains has been modified to meet the comprehension capacity and domain relevance of each group. This approach is unique among SWB scales, and is particularly advantageous in the field of intellectual disability. While other scales have been developed for this group, such as the Lifestyle Satisfaction Scale (Heal & Chadsey-Rusch, 1985) and the Quality of Life Scale (Schalock & Keith, 1993), the results from these scales cannot be norm-referenced back to the general population. The PWI overcomes this problem. The parallel versions permit a comparison of the PWI scores of people who are intellectually disabled with those of the general public.

The PWI-A has been used extensively within the Australian population. It is used as part of the Australian Unity Wellbeing Index, a project funded by Australian Unity, and managed by the Australian Centre on Quality of Life (ACQOL) at Deakin University. The project involves regular surveys of the Australian general population. Raw data from these surveys and the associated reports are available from the ACQOL website.

The PWI is also now used by a growing community of scholars in more than 50 countries (International Wellbeing Group, 2006). Index translations and the names of these scholars are available from the ACQOL website.

The Personal Wellbeing Index – Intellectual Disability (PWI-ID)

The PWI-ID is designed as a parallel version of the adult scale. It therefore uses the same theoretical basis and domain structure as the PWI-A, with the exception of the eighth domain of religion/spirituality, which has not yet been included. The PWI-ID also includes important modifications, which augment its suitability for respondents with a cognitive disability. These modifications are designed to increase the likelihood of data validity and reliability. They are as follows:

(a) *Item wording*: The wording of each item is simpler and more concrete than the original, and the term "satisfaction" is substituted by the word "happiness." For example, the question in the PWI-A "How satisfied are you with your health," has been simplified in the PWI-ID to "How happy do you feel about how healthy you are?" The PWI-ID questions are listed in Table 3.1.

These modifications are problematic for two reasons. The first is the uncertain extent to which they represent the construct of the original wording. The second is that, since they are more concrete and specific, they are further away from being a valid measure of SWB. Nevertheless, despite these two concerns, the Index does produce data very similar to those of the PWI-A, as is shown later.

(b) *Response choice*: A further modification is the availability of reduced-choice formats (5-, 3-, and 2-point scales) for those who cannot cope with the standard 11-point scale. This reduced-choice format is pictorial, represented by a series of outline faces (from very happy to sad) to enhance comprehension (Fig. 3.1).

Despite the use of these simplifying procedures, there is a minimum level of cognitive abstraction that is required to respond validly to the scale. In practice we have found that the PWI-ID is appropriate for people with a mild or upper-moderate level of cognitive impairment. It cannot be reliably used to test anyone with a severe or profound level of disability. Such people do not have the ability to provide valid self-reports of this type (Chadsey-rusch, DeStefano, O'Reilly, Gonzalez, & Coller-Klingenberg, 1992).

Table 3.1 The PWI-ID questions and the life domains they represent

Life domains	PWI-ID questions
	How happy do you feel about . . .?
Standard of living	The things you have? Like the money you have and the things you own?
Personal health	How healthy you are?
Life achievement	The things you make or the things you learn?
Personal relationships	Getting on with the people you know?
Personal safety	How safe you feel?
Community connectedness	Doing things outside your home?
Future security	How things will be later in your life?

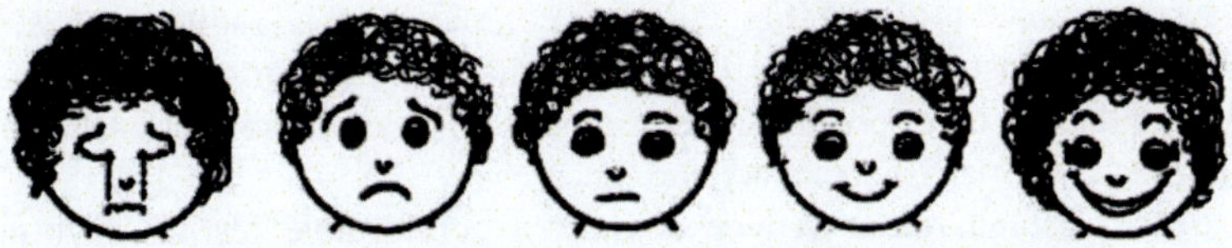

Fig. 3.1 The reduced-choice formats of the PWI-ID represented by outline faces

(c) *Pre-testing*: A unique feature of the PWI-ID is a pre-testing protocol, designed to include only those people who can respond validly to such scales. This protocol includes an initial test for acquiescent responding. If people are found to display this characteristic, testing is terminated. Testing for acquiescent responding and Likert scale competence is important because people with an intellectual or cognitive disability are likely to answer in ways they perceive are desired by the interviewer. See Cummins and Lau (2005) for further information about the test procedure methodology.

If respondents do not show acquiescent responding, they are tested for response-scale competence on the 0–10 scale format. This involves assessing whether they can count to 10 and, if they can, they are asked various questions to establish whether they can reliably respond to this scale format.

If they are unable to count to 10, or fail to provide a reliable response to questions using the 0–10 scale, they are tested for their ability to use the alternative reduce-choice formats using the faces in Fig. 3.1. These scales can present five, three, or two faces as choices.

The pre-testing protocol is a unique feature of the PWI-ID. It is notable that studies using other scales rarely provide clear information about the method they used, if any, to exclude participants with severe cognitive impairment (e.g., Reed & Roskell-Payton, 1996; Riemsma, Forbes, Glanville, Eastwood, & Kleijnen, 2001). Others have used unreliable exclusion methods, such as subjective decisions made by a third party informant (e.g., staff members of a nursing home: Bland, 1996). Such procedures may well result in the inappropriate omission of people who are, in fact, capable of rating their own SWB.

If people are found to respond reliably, using even the two-faces scale, then assessment can proceed. Otherwise testing is terminated, and this gives rise to the question of how to assess the SWB of people who lack the capacity to respond for them selves.

Our advice is that SWB cannot be validly measured for such people (but see Finlay and Lyons, 2001, for an alternative methodology). Notably, some scales recommend the use of proxy responding, which involves the provision of responses by another person on behalf of the person who is disabled. We do not recommend this technique for the reasons stated earlier.

Scale Administration

The administration of the scale, both for the pre-testing phase and for the scale itself, follows a determined protocol (Fig. 3.2). It is completed on an individual basis with only the test administrator and the person responding to the items being present. We recommend that no other person should be present, unless absolutely necessary, in order to reduce the risk of social acquiescence.

As further safeguards to reduce anxiety, a comfortable testing environment should be provided and all possible measures should be taken to reduce the perception of a power differential between interviewer and interviewee. For example,

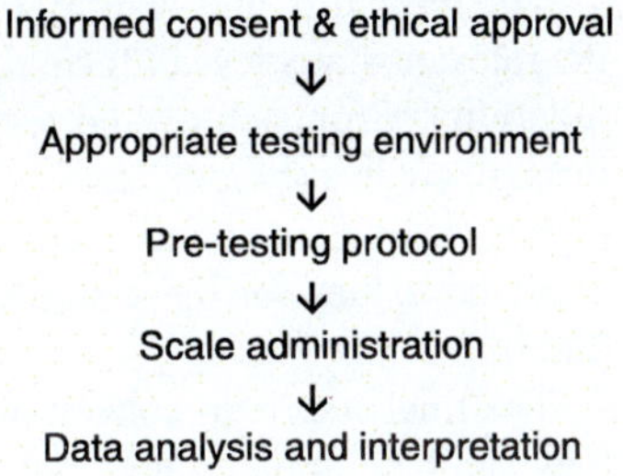

Fig. 3.2 A summary of the scale's administration procedure. See Cummins and Lau (2005) for further information

the interview can be conducted in a setting that is familiar to the respondent; the interviewer should dress in an appropriate manner, portray friendly or neutral mannerisms, and engage in social rituals, such as having a cup of tea, or meeting other members of the household before testing takes place.

There should also be attention to the ethical considerations of testing. Consent must be obtained from the interviewee or, when necessary, their parent or guardian. If testing is part of a research project, the aims, methods, possible outcomes, potential benefits or risks, etc. should be fully explained, along with the person's rights with respect to declining or agreeing to participate. It is important also to assess whether the interviewee has understood this information by, for example, asking appropriate questions (Arscott, Dagnan, & Kroses, 1998). The interviewer or principal researcher may need to obtain appropriate ethics approval from the relevant authority under which they are working, such as their university or departmental ethics committees.

Data Analysis

A crucial aspect of raw data processing, prior to running analyses to test hypotheses, is to thoroughly check the raw data for aberrant values. It is disturbing to note how rarely this procedure is reported in the empirical literature, even though it is an essential step when dealing with data from the PWI or other subjective data. Even with the full pre-testing protocol in place as a screening device, we still find a high incidence of aberrant data, relative to data collected from the general population. There are various ways through which such checks can be made.

First, the data should be checked for response sets. These are most evident when a respondent scores at the top or the bottom of the scale for all domains. When someone does this, their reason for doing so is uncertain, and so there is a slight possibility that the data are valid. However, there is a much higher probability that they are not and that the respondent is engaging in "yea-saying" or, much more rarely, "nay-saying." Such response patterns are extremely rare in general population samples but can be present in up to 30% of responses from people with an intellectual disability (Sigelman & Budd, 1986; Sigelman, Budd, Spanhel, & Schoenrock, 1981). Such responses, if included, will seriously change the values of the combined data set from the sample.

The reliability and validity of the data should be also determined to ensure that the relevant statistics conform to expectation. Reliability methods include split-half reliability, Cronbach α, and test–retest, if this is available. Validity is determined through such techniques as factor analysis and multiple regression. The validation process is explained and exemplified in further detail by Lau et al. (2005) and the expected values for these statistics are provided in the manual (Cummins & Lau, 2005).

The final step is to convert all scores into a standard 0–100 scale format so that they can be compared both with other studies of people with ID and, most importantly, with general population norms. These norms are reported in both the PWI-A and the PWI-ID manuals. These norms are presented as ranges of scores both from individual respondents and for group means. They are mainly based on Australian and Hong Kong data, so due care must be taken when using data from other cultures. This is discussed in more detail below.

In general, PWI-A data show good psychometric properties as determined from a range of western and Asian data (e.g., Lau et al., 2005). Fewer studies have used the PWI-ID, although studies are beginning to emerge, and the results are promising. In Australia and Hong Kong, the scale has yielded a Cronbach α of 0.76 and 0.68, respectively, and the domains form a single stable factor that predicts over 50% of the variance in "satisfaction with life as a whole" (McGillivray, Lau, Cummins, & Davey, 2009). These values mirror those obtained previously in the general population.

The Subjective Wellbeing of People with an Intellectually Disability

There has been a paucity of research on the SWB of people with an intellectual disability. This is of concern because ensuring that such people have normal levels of SWB, and identifying the variables which influence it, is essential. While the assumption of simple extrapolation from general population data is likely to be mainly valid, this group, of course, has special needs, and so complete congruence between the two populations is most unlikely.

It is likely, however, that the same theoretical principles derived from the SWB of general population adults will apply universally. Indeed, should it be found otherwise, the general theory would need revision. So, calling on the theory of SWB Homeostasis, various predictions can be made.

First, since people with an intellectual disability carry a psychological, and often a physical burden imposed by their disability, this is an added source of stress, which non-disabled people do not have. This, then, predicts that all people who have a disability will, on average, be less resilient than normal. The reason is that their homeostatic system is being forced to cope with a constant background level of challenge, thereby leaving less capacity to deal with other challenges. This, in turn, predicts that the level of SWB experienced by people with an intellectual disability will be normal range provided that they are receiving the level of support resources

Table 3.2 PWI-ID values from Australia and Hong Kong

	Australia		Hong Kong	
	M	SD	*M*	SD
Life domains Satisfaction with				
Standard of living	75.18	26.86	61.52	33.98
Personal health	70.49	26.39	61.05	33.66
Life achievement	79.30	26.05	66.98	31.76
Personal relationships	82.06	24.19	73.69	28.68
Personal safety	79.25	23.12	66.00	30.78
Community connectedness	81.84	23.10	65.40	32.20
Future security	72.41	26.44	52.99	34.05
Personal wellbeing index	77.08	16.64	63.99	18.86

that they require. However, being more prone than normal to homeostatic failure due to this background stress, they will be more likely to have below normal range SWB. There is evidence to support this view (e.g., Ahlsiö, Britton, Murray & Theorell, 1984; Viitanen, Fugl-Meyer, Bernspang, & Fugl-Meyer, 1988).

The determination of this normal SWB range depends, of course, on the availability of data. At the most approximate levels of estimation, early reports used published population mean scores as data. These estimated the normal range, as two standard deviations on either side of the grand mean, at 70–80 points for western populations, and 60–80 points for broader international data (Cummins, 1995, 1998), based on the 0–100 point scale. These estimates have been refined for two countries. In Australia, the population mean scores from 18 surveys has yielded a normal range of 73.4–76.4 points (Cummins et al., 2008 – Report 18.0). In Macau (2007), four population surveys conducted in each quarter during 2007 have yielded values that range from 63.4 to 64.4 points. Each of these reports shows a very steady estimate and one that reflects the approximately 10-point cultural response bias that has been reported elsewhere (Lau et al., 2005).

In terms of the PWI-ID, mean scores from Australia (77.08) and Hong Kong (63.99), as well as the individual domain mean scores (Table 3.2), approximate the normative population range. That the PWI-ID score is not compromised refutes the view that people with cognitive impairment have a level of SWB that is necessarily lower than the normative range. These results also indicate an appropriate level of support for the people in these samples from both countries.

These results are shown in Table 3.2. The domain and PWI-ID scores (measured on a 0–100 scale) are drawn from an Australian and Hong Kong sample (McGillivray et al., 2009).

Conclusions

From the description that has been offered it seems that the PWI-ID fulfills the statistical requirements of being reliable and valid. The particular strengths of this scale are that its construction is theoretically embedded and that its output can be compared with normative values. It is also unique among scales of this type in having a pre-testing protocol that attempts to ensure that the people who complete the questions of satisfaction have the cognitive capacity to do so reliably. Finally, the data that are produced can be interpreted with the assistance of SWB homeostasis theory. In sum, the PWI-ID represents the state of the art for the measurement of SWB for people with an intellectual disability.

References

ACQOL. (2008). Deakin University. Retrieved 2 May, 2008, from http://www.deakin.edu.au/research/acqol/instruments/index.htm

Ahlsiö, B., Britton, V., Murray, V., & Theorell, T. (1984). Disablement and quality of life after stroke. *Stroke, 15*, 886–890.

Andrews, F. M., & Withey, S. B. (1976). *Social indicators of well-being: American's perceptions of life quality*. New York: Plenum Press.

Arscott, K., Dagnan, D., & Kroses, B. S. (1998). Consent to psychological research by people with an intellectual disability. *Journal of Applied Research in Intellectual Disabilities, 11*(1), 77–83.

Bland, R. (1996). *Episodic care of people with a mental illness*. In Towards A National Agenda for Carers: Workshop Papers: Australia Government Publishing Services Aged and Community Care Division, DHSH. Canberra, Australia.

Budd, E. C., Sigelman, C. K., & Sigelman, L. (1981). Exploring the outer limits of response bias. *Sociological Focus, 14*(4), 297–307.

Campbell, A., Converse, P. E., & Rodgers, W. L. (1976). *The quality of American life: Perceptions, evaluations, and satisfactions*. New York: Russell Sage Foundation.

Chadsey-rusch, J., DeStefano, L., O'Reilly, M., Gonzalez, P., & Coller-Klingenberg, L. (1992). Assessing the loneliness of workers with mental retardation. *Mental Retardation, 2*, 85–92.

Cummins, R. A. (1995). On the trail of the gold standard for life satisfaction. *Social Indicators Research, 35*, 179–200.

Cummins, R. A. (1996). The domains of life satisfaction: An attempt to order chaos. *Social Indicators Research, 38*, 303–332.

Cummins, R. A. (1997). Self-rated quality of life scales for people with an intellectual disability: A review. *Journal of Applied Research in Intellectual Disability, 10*, 199–216.

Cummins, R. A. (1998). The second approximation to an international standard of life satisfaction. *Social Indicators Research, 43*, 307–334.

Cummins, R. A. (2002a). Proxy responding for subjective well-being: A review. *International Review of Research in Mental Retardation, 25*, 183–207.

Cummins, R. A. (2002b). *Vale ComQol: Caveats to using the comprehensive quality of life scale. Welcome: the personal wellbeing index*. Deakin University, Retrieved 2 May, 2008, from http://www.deakin.edu.au/research/acqol/instruments/ValeComQol.doc

Cummins, R. A. (2003). Normative life satisfaction: Measurement issues and a homesotatic model. *Social Indicators Research, 64*, 225–256.

Cummins, R. A. (2005a). Instruments assessing quality of life. In J. Hogg & A. Langa (Eds.), *Approaches to the assessment of adults with intellectual disability: A service provider's guide* (pp. 118–137). London: Blackwell Publishing.

Cummins, R. A. (2005b). Issues in the systematic assessment of quality of life. In J. Hogg & A. Langa (Eds.), *Approaches to the assessment of adults with intellectual disability: A service provider's guide* (pp. 9–22). London: Blackwell Publishing.

Cummins, R. A., Eckersley, R., Pallant, J., Van Vugt, J., & Misajon, R. (2003). Developing a national index of subjective wellbeing: The Australian Unity Wellbeing Index. *Social Indicators Research, 64*, 159–190.

Cummins, R. A., Gullone, E., & Lau, A. L. D. (2002). A model of subjective well being homeostasis: The role of personality. In E. Gullone & R. A. Cummins (Eds.), *The universality of subjective wellbeing indicators: Social indicators research series* (pp. 7–46). Dordrecht: Kluwer.

Cummins, R. A., & Lau, A. L. D. (2005). Quality of Life Measurement. In R. Norman & D. Currow (Eds.), *Supportive care of the urology patient* (pp. 5–23). Oxford: Oxford University Press.

Cummins, R. A., Lau, A. L. D., & Stokes, M. (2004). HRQOL and subjective wellbeing: noncomplementary forms of outcome measurement. *Expert Reviews in Pharmacoeconomics Outcomes Research, 4*, 413–420.

Cummins, R. A., McCabe, M. P., Romeo, Y., Reid, S., & Waters, L. (1997). An initial evaluation of the comprehensive quality of life scale – Intellectual disability. *International Journal of Disability Development and Education, 44*, 7–19.

Cummins, R. A., Woerner, J., Tomyn, A., Gibson, A., Lai, L., & Collard, J. (2008). *Australian unity wellbeing index: Report 18 – The wellbeing of Australians – Changing conditions to make life better*. Australian Centre on Quality of Life, School of Psychology, Deakin University, ISBN 978 1 74156 101 2, Retrieved 2 May, 2008, from http://www.deakin.edu.au/research/acqol/index_wellbeing/index.htm

De Fraine, B., Van Landeghem, G., Van Damme, J., & Onghena, P. (2005). An analysis of wellbeing in secondary school with multilevel growth curve models and multilevel multivariate models. *Quality & Quantity, 39*, 297–316.

Diener, E. (2006). Guidelines for national indicators of subjective well-being and ill-being. *Journal of Happiness Studies, 7*, 397–404.

Evans, M. G. (1991). The problem of analyzing multiplicative composites. *American Psychologist, 46*(1), 6–15.

Finlay, W. M. L., & Lyons, E. (2001). Methodological issues in interviewing and using self-report questionnaires with people with mental retardation. *Psychological Assessment, 13*(3), 319–335.

Hagerty, M. R., et al. (2001). Quality of life indexes for national policy: review and agenda for research. *Social Indicators Research, 55*, 1–91.

Heal, L. W., & Chadsey-Rusch, J. (1985). The lifestyle satisfaction scale (LSS): Assessing individuals' satisfaction with residence, community setting, and associated services. *Applied Research in Mental Retardation, 6*, 475–490.

International Wellbeing Group. (2006). *Personal wellbeing index* (4th ed.). Melbourne, Australian Centre on Quality of Life, School of Psychology, Deakin University, ISBN 1 74156 048 9. Retrieved 25 June, 2007, from http://www.deakin.edu.au/research/acqol/instruments/wellbeing_index.htm

Lau, A. L. D., Cummins, R. A., & McPherson, W. (2005). An investigation into the cross-cultural equivalence of the personal wellbeing index. *Social Indicators Research, 72*, 403–430.

Macau. (2007). *The Macau quality of life report, number 4*. Retrieved 2 May, 2008, from http://www.iium.edu.mo/index.php?option=com_content&task=view&id=618&Itemid=1399

McGillivray, J. A., Lau, A. L. D., Cummins, R. A., & Davey, G. (2009). The utility of the personal wellbeing index intellectual disability scale (PWI-ID) in an Australian sample. *Journal of Applied Research in Intellectual Disability, 22*, 276–286.

McHorney, C. A., Ware, J. E., Jr., Lu, J. F. R., & Sherbourne, C. D. (1994). The MOS 36-item Short-Form Health Survey (SF-36): III. Tests of data quality, scaling assumptions, and reliability across diverse patient groups. *Medical Care, 32*, 40–66.

Ott, J. (2005). Level and inequality of happiness in nations: Does greater happiness of a greater number imply greater inequality in happiness? *Journal of Happiness Studies, 6*, 397–420.

Perkins, A. (2007). Self- and proxy reports across three populations: Older adults, persons with Alzheimer's disease, and persons with intellectual disabilities. *Journal of Policy and Practice, 4*(1), 1–10.

Perry, J., & Felce, D. (2003). Quality of life outcomes for people with intellectual disabilities living in staffed community housing services: A stratified random sample of statutory, voluntary and private agency provision. *Journal of Applied Research in Intellectual Disabilities, 16*, 11–28.

Reed, J., & Roskell-Payton, V. (1996). Constructing familiarity and managing the self: Ways of adapting to life in nursing and residential homes for older people. *Ageing Society*, *16*, 543–560.
Riemsma, R. P., Forbes, C. A., Glanville, J. M., Eastwood, A. J., & Kleijnen, J. (2001). General health status measures for people with cognitive impairment: learning disability and acquired brain injury. *Health Technology Assessment*, *5*(6), 1–100.
Ryff, C. D. (1989). Happiness is everything, or is it? Explorations on the meaning of psychological well-being. *Journal of Personality and Social Psychology*, *57*, 1069–1081.
Schalock, R. L., & Keith, K. D. (1993). *Quality of life questionnaire manual*. Worthington, OH: IDS Publishing Corporation.
Sigelman, C. K., & Budd, E. C. (1986, March). Pictures as an aid in questioning mentally retarded persons. *Rehabilitation Counselling Bulletin*, *29*, 173–181.
Sigelman, C. K., Budd, E. C., Spanhel, C. L., & Schoenrock, C. J. (1981). When in doubt, say yes: Acquiescence in interviews with mentally retarded persons. *Mental Retardation*, *19*, 53–58.
Stancliffe, R. J. (1999). Proxy respondents and the reliability of the quality of life questionnaire empowerment factor. *Journal of Intellectual Disability Research*, *43*, 185–193.
The Council on Quality and Leadership. (2005). *Personal outcome measures: Measuring personal quality of life*. Towson, USA: The Council on Quality and Leadership.
Trauer, T., & Mackinnon, A. (2001). Why are we weighting? The role of importance ratings in quality of life measurement. *Quality of Life Research*, *10*, 579–585.
Verdugo, M. A., Gomez, L. E., & Martinez, B. A. (2007, December 6–9). *Validation of the eight-domain model of quality of life*. Paper presented at the Conference of the International Society for Quality of Life Studies, San Diego, CA.
Viitanen, M., Fugl-Meyer, K. S., Bernspang, B., & Fugl-Meyer, A. R. (1988). Life satisfaction in long-term survivors after stroke. *Scandinavian Journal of Rehabilitation Medicine*, *20*, 17–24.
Wills, E. (2009). Spirituality and subjective wellbeing: Empirical evidences for a new domain in the PWI index. *Journal of Happiness Studies*, *10*, 49–69.

Chapter 4
The Integral Quality of Life Scale: Development, Validation, and Use

Miguel Á. Verdugo, Laura E. Gómez, Benito Arias, and Robert L. Schalock

Introduction

Although the concept of quality of life (QOL) is not new, the professional or academic approach to its conceptualization and measurement in the field of intellectual disabilities (ID) is relatively recent. Even though the conceptualization and measurement of QOL is a complex process, there is an emerging consensus that one's quality of life has both subjective and objective aspects. However, it is not easy to find a QOL instrument, which has been developed from this perspective. The two purposes of this chapter are to: (a) present the QOL conceptual and measurement framework that is currently being used to implement QOL-related program practices, to assess and report personal outcomes, to guide quality improvement strategies, and to evaluate the effectiveness of those practices and strategies (Schalock, Bonham, & Verdugo, 2008); and (b) present a QOL questionnaire, the QOL Integral Scale (Verdugo, Gómez, Arias, & Schalock, 2010) developed by the Institute on Community Integration (INICO, University of Salamanca, Spain), using that theoretical framework.

The content of this chapter is primarily relevant to professionals working in the field of intellectual disabilities who are interested on implementing QOL focused program practices and individualized supports, and to those who would like to apply quality of life enhancement strategies at the individual (micro-system) level. In the same way, it is very helpful for guiding organization, policies, and practices (meso- and macro-system). Moreover, it will be of great interest to those researches working at a more theoretical level who are concerned about impacting the QOL field, and moving from a QOL conceptual framework toward a real QOL theory with identified mediators and moderators and with clear relationships among its components (Kalafat, Illback, & Sanders, 2007).

M.Á. Verdugo (✉)
School of Psychology-University of Salamanca, Institute on Community Integration, University of Salamanca, Salamanca, Spain
e-mail: verdugo@usal.es

R. Kober (ed.), *Enhancing the Quality of Life of People with Intellectual Disabilities*, Social Indicators Research Series 41, DOI 10.1007/978-90-481-9650-0_4,

Table 4.1 Domains and core indicators of quality of life

Domains	Core indicators
Self-determination	Autonomy; decisions; choices; goals; and personal preferences
Rights	Human; legal
Emotional wellbeing	Absence of negative feelings; self-concept; satisfaction with life
Social inclusion	Integration; participation; supports
Personal developmental	Work; education, activities of daily life
Interpersonal relationships	Family relationships; social relationships
Material wellbeing	Incomes; possessions; conditions of housing, conditions of workplace
Physic wellbeing	General health; health (consequences); sanitary attention; sleep

Conceptual Framework

The present work is based on the initial framework of Schalock & Verdugo (2002) and subsequent work regarding its validation and cross-cultural use (Jenaro et al., 2005; Schalock et al., 2005, 2008; Verdugo & Schalock, 2001; Verdugo, Arias, & Gómez, 2006; Verdugo, Gómez, Arias, & Martin, 2006). According to this framework, QOL is defined as a concept that (a) is multidimensional; (b) has etic (universal) and emic (culture-bound) properties; (c) has objective and subjective components; and (d) is influenced by personal and environmental factors. QOL is composed of eight domains (listed in Table 4.1) that emerged as a result of a very exhaustive review of international QOL literature in the areas of education, special education, intellectual disabilities, mental health, and aging (Schalock & Verdugo, 2002). From this review the core indicators listed in Table 4.1 also emerged. Core indicators are QOL-related perceptions, behaviors, and conditions that define operationally each domain. These domains and indicators were seen as stable and were validated in a series of cross-cultural studies (Bonham et al., 2004; Gómez, Verdugo, & Arias, 2007; Jenaro et al., 2005; Schalock et al., 2005; Verdugo, Gómez, et al., 2006). The indicator measurement results in personal outcomes that can be used for both reporting purposes and guiding organization improvements (Keith & Bonham, 2005; Langberg & Smith, 2006; Schalock & Bonham, 2003; Schalock et al., 2008; Veerman & van Yperen, 2007).

This framework has been developed over the last two decades using three sequential steps (Schalock & Verdugo, 2007; Shoemaker, Tankard, & Lasorsa, 2004). The first step was observing and describing the phenomenon; the second consisted in concept mapping; finally, the third step was empirically testing the framework (Carlisle & Christensen, 2006; Hughes, Hwang, Kim, Eisenman, & Killian, 1995; Poole, Duvall, & Wofford, 2006; Schalock & Verdugo, 2002, 2007; Schalock et al., 2008; Shoemaker et al., 2004; Sutherland & Katz, 2005).

Measurement Framework

Measuring personal outcomes related to QOL is currently a clear conceptual and psychometric process. Developing and assessing an instrument must be carried out within a conceptual framework that defines clearly the construct to be measured. The framework also should specify the observable behaviors related to the construct through semantic definitions. The aspects referenced to these behaviors must be reflected by the items that compose the instrument. According to this, the approach to QOL measurement is based on the assessment of indicator items associated with the domains and core indicators listed in Table 4.1.

The next step in developing an assessing instrument is defining the assessment purpose. Depending on the purpose and the perspective of the instrument developed, indicator items will be used to assess either person's perceived wellbeing on the item ("self-report") or the person's life experiences and circumstances ("direct observation") (Schalock et al., 2008). In this sense, we can speak about objective and subjective questionnaires depending on their purpose, content, and respondent (Brown, 1997; Cummins, 1997; Perry & Felce, 1995, 2005; Schalock, Keith, Verdugo, & Gómez, 2010; Verdugo, Arias, Gómez, & van Loon, 2007). When the goal is program evaluation or quality improvement implementation, applying objective questionnaires based on the direct observation of personal experiences and circumstances is recommended. On the contrary, if the evaluator desires to assess personal outcomes and is interested in developing person-centered planning, subjective Likert-type scales answered by the person with disabilities should be used (Schalock & Felce, 2004). Nevertheless, a general agreement exists at the present time, about the urgent need of investigating the best ways of measuring and evaluating the QOL concept, lending special attention to both objective and subjective circumstances (Anderson & Burckhardt, 1999; Cummins, 1996; Gómez et al., 2007; Goodley, Armstrong, Sutherland, & Laurie, 2003; Schalock & Felce, 2004; Schalock & Verdugo, 2002; Schalock et al., 2010; Verdugo, Gómez, et al., 2006). As discussed later the QOL Integral Scale was developed to serve this purpose.

Once the conceptual and measurement framework has been defined and the goal of the assessment has been specified, the next step in the development of an instrument consists in selecting representative items. A concept mapping approach is typically used to select specific items (Schalock et al., 2010). In this sense, the process used to develop the GENCAT Scale (Verdugo, Arias, Gómez, & Schalock, 2008) –an objective QOL questionnaire for users of social services in Catalonia, Spain serves nationally and internationally as a model to develop multidimensional QOL scales focusing on the context (Schalock et al., 2010; Van Loon, Van Hove, Schalock, & Claes, 2008; Verdugo, Schalock, Gómez, & Arias, 2007). This process includes several steps that are summarized in Fig. 4.1.

The Integral Quality of Life Scale

The development of the *Integral QOL Scale* was based on the model summarized in Fig. 4.1 and involved the following steps (with the exception of the focus group step): (a) review of QOL previous research and literature; (b) development of a pool of items based on that review; (c) organizing the selected items by domains and indicators, and selecting the most representative; (d) creating new items for each indicator when it was necessary (there should be at least two items by indicator); (e) once all domains and indicators were represented by several items, expert judges

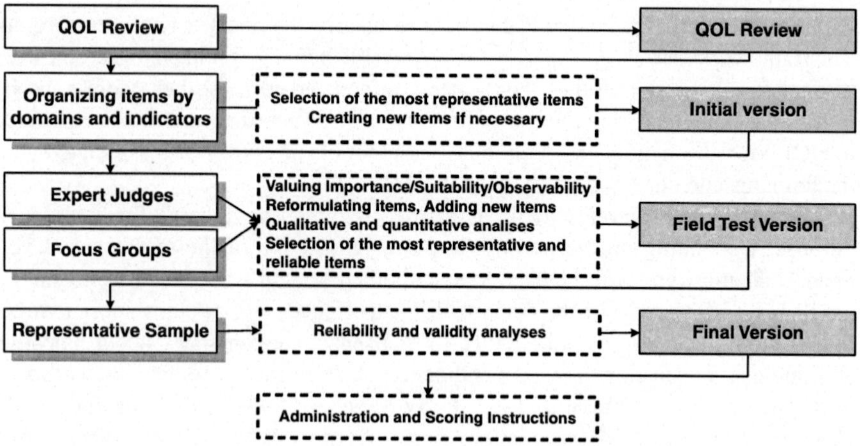

Fig. 4.1 Model to develop multidimensional QOL scales focusing on the context

in the field evaluated each item and reformulated items and suggested new ones for each domain; (f) selection of the most reliable and valid items was made based on quantitative and qualitative analysis of concordance among judges; (g) a field-test scale was developed based on the analysis of obtained information from experts; (h) application of the field-test scale to a representative sample of the population in Spain; (i) determining psychometric properties of the instrument; and (j) finalizing administration and scoring instructions.

The Objective Subscale

This scale is considered objective for three reasons: first, because it measures objective and observable aspects of QOL, second because of its "yes/no" answer format, and third because it captures the point of view of an external observer and specifically the staff who work with the person with intellectual disabilities. It consists of a listing of 29 items, formulated as third person statements. Also, the professional is required to value the quality of life of the person with disabilities in a general way by using a 5-point Likert scale (choosing among "very high," "high," "average," "low," and "very low").

The Subjective Subscale

This subscale is considered subjective for three reasons: first, because it assesses subjective aspects of QOL, second, because of its Likert-type scale, and third because it reflects the point of view of the person with intellectual disabilities. Although it is a self-reported instrument, a face-to-face interview is highly recommended to guarantee a total understanding of the instructions, the items, and the Likert-type scale. For this reason, the listing of items is preceded by instructions for the interviewer and the person being interviewed. The questionnaire consists of 47 items with a 4-point Likert scale ("strongly disagree," "disagree," "agree," and "totally agree"). The subjective scale also includes two questions more. In the first one, the person has to value his/her general QOL, choosing among five options ("very high," "high," "average," "low," "very low"). In the second, the person has to order the eight QOL domains according to its importance.

The originality and importance of the present validation research lies in that *The Integral Scale*: (a) is based on the current theoretical framework; (b) overcomes some of the limitations found in previous QOL instruments; and (c) allows an integral (i.e., subjective and objective) assessment of QOL. The result is that *the Integral QOL Scale* allows one to measure QOL from an objective and a subjective perspective, to determine if discrepancies among both perspectives exist, and, if they do, it allows one to compare and interpret them. It also serves as a guide of improvement for staff, services, and politics.

Testing the Scale's Conformity to the QOL Framework

Once the questionnaire was developed and its reliability was determined, testing the Scale's conformity with the proposed QOL conceptual framework was the next goal. In order to corroborate the factorial structure of the eight-domain model, the Integral QOL Scale was applied to 413 adults with intellectual disabilities in Spain. In this analysis, factorial analysis was combined with innovative analysis such as self-organizing maps (SOM), generative topographic mapping (GTM), and non-metric multidimensional scaling. These latter three methods have not typically been used in the psychology and education field until the work described below.

To test the factorial structure of the QOL conceptual framework, first-level confirmatory factorial analysis was carried out with the subjective scale following the recommendations for ordinal data analysis suggested by Jöreskog (1993, 2002). The *Satorra-Bentler Scaled Chi-Squared* statistic (Satorra & Bentler, 1988) – typically used to assess the goodness of fit of the model – showed that there were differences between matrixes of observed (by the data) and predicted (by the model) variances–covariances. However, to better evaluate the goodness of fit of the model, several

Table 4.2 Composed reliability and extracted variance of the subjective scale

Domains	Composed reliability (ρ_c)	Extracted variance (ρ_v)
Self-determination	0.71	0.24
Rights	0.66	0.34
Emotional wellbeing	0.80	0.52
Social inclusion	0.65	0.25
Personal development	0.49	0.26
Interpersonal relationships	0.73	0.31
Material wellbeing	0.88	0.52
Physical wellbeing	0.80	0.38

additional indexes were also provided (Table 4.2): the *root mean squared error of approximation* (RMSEA; Steiger, 1990), the *standardized root mean squared residual* (SRMSR; Jöreskog & Sörbom, 1996), the *goodness-of-fit index* (GFI; Tanaka & Huba, 1985), and the *comparative fit index* using the independence model as baseline (CFI: Bentler, 1990). Adequate to good fit is suggested by RMSEA and SRMSR values approaching 0.05. For the GFI and the CFI indexes, values between 0.80 and 1.00 indicate adequate to good fit. As it is shown in the next table, the additional indexes were adequate. For this reason, it can be concluded that quality of life is a multidimensional concept composed of eight domains: emotional wellbeing, physical wellbeing, material wellbeing, personal development, self-determination, social inclusion, interpersonal relationships, and rights. Figure 4.2 represents the standardized solution, and indicates that the data fit the model.

Our next challenge was to determine how the items were distributed in an *n*-dimensional space using neural networks. The methodology of artificial neural networks allows us to determine in an automatic way (without the intervention of the user) possible subjacent structures. Three types of artificial neural networks were used: *non-metric multidimensional scaling* (NMDS; Kruskal, & Wish, 1978; Wilkinson et al., 1992), *self-organizing maps* (SOM; Kohonen, 1990, 2001), and *generative topographic mapping* (GTM; Bishop, Svensén, & Williams, 1996; Nabney, 2004; Svensén, 1998). The methods consist in projecting the data – in this case, the items of the subjective scale – on a low-dimensional representation. The goal was testing if the items are presented as groups in the projection space.

As an example of innovator representation of data in our field, Fig. 4.3 shows the SOM for the subjective scale. Kohonen's SOM is an unsupervised neural network providing a mapping from a high-dimensional input space to a low-dimensional output space while preserving topological relations as faithfully as possible. According to this method, the relationships are shown between the items according to distance among them. So, projected data in close proximities are similar and so grouped. As the standardized solution did, SOM figure shows that the eight domains were projected on to the 2D space and that there were also some isolated items.

SOM has some limitations that were highlighted by Kohonen (2005). Chief among these are: (a) the absence of a cost function, (b) the lack of a theoretical basis for choosing learning rate parameter schedules and neighborhood parameters to ensure topographic ordering, (c) the absence of any general proofs of convergence, and (d) the fact that the model dos not define a probability density. For this reason, the GTM model was also used since it overcomes most of the limitations of the SOM while introducing no significant disadvantages. The GTM model is defined in terms of a mapping from the latent space into the data space. For the purposes of data visualization, the mapping is then inverted using Bayes' theorem, giving rise to a posterior distribution in latent space. As it can be observed in Fig. 4.4, the items were grouped in the eight domains, and so the proposed model was also confirmed by this method.

Beyond this conclusion, it was also determined through a 3D SOM model that there could be a subjacent structure. In Fig. 4.5, the reader can observe that the

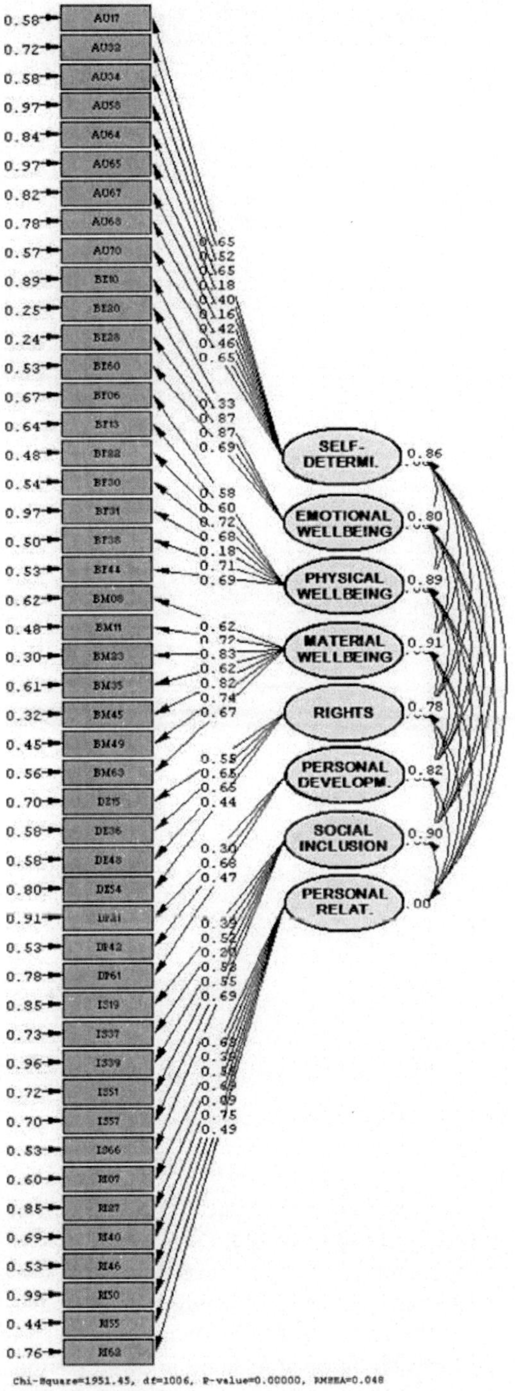

Fig. 4.2 Subjective scale standard solution

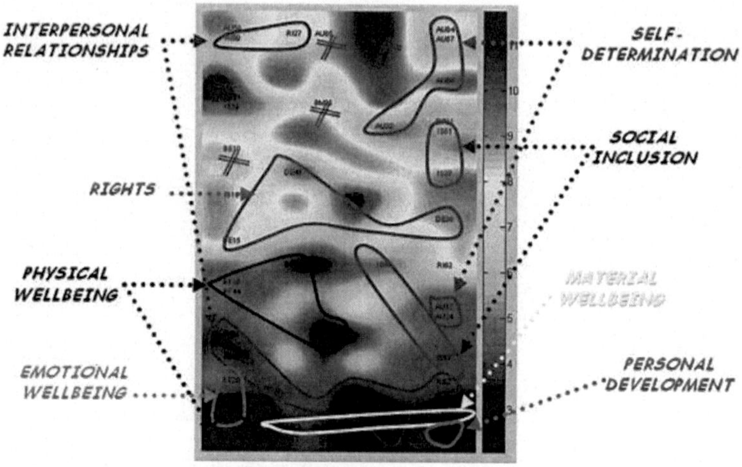

Fig. 4.3 Bi-dimensional SOM for the subjective scale

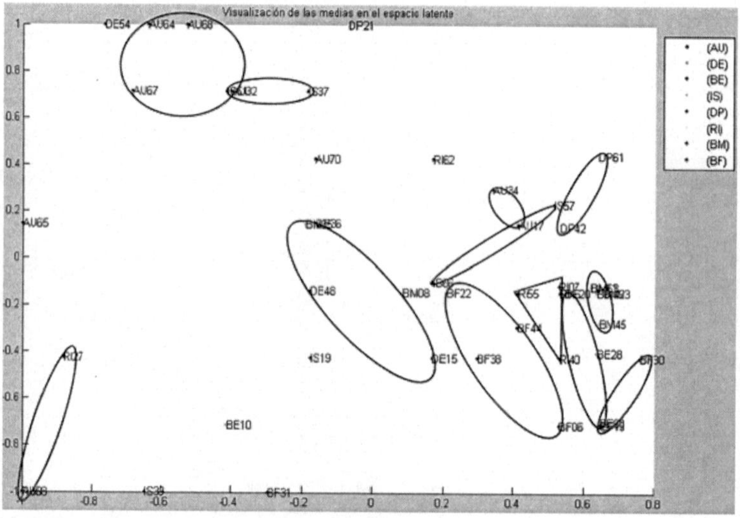

Fig. 4.4 GTM for the subjective scale

eight domains might be reduced to four bigger areas, and therefore, to four potential second-level factors of QOL.

In summary, eight first-level factors of QOL were confirmed, although some items appeared isolated from their domains. Moreover, four bigger factors potentially could be seen in the projection. This finding encourages further studies that focus on the need to study in depth the theoretical framework of QOL so that

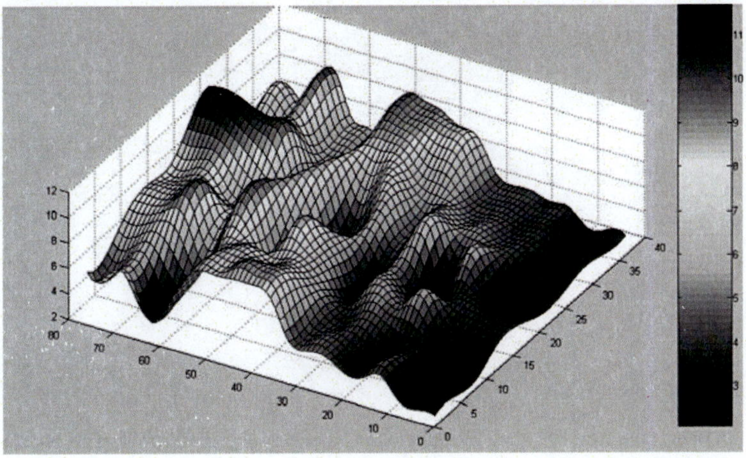

Fig. 4.5 Bi-dimensional SOM for the subjective scale

we will be able to move toward from a framework to a more detailed model of QOL (Schalock et al., 2008).

Preliminary Psychometric Studies

Concerning to the composed reliability of the latent variables (construct reliability) and the extracted mean variance, Table 4.2 shows that the obtained values indicated an adequate reliability, especially material wellbeing, physical wellbeing, and emotional wellbeing ($\rho_c > 0.80$). The less reliable domain was personal development ($\rho_c = 0.49$).

Scale Validation and Framework Confirmation

At present, we have two research goals: to validate the *Integral QOL Scale* and to confirm the QOL framework. To achieve these goals, the first task was to apply the *Integral Scale* to a larger and more representative sample in Spain. The sample was composed of 861 people with intellectual disabilities from different counties in Spain. As shown in Fig. 4.6, not only most of the participants were from the north west, but also an important number of people were from the south. Almost 60% of the people were male. In relation to their age, most of them were among the 31–40 years old. Concerning to their civil state, 98% were single. Most had a middle socioeconomic level, lived in the family house, and were in sheltered works.

At this moment, we are working on the analysis of the data, applying methods such as structural equation model (SEM) and item response theory (IRT). The

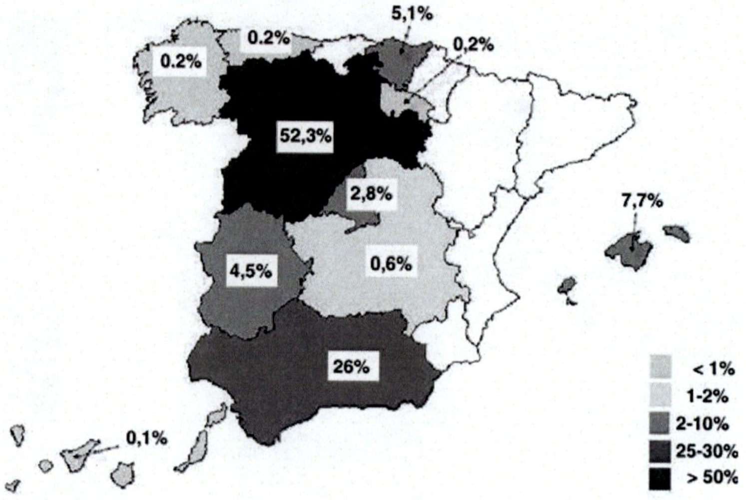

Fig. 4.6 Geographic distribution of the Spanish sample

authors expect to achieve the final version of the instrument in the very near future. This finalization will allow using the scale in our on-going work on QOL theory construction and model development.

Adaptation to Other Cultures

The Integral QOL Scale has been widely accepted not only nationally, but also internationally. The authors are currently collaborating with researchers from several countries to adapt and validate the instrument for their respective cultures. One of the geographical areas where its being applied is Europe, including The Netherlands, Belgium, Ireland, and Portugal. In the Netherlands, there is a Dutch version of the questionnaire (Verdugo, Arias, Gómez, & van Loon, 2007) that has been applied to 35 clients with a mild intellectual disability and severe challenging behavior. It will be applied to a bigger sample in the next few months and it is being considered for application to people with mental health problems. In Belgium, a French version of the questionnaire has already been applied to 30 people with intellectual disabilities, with a larger sample included in the near future. In Ireland and Portugal, the *Integral QOL Scale* is being adapted to be applied to a significant number of persons with intellectual disabilities.

The second geographical area where the questionnaire is being applied is South America, including Colombia, Brazil, and Argentina. In Brazil, the Portuguese version of the instrument is being used and applied to 205 people with intellectual disabilities (Moreno et al., 2005). In Colombia ($N = 152$) and Argentina ($N = 324$), the Spanish version has been used after confirming the relevance of the respective items.

Discussion

The present chapter has described a recently developed instrument to assess QOL of persons with intellectual disabilities in a comprehensive way. There are two characteristics that make the instrument innovative for the field. The first aspect is that it is composed of two scales that allow both objective and subjective assessment of QOL. And second, it is based on the theoretical framework of eight core domains and associated indicators proposed by Schalock and Verdugo (2002). Preliminary studies on the psychometric properties of the *QOL Integral Scale* indicate that the instrument is reliable and valid, and therefore, the Scale can serve as a basis for the development of both person-centered plans and quality improvement strategies in organizations.

Analysis of the data collected to date indicates that there is a very low relationship between the subjective and objective data obtained from the scale. This result is consistent with what has been found in other studies and we agree with them when they conclude that the discrepancies between both perspectives must not be understood as a non-desirable result, but differences can contribute more information for evaluation and care provision (Olson & Schober, 1993; Perry & Felce, 2005; Janssen, Schuengel, & Stolk, 2005). Since they are different, the necessity and the utility of having an instrument like the *Integral Scale* is evident, and so we encourage the research community to study such discrepancies and to develop more adjusted programs to individuals' perceptions and needs. *The Integral Scale* constitutes a useful tool to achieve these goals.

After three decades of researching and making progress in the field, we can say that we are living an exciting time for researches and practitioners in which the concept of QOL is evolving from an idea that just describes the reality to an action-oriented change agent that suggest how to improve the life of people with intellectual disabilities and how to improve program practices. As part of this effort, *The Integral Scale* can serve to contribute to the important and interesting task we face nowadays: to evolve from a conceptual framework to a detailed model of QOL, a model in which a mixture of causal and indicator variables are comprised and a model in which inputs, outputs, and a clear delineation of mediator and moderator variables are included (Schalock et al., 2010). Teti (2005) has stated that the important difference between theories and models is that the first is explanatory as well as descriptive, while the second is only descriptive. Theories are important to intervention and evaluation research because they guide the development of the intervention and the design and conduct of the study, and attempt to explain how the intervention works and which factors facilitate or inhibit the effectiveness of the intervention. The authors, together with other colleagues of the Institute on Community Integration (INICO; University of Salamanca, Spain), want to be part of the process of the next phase in the field's evolution: theory construction and model development. For this reason, we hope this instrument contributes to making progress in the field and other researches find it also useful to achieve this and other goals.

References

Anderson, K., & Burckhardt, C. (1999). Conceptualization and measurement of quality of life as an outcome variable for health care intervention and research. *Journal of Advanced Nursing, 29*, 298–306.

Bentler, P. M. (1990). Comparative fit indexes in structural models. *Psychological Bulletin, 107*, 238–246.

Bishop, C. M., Svensén, M., & Williams, C. K. I. (1996). A fast EM algorithm for latent variable density models. In D. S. Touretzky, M. C. Mozer, & M. E. Hasselmo (Eds.), *Advances in neural information processing systems* (8, pp. 465–471). Cambridge, MA: MIT Press.

Bonham, G. S., Basehart, S., Schalock, R. L., Marchand, C. G., Kirchner, N., & Rumenap, J. M. (2004). Consumer-based quality of life assessment: The Maryland Ask Me! Project. *Mental Retardation, 42*(5), 338–355.

Brown, R. I. (1997). *Quality of life for people with disabilities: Models research and practice* (2nd ed.). Cheltenham: Stanley Thornes.

Carlisle, P. R., & Christensen, C. M. (2006). *The cycles of theory building in management research*. Boston: School of Management-Boston University and Harvard Business School.

Cummins, R. A. (1996). Quality of life and disability. In P. O'Brien & R. Murray (Eds.), *Human services: towards partnership and support* (pp. 255–268). Auckland: Dunmore.

Cummins, R. A. (1997). *The comprehensive quality of life scale – Adult (ComQOl-A5)* (5th Ed.). Melbourne: School of Psychology, Deakin University.

Goodley, D., Armstrong, D., Sutherland, K., & Laurie, L. (2003). Self-advocacy, learning difficulties, and the social model of disability. *Mental Retardation, 43*(3), 149–160.

Gómez, L. E., Verdugo, M. A., & Arias, B. (2007). *Validation of the eight-domain model of quality of life*. Presentation at the ISQOL Conference: International Society for Quality-of-Life Studies. San Diego, CA, December 6–8.

Hughes, C., Hwang, B., Kim, J. H., Eisenman, L. T., & Killian, D. J. (1995). Quality of life in applied research: A review and analysis of empirical measures. *American Journal on Mental Retardation, 99*, 623–641.

Janssen, C., Schuengel, C., & Stolk, J. (2005). Perspectives on quality of life of people with intellectual disabilities: the interpretation of discrepancies between clients and caregivers. *Quality of Life Research, 14*(1), 57–69.

Jenaro, C., Verdugo, M. A., Caballo, C., Balboni, G., Lachapelle, Y., Otrebski, W., et al. (2005). Cross-cultural study of person-centred quality of life domains and indicators: a replication. *Journal of Intellectual Disability Research, 49*(10), 734–739.

Jöreskog, K. G. (1993). *LISREL 8: User's reference guide*. Chicago: Scientific Software International.

Jöreskog, K. G. (2002). *Structural equation modeling with ordinal variables using LISREL*. Available at http://www.ssicentral.com/lisrel/ordinal.htm

Jöreskog, K. G., & Sörbom, D. (1996). *LISREL 8: User's reference guide*. Chicago: Scientific Software International.

Kalafat, J., Illback, R. J., & Sanders, D., Jr. (2007). The relationship between implementation fidelity and educational outcomes in school-based family support program: Development of a model for evaluating multidimensional full-service programs. *Evaluation and Program Planning, 30*(2), 136–148.

Keith, K. D., & Bonham, G. S. (2005). The use of quality of life data at the organization and systems level. *Journal of Intellectual Disability Research, 49*(10), 799–805.

Kohonen, T. (1990). The self-organizing map. *Proceedings of the IEEE, 78*, 1464–1480.

Kohonen, T. (2001). *Self-organizing maps*. (3rd ed.). Berlin: Springer.

Kohonen, T. (2005). *Self-organizing maps*. Berlin: Heidelberg.

Kruskal, J. B., & Wish, M. (1978). *Multidimensional scaling*. Beverly Hills, CA: Sage.

Langberg, J. M., & Smith, B. H. (2006). Developing evidence-based intervention for deployment into school settings: A case example highlighting key issues of efficacy and effectiveness. *Evaluation and Program Planning, 29*(4), 323–334.

Moreno, M., Verdugo, M. A., Gómez, L. E., Arias, B., Mendonça, K., & Holanda, M. (2005). *Adaptation of the quality of life scale for adults with intellectual disabilities for being applied in Brazil*. Presentation at the II Congresso Brasileiro de Educaçao Especial e II Encontro da Associaçao Brasileira de Pesquisadores em Educaçao Especial, Sao Carlos, Brasil, November 5.

Nabney, I. T. (2004). *NETLAB: Algorithms for pattern recognition* (3rd ed.). Berlin: Springer.

Olson, G. I., & Schober, B. I. (1993). The satisfied poor. Development of an intervention-oriented theoretical framework to explain satisfaction with a life in poverty. *Social Indicators Research, 28*, 173–193.

Perry, J., & Felce, D. (1995). Objective assessments of quality of life: How much do they agree with each other? *Journal of Community and Applied Social Psychology, 5*(1), 1–19.

Perry, J., & Felce, D. (2005). Correlation between subjective and objective measures of outcome in staffed community housing. *Journal of Intellectual Disability Research, 49*, 278–287.

Poole, D. L., Duvall, D., & Wofford, B. (2006). Concept mapping key elements and performance measures in a state nursing home-to-community transition project. *Evaluation and Program Planning, 29*(1), 10–22.

Satorra, A., & Bentler, P. M. (1988). *Scaling corrections for chi-square statistics in covariance structure analysis*. Proceedings of the American Statistical Association, 308–313.

Schalock, R. L., & Bonham, G. S. (2003). Measuring outcomes and managing for results. *Evaluation and Program Planning, 26*(3), 229–235.

Schalock., R. L., Bonham, G. S., & Verdugo, M. A. (2008). The conceptualization and measurement of quality of life: Implications for program planning and evaluation in the field of intellectual disabilities. *Evaluation and Program Planning, 31*, 181–190.

Schalock, R. L., & Felce, D. (2004). Quality of life and subjective well-being: conceptual and measurement issues. In E. Emerson, C. Hatton, T. Thompson, & T. R. Parmenter (Eds.)., *The international handbook of applied research in intellectual disabilities* (pp. 261–279). London: Wiley.

Schalock, R. L., Keith, K. D., Verdugo, M. A., & Gómez, L. E. (2010). Quality of life theory construction and model development in the field of intellectual disabilities. In R. Kober (Ed.), *Enhancing quality of life for people with intellectual disability: From theory to practice* (pp. 17–32). New York: Springer.

Schalock, R. L., & Verdugo, M. A. (2002). *Handbook on quality of life for human service practitioners*. Washington, DC: American Association on Mental Retardation.

Schalock, R. L., & Verdugo, M. A. (2007). The concept of quality of life in services and supports for people with intellectual disabilities. *Siglo Cero, 38*(4), 21–36.

Schalock, R. L., Verdugo, M. A., Jenaro, C., Wang, M., Wehmeyer, M., Jiancheng, X., et al. (2005). A cross-cultural study of QOL indicators. *American Journal on Mental Retardation, 110*(4), 298–311.

Shoemaker, P. J., Tankard, J. W., Jr., & Lasorsa, D. L. (2004). *How to build social service theories*. Thousand Oaks, CA: Sage Publications.

Steiger, J. H. (1990). Structural model evaluation and modification: An interval estimation approach. *Multivariate Behavioral Research, 25*(2), 173–180.

Sutherland, S., & Katz, S. (2005). Concept mapping methodology: a catalyst for organizational learning. *Evaluation and Program Planning, 28*, 257–269.

Svensén, M. (1998). *GTM: The generative topographic mapping*. Ph.D. thesis. Aston University, Birmingham.

Tanaka, J. S., & Huba, G. J. (1985). A fit Index for covariance structure models under arbitrary GLS estimation. *British Journal of Mathematical and Statistical Psychology, 38*, 197–201.

Teti, D. M. (Ed.). (2005). *Handbook of research methods in developmental science*. Cambridge, MA: Blackwell.

Van Loon, J., Van Hove, J., Schalock, R. L., & Claes, C. (2008). *Personal outcomes scale*. Gent: Stichting Arduin, Universiteit Gent.

Veerman, J. W., & van Yperen, T. A. (2007). Degrees of freedom and degrees of certainty: A developmental model for the establishment of evidence-based youth care. *Evaluation and Program Planning, 30*(2), 136–148.

Verdugo, M. A., Arias, B., & Gómez, L. E. (2006). Escala integral de medición subjetiva y objetiva de la calidad de vida en personas con discapacidad intelectual. In M. A. Verdugo (Dir.), *Como mejorar la calidad de vida de las personas con discapacidad. Instrumentos y estrategias de evaluación* (pp. 417–448). Salamanca: Amarú.

Verdugo, M. A., Arias, B., Gómez, L. E., & van Loon, J. (2007). *Schaal Voor Kwaliteit Van Bestaan Voor Mensen Met Een Verstandelijke Beperking [QOL Integral Scale]*. Holland: Stichting Arduin.

Verdugo, M. A., Arias, B., Gómez, L. E., & Schalock, R. L. (2008). *Formulari de l'Escala Gencat de Qualitat de vida. Manual d'aplicació de l'Escala Gencat de Qualitat de vida*. Departamento de Acción Social y Ciudadanía. Generalitat de Cataluña.

Verdugo, M. A., Gómez, L. E., Arias, B., & Martin, J. C. (2006). *Validation of the eight domain model of quality of life*. Presentation at the symposium on quality of life outcomes: Their empirical development, verification, and use. International symposium on social inclusion, Montreal, CA, May 2–6.

Verdugo, M. A., Gómez, L. E., Arias, B., & Schalock, R. L. (2009). *Quality of life integral scale*. Madrid: CEPE.

Verdugo, M. A., & Schalock, R. L. (2001). *Cross-cultural survey of quality of life indicators*. Salamanca: Institute on Community Integration, Faculty of Psychology, University of Salamanca.

Verdugo, M. A., Schalock, R. L., Gómez, L. E., & Arias, B. (2007). Developing multi-dimensional quality of life scales focusing on the context: The GENCAT scale. *Siglo Cero, 38*(4), 57–72.

Wilkinson, L., Hill, M., & Vang, E. (1992). *SYSTAT: Statistics*. Evanston, IL: SYSTAT.

Chapter 5
Using Quality of Life to Assess Performance of Agencies Assisting People with Intellectual Disabilities

Ralph Kober and Ian R.C. Eggleton

Measurement of performance in the disability services sector is extremely important in terms of measuring the efficiency and effectiveness of organizations in achieving their goals. Performance indicators assist management in strategic decision-making and in fulfilling their accountability obligations to funders, purchasers, consumers, and other stakeholder groups for the best use of limited resources (Eggleton, Silalahi, Chong, & Kober, 2005). In this chapter we argue that agencies assisting people with intellectual disabilities can use quality of life as one of a suite of measures to assess performance at the individual consumer, program, and/or agency level. This will be demonstrated with reference to research conducted in the intellectual disability employment sector.

Performance Measurement Framework

To illustrate how quality of life can be used to measure performance in the disability sector, it is important, first, to have an understanding of the different aspects of performance measurement. To do this we will use Eggleton (1991) performance measurement framework, which is depicted in Fig. 5.1. The framework can be viewed as a cascading hierarchy in that, first, the mission statement (which identifies the agency's purpose in terms of the social function or need for which it has been created to fulfill) guides the formulation of the agency's goals (which should explicitly state what outcomes the agency plans to achieve for its consumers). Next, the goals guide formulation of the agency's operationalized objectives (which identify more specifically – through quantification – the particular outputs the agency plans to deliver in pursuing its outcome focused goals). Once the operationalized objectives have been set, they determine the expected costs of inputs (which are the

R. Kober (✉)
Department of Accounting and Finance, Monash University, Caulfield East, VIC 3145, Australia
e-mail: ralph.kober@monash.edu

This chapter is an updated and edited version of the article Kober and Eggleton (2006). We thank the publisher for granting us permission to edit and update the article for inclusion in this book.

R. Kober (ed.), *Enhancing the Quality of Life of People with Intellectual Disabilities*, Social Indicators Research Series 41, DOI 10.1007/978-90-481-9650-0_5,

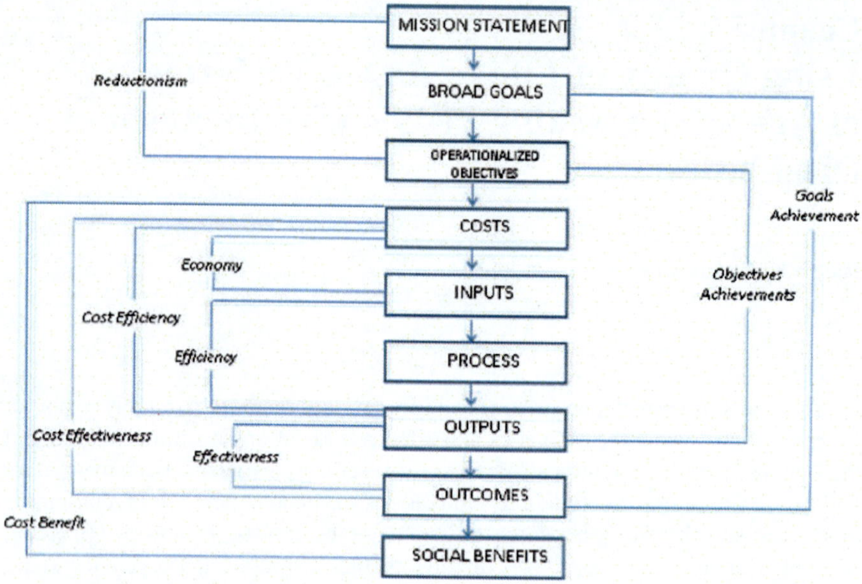

Fig. 5.1 Partial replication of Eggleton (1991) basic performance measurement framework

resources both human and physical) required to undertake the processes that deliver the outputs and outcomes specified in their operationalized objectives and goals, respectively.

An important aspect of the framework is the distinction made between outputs and outcomes. Outputs are the goods and services produced by the agency through the conversion process applied to its inputs (Eggleton, 1991). For example, in relation to a disability employment agency, the main outputs are the hours of job search and job support provided to job seekers and placed workers, respectively. In contrast, outcomes refer to impacts that agency outputs have on users of services (Eggleton, 1991; Miller, Copper, Cook, & Petch, 2008). In relation to a disability employment agency, outcomes for the job seeker may include the acquisition of interviewing skills, greater confidence, and a job; for the worker, outcomes may include continuing employment, take-home pay, higher self-esteem, job satisfaction, and increased quality of life. Modell (2005) notes that compared with outputs, outcomes may be more indirect or accrue over long periods. Outcomes may also accrue to stakeholders other than job seekers and workers. Family members and carers, for example, may have more time for respite; employers may gain a more diverse workforce and associated benefits in the form of higher productivity levels, lower absenteeism rates, etc. Broader societal outcomes may also be identified, such as greater levels of participation of people with intellectual disabilities in the workforce, changes in citizens' attitudes toward people with disabilities, removal of impediments so as to enhance access to public buildings, modifications to pavements to improve mobility, and greater inclusion of people with disabilities in other socially valued roles. Modell (2005) argues that as

> the ultimate objectives of public sector operations are typically related to the enhancement of the usefulness of services to beneficiaries and citizens rather than the maximization of service provision (outputs) or efficiency aspects, adequate measures of outcomes are pivotal for ascertaining the effectiveness of public sector organizations (Modell, 2005, p. 3).

Eggleton (1991) performance measurement framework pivots around the *three e's* of *economy*, *efficiency*, and *effectiveness*, and explicitly links these performance measures to the main stages of the framework involving the purchase of inputs, the conversion of these to outputs, and the outcomes thereby accruing to consumers and other stakeholders. From the framework it can be seen that *economy* is the cost per unit of input (or units of input per dollar), *efficiency* is the output per unit of input (or inputs per unit of outputs), and *effectiveness* is the process success rate (or impact) in terms of outputs being converted to successful outcomes. Whether the agency's goals (and hence mission) are accomplished is measured in terms of objectives and goal achievement indicators.[1] As noted by Kober and Eggleton (2009), Eggleton (1991) framework also clearly reveals that cost-efficiency is output per dollar (or dollars per unit of output) (*e.g.,* (*cost of all hours worked by job support employee*)/(*hours worked by job support employees which can be directly allocated to a job seeker of worker*)) and cost-effectiveness is the outcome per dollar (or dollars per unit of outcome) (*e.g., cost of finding and supporting a worker in a job*). Furthermore, Kober and Eggleton (2009, p. 43) highlight that "these performance indicators may be computed at both the individual job seeker or worker level, and at the service provider level (*e.g., for a service providers' overall cost effectiveness: the average cost of finding and supporting their workers in a job*)."

Why Use Quality of Life as an Outcome Measure?

Calls for consumer-referenced outcomes in the disability services sector in general have been made by several researchers. Cummins and Baxter (1994) argued that the measurement of objective (output) variables alone would not reflect the value of a service to recipients, and they asserted that the only way such value could be appropriately reflected was through the use of subjective, consumer-focused outcome measures. Similarly, Wehmen et al. (1987), in relation to employment programs, noted the need for non-monetary, consumer-focused outcome evaluations, which they stated were far more important to consumers than monetary outcomes. They argued that to ignore such non-monetary, consumer-focused measures would be an injustice to the consumers of disability employment agencies. Furthermore, as evidence from Miller et al. (2008) indicates, when asked, people with intellectual disabilities report that quality of life outcomes are important to them. DeStefano (1990) specifically noted that an assessment of quality of life was an essential part of any comprehensive outcome evaluation. As stated by Landesman (1986, p. 142)

[1]For a more detailed explanation of the modified Eggleton (1991) framework refer to Kober and Eggleton (2009).

> To judge the effectiveness of any ... [program], we must establish evaluative standards. Despite the tremendous concern with accountability, we have failed to develop clear procedures for measuring the "success" of a given program *at an individual level*, that is, sensitive to a person's own perceptions of quality of life ....

Baker and Itagliata (1982) identified five reasons why an agency involved in the provision of services to people with intellectual disabilities should focus on quality of life rather than other outcome measures. They termed the first reason *comfort rather than cure*, since intellectual disability is not a curable condition and quality of life defines the individual's condition in positive terms, not in terms of symptoms or absence of symptoms (Murrell & Norris, 1983). Their second reason was that *complex programs require complex outcome measures*. A complex set of interventions is involved in the provision of different methods of employment. The outcomes of these programs are complicated and difficult to measure; as such, a multi-dimensional variable such as quality of life serves to offer the hope of assessing the synergistic interaction of a number of smaller, less powerful outcome variables. The third reason was the desirability of *keeping the customer happy*. If the method of employment (open employment[2] or sheltered employment[3]), does not in some way improve consumer outcomes, such as self-worth, job satisfaction, or quality of life, etc., it is hard to justify the placement. *Re-emergence of the holistic perspective* was their fourth reason. Quality of life offers a way to look at the whole life situation of a person as opposed to narrowly focusing on one aspect. As noted by Kober and Eggleton (2009, p. 41), this "holistic approach is in keeping with the World Health Organization's International Classification of Functioning, Disability, and Health (ICF), which takes into account the social aspects of disability and does not view disability as solely a medical or biological dysfunction (World Health Organization, 2001)." The final reason Baker and Intagliata (1982) identified was that *quality of life is good politics*. It is part of our current western cultural philosophy that a person should be able to enjoy their life, and hence it is politically sound for governments to attempt to increase enjoyment of life by people with intellectual disabilities.

We believe four more reasons can be identified for supporting the use of quality of life as an outcome measure. First, Schalock (1999, 2004) noted that the quality revolution of the 1980s and the public sector reform movement of the 1990s has caused a significant change in how the public views the purposes, characteristics, responsibilities, and desired outcomes of social service programs. There has been a change in focus from inputs to outcomes (Schalock, 2004), clients have been redefined as either consumers or customers, citizens have become more empowered

---

[2] *Open employment* is where people with intellectual disabilities work alongside people without disabilities in integrated, meaningful employment in a community setting, supported by their employment agency. The alternative terms of *competitive employment* or *supported employment* are also often used.

[3] *Sheltered employment* refers to the situation where people with intellectual disabilities work alongside other people with a disability in a segregated, specially tailored setting. Typically, in this setting, the only people without disabilities in the workplace with whom people with intellectual disabilities would interact would be their supervisors.

(Kaul, 1997; Schalock, 1999), and the expectation now is that agencies are guided by goals related to person-referenced outcomes (Schalock, 2004). Given this expectation of focusing on person-referenced outcomes, it is understandable, as noted by McVilly and Rawlinson (1998) and Schalock (1999), that both society as a whole and individual consumers prefer the measurement of agencies' achievements to be person-referenced. As such, a person-referenced measure of quality of life would be ideal in serving such a purpose. Second, having a low quality of life does not stigmatize the individual as having any sort of deficit; rather it suggests that the individual is not well-suited to his or her current environment (Murrell & Norris, 1983). Third, as noted by Fabian (1991), quality of life can also be used as a needs assessment tool, particularly for broad-scoped programs like disability employment programs. Finally, widespread adoption by disability employment agencies of quality of life as an outcome measure would facilitate benchmarking processes and the identification of best practice agencies (and their related strategies and processes) (Camp, 1989; Eggleton, 1994).

An Example Using the Disability Employment Sector

The disability employment sector is an ideal sector in which to highlight how quality of life can be used as an outcome measure to determine the effectiveness of different methods of employment for people with intellectual disabilities. The overriding issues today are economic, and the major issue for agencies assisting people with intellectual disabilities is to demonstrate their efficiency and effectiveness (Kober & Eggleton, 2009; Shalock & Lilley, 1986). That is, agencies must demonstrate measurability of outcomes, reportability, and accountability.

Within the disability sector, and specifically the disability employment sector, there have been calls for non-financial performance measures to assess performance (Inge, Banks, Wehman, Hill, & Shafer, 1988; Parmenter, 1990; Wehman, Kregel, Banks, Hill, & Moon, 1987). Inge et al. (1988) contend that although open employment has been shown to result in positive financial outcomes (e.g., Conley, Rusch, McCaughrin, & Tines, 1989; Hill & Wehman, 1983; Hill et al., 1987; McCaughrin, Ellis, Rusch, & Heal, 1993; Noble, Conley, & Banerjee, 1991; Rusch, Conley, & McCaughrin, 1993; Shearn, Beyer, & Felce, 2000; Tines, Rusch, McCaughrin, & Conley, 1990; Tuckerman, Smith, & Borland, 1999), it is equally important to determine whether open employment has a positive effect on the lives of individuals.

To demonstrate how quality of life can be used as a measure of performance we refer to Kober (2006) who assessed the effectiveness of different methods of employment for people with intellectual disabilities, using quality of life as one of the outcome measures.[4] Using Eggleton (1991) performance measurement framework, effectiveness was viewed in terms of the effect that the different methods

[4]The results relating to quality of life from Kober (2006) are partially reported in Kober and Eggleton (2005).

of employment (open employment and sheltered employment, which are different service delivery processes) had on the quality of life (the outcome measure) of the participating individuals.

Kober (2006) interviewed 117 people with intellectual disabilities participating in either open employment (64 people) or sheltered employment (53 people), using the Schalock and Keith (1993) quality of life questionnaire (QOL.Q), which, in addition to the calculation of an overall quality of life score, allows the computation of scores for four sub-dimensions (factors): (1) personal life satisfaction, (2) individual competence and productivity at work, (3) feelings of empowerment and independence in the living environment, and (4) feelings of belonging and community integration. In addition to conducting an analysis for the entire sample, Kober (2006) also conducted an analysis based on a participants level of functional work ability,[5] separating the sample into people with high levels of functional work ability and those with low levels of work ability.

The results of Kober (2006), which are partially reported in Kober and Eggleton (2005) and shown in Table 5.1, reveal that participants with high levels of functional work ability report statistically significantly higher scores in open employment compared with sheltered employment for the factors *empowerment/independence* and *social belonging/community integration*, as well as total *quality of life* (Panel A, Table 5.1). For people with low levels of functional work ability, Kober (2006) reports no difference in the outcomes in relation to quality of life or any of the four factors based on method of employment (Panel B, Table 5.1). The results of Kober (2006) therefore indicate that for people with low functional work ability, there is no difference in the effectiveness of open employment compared with sheltered employment. However, for participants with high functional work ability, open employment appears to have a higher degree of effectiveness than sheltered employment.

These results would support people with intellectual disabilities with a high level of functional work ability being placed in open employment rather than in sheltered employment. However, it should be noted that to make any recommendation that would force people of a certain level of functional work ability to partake in one method of employment at the exclusion of the other would only serve to disempower people with intellectual disabilities by further reducing their power of choice with respect to the method of employment preferred. Rather, a preferable outcome would be to provide the above results concerning the effectiveness of the different methods of employment to people with intellectual disabilities and their parents/guardians to aid their decision whether they would prefer placement in open or sheltered employment.

[5]Functional work ability was measured by the functional assessment inventory (FAI) (Crewe & Athelstan, 1984). The FAI consists of 30 behaviorally anchored rating items, ranging from 0 (no significant impairment) to 3 (severe impairment), which assess a person's work capabilities and deficiencies, thus giving a theoretical range of 0–90; the higher the score, the lower the person's functional work ability. Low functional work ability was defined as a score of equal to or greater than 26, with high functional work ability defined as a score of 20 or less. These cut-off scores were selected as they represented approximately the top and bottom 40% of the sample, respectively.

Table 5.1 Differences in quality of life scores between open employment and sheltered employment

	Satisfaction	Competence/ productivity	Empowerment/ independence	Social belonging/ community integration	QOL
Panel A: Participants with high functional work ability ($n = 48$)					
Open employment ($n = 36$)	23.94	24.50	26.44	22.42	97.31
Sheltered employment ($n = 12$)	23.67	25.08	22.75	20.33	91.83
Z	−0.937	−0.383	−3.446[a]	−2.272[b]	−2.291[b]
Significance (p)	0.349	0.702	0.001	0.023	0.022
Open employment ($n = 20$)	24.85	26.20	23.65	22.30	97.00
Panel B: Participants with low functional work ability ($n = 51$)					
Sheltered employment ($n = 31$)	24.52	25.65	21.87	21.74	93.77
Z	−0.340	−0.633	−1.869	−0.786	−1.276
Significance (p)	0.734	0.527	0.062	0.432	0.202

[a]Significant at the 1% level
[b]Significant at the 5% level
Source: Figures obtained from Tables 1 and 2 of Kober and Eggleton (2005)

Conclusion

This chapter has argued that for agencies serving people with intellectual disabilities, quality of life can be used as one measure to assess the performance of the agencies and/or their programs. With reference to Eggleton (1991) performance measurement framework, it was argued that quality of life would be a suitable outcome measure for agencies serving people with intellectual disabilities. How this can be done was illustrated using the results of Kober (2006), who used quality of life as one of the outcome measures to assess the effectiveness of different methods of employment for people with intellectual disabilities. It was shown how performance could be assessed by use of statistical analysis, comparing the quality of life scores between the two methods of employment.

However, it would not be appropriate to use only quality of life to assess the effectiveness of agencies that serve people with intellectual disabilities since, as mentioned above, public sector agencies, including those assisting people with intellectual disabilities, serve a wide variety of stakeholders, and not just the person with the intellectual disability. Other stakeholders of such agencies include family members and carers of people with intellectual disabilities, employers of people with intellectual disabilities, and the broader community. As such, any comprehensive evaluation of the effectiveness of agencies that serve people with intellectual disabilities also needs to be conducted with reference to additional performance measures that would reflect outcomes achieved for these other stakeholders.

Furthermore, there may also be other person-referenced outcome measures, in addition to quality of life, which may be useful in assessing the effectiveness of agencies that serve people with intellectual disabilities. For example, in relation

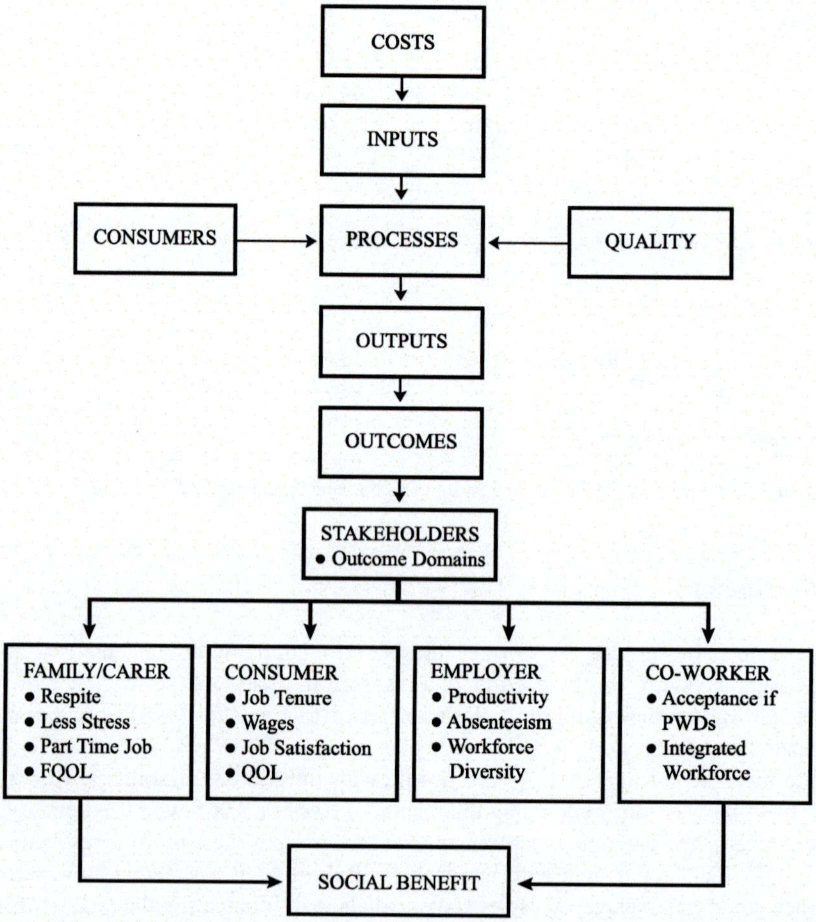

Fig. 5.2 Example of the modified Eggleton (1991) framework (Notes: (1) Source: Kober and Eggleton (2009). (2) The linkages of economy, efficiency, effectiveness, cost-efficiency, and cost-effectiveness apply equally in this modified performance framework as they do in the framework shown in Fig. 5.1. They have been omitted from this figure due to presentational ease. (3) The stakeholders shown in this figure are by no means comprehensive and are used solely to illustrate one potential manner in which Eggleton (1991) framework could be modified to incorporate various stakeholders.)

to agencies that place people into employment, the benefits of employment that accrue to the individual may also include shorter-term outcomes such as feelings of self-esteem and job satisfaction. Reporting these outcomes would complement the longer-term outcomes associated with enhanced quality of life, and should also be included in any assessment of agency or program effectiveness. Kober and Eggleton (2009) show how this can be done within Eggleton (1991) framework and provide an example of a modified framework that incorporates multiple outcomes that accrue to multiple stakeholders (shown in Fig. 5.2).

As such, we believe that while quality of life is an important outcome measure that needs to be assessed in determining the effectiveness of agencies or programs that serve people with intellectual disabilities, it should be one of a number of performance measures used as part of a comprehensive multi-stakeholder assessment.

References

Baker, F., & Intagliata, J. (1982). Quality of life in the evaluation of community support systems. *Evaluation and Program Planning*, *5*, 69–79.

Camp, R. C. (1989). *Benchmarking: The search for industry best practices that lead to superior performance*. Milwuakee, WI: Quality Press.

Conley, R. W., Rusch, F. R., McCaughrin, W. B., & Tines, J. (1989). Benefits and costs of supported employment: An analysis of the Illinois supported employment project. *Journal of Applied Behavior Analysis*, *22*, 441–447.

Crewe, N. M., & Athelstan, G. T. (1984). *Functional assessment inventory manual*. Menomonie, WI: Stout Vocational Rehabilitation Institute, University of Wisconsin-Stout.

Cummins, R. A., & Baxter, C. (1994). Choice of outcome measures in service evaluations for people with an intellectual disability. *Evaluation Journal of Australasia*, *6*, 22–30.

DeStefano, L. (1990). Designing and implementing program evaluation. In F. Rusch (Ed.), *Supported employment: Models, methods, issues* (pp. 229–246). Sycamore, IL: Sycamore Publishing Company.

Eggleton, I. R. C. (1991). *Performance measurement for public sector organisations*. Perth, WA: Decision Consulting Training and Research/New Zealand Society of Accountants.

Eggleton, I. R. C. (1994). *A benchmarking methodology for the Australian water industry* (Urban Water Research Association of Australia, Research Report No. 77, Melbourne, Victoria, Australia).

Eggleton, I. R. C., Silalahi, S., Chong, V. K., & Kober, R. (2005). *Antecedents and consequences of performance indicators in the public sector.* Working Paper, Waikato Management School, University of Waikato, Hamilton, New Zealand.

Fabian, E. S. (1991). Using quality-of-life indicators in rehabilitation program evaluation. *Rehabilitation Counseling Bulletin*, *34*, 344–356.

Hill, M. L., Banks, P. D., Handrich, R. R., Wehman, P. H., Hill, J. W., & Shafer, M. S. (1987). Benefit-cost analysis of supported competitive employment for persons with mental retardation. *Research in Developmental Disabilities*, *8*, 71–89.

Hill, M., & Wehman, P. (1983). Cost benefit analysis of placing moderately and severely handicapped individuals into competitive employment. *TASH Journal*, *8*, 30–38.

Inge, K. J., Banks, P. D., Wehman, P., Hill, J. W., & Shafer, M. S. (1988). Quality of life for individuals who are labelled mentally retarded: Evaluating competitive employment versus sheltered workshop employment. *Education and Training in Mental Retardation*, *23*, 97–104.

Kaul, M. (1997). The new public administration: management innovations in government. *Public Administration and Development*, *17*, 13–26.

Kober, R. O. (2006). *The effectiveness of different methods of employment for people with intellectual disabilities*. PhD thesis, The University of Western Australia, Crawley, Western Australia, Australia.

Kober, R., & Eggleton, I. (2005). The effects of different types of employment on quality of life. *Journal of Intellectual Disability Research, 49*, 756–760.

Kober, R., & Eggleton, I. R. C. (2006). Using quality of life to assess performance in the disability services sector. *Applied Research in Quality of Life, 1*, 63–77.

Kober, R., & Eggleton, I. R. C. (2009). Using quality of life to evaluate outcomes and measure effectiveness. *Journal of Policy and Practice in Intellectual Disability, 6*, 40–51.

Landesman, S. (1986). Quality of life and personal life satisfaction: Definition and measurement. *Mental Retardation, 33*, 141–143.

McCaughrin, W. B., Ellis, W. K., Rusch, F. R., & Heal, L. W. (1993). Cost-effectiveness of supported employment. *Mental Retardation, 31*, 41–48.

McVilly, K. R., & Rawlinson, R. B. (1998). Quality of life issues in the development and evaluation of services for people with intellectual disability. *Journal of Intellectual and Developmental Disability, 23*, 199–218.

Miller, E., Copper, S., Cook, A., & Petch, A. (2008). Outcomes important to people with intellectual disabilities. *Journal of Policy and Practice in Intellectual Disabilities, 5*, 150–158.

Modell, S. (2005). Performance management in the public sector: past experiences, current practices and future challenges. *Australian Accounting Review, 37*, 56–66.

Murrell, S. A., & Norris, F. H. (1983). Quality of life as the criterion for need assessment and community psychology. *Journal of Community Psychology, 11*, 88–97.

Noble, J. H., Conley, R. W., & Banerjee, S. (1991). Supported employment in New York state: A comparison of benefits and costs. *Journal of Disability Policy Studies, 2*, 39–71.

Parmenter, T. R. (1990). Evaluation and service delivery research in the area of severe intellectual disability in Australia. *Australia and New Zealand Journal of Developmental Disabilities, 16*, 187–193.

Rusch, F. R., Conley, R. W., & McCaughrin, W. B. (1993). Benefit-cost analysis of supported employment in Illinois. *Journal of Rehabilitation, 59*, 31–36.

Schalock, R. L. (1999). Could Mother Teresa survive an outcomes-oriented world? *Australian Society for the Study of Intellectual Disability Conference*, Sydney.

Schalock, R. L. (2004). The concept of quality of life: What we know and do not know. *Journal of Intellectual Disability Research, 48*, 203–216.

Schalock, R. L., & Keith, K. D (1993). *Quality of life manual*. Nebraska: Self published.

Schalock, R. L., & Lilley, M. A. (1986). Placement from community-based mental retardation programs: How well do clients do after 8 to 10 years. *American Journal of Mental Deficiency, 90*, 669–676.

Shearn, J., Beyer, S., & Felce, D. (2000). The cost-effectiveness of supported employment for people with severe intellectual disabilities and high support needs: A pilot study. *Journal of Applied Research in Intellectual Disabilities, 13*, 29–37.

Tines, J., Rusch, F. R., McCaughrin, W., & Conley, R. W. (1990). Benefit-cost analysis of supported employment in Illinois: A statewide evaluation. *American Journal on Mental Retardation, 95*, 44–54.

Tuckerman, P., Smith, R., & Borland, J. (1999). The relative cost of employment for people with a significant intellectual disability: The Australian experience. *Journal of Vocational Rehabilitation, 13*, 109–116.

Wehman, P., Kregel, J., Banks, P. D., Hill, M., & Moon, M. S. (1987). Sheltered versus supported work programs: A second look. *Rehabilitation Counseling Bulletin, 31*, 42–53.

World Health Organization. (2001). *International classification of functioning, disability and health*. Geneva: World Health Organization.

Part II
Literature Reviews

Chapter 6
Quality of Life for Persons with Intellectual Disabilities: A Review of the Literature

Gordon Lyons

Introduction

Strauss and Corbin's (1994) rationales for reviewing literature guided this review, i.e., (a) knowledge of philosophy and existing theories assists in identifying appropriate methods of inquiry, (b) an understanding of the extant literature aids in the generation of questions for enquiry, and (c) familiarity with the literature enhances researcher sensitivity to data and emerging concepts. This review ventured eclectically but pragmatically into the fields of sociology, psychology, philosophy, disability studies, education, nursing, and research methodology.

The review opens with a brief contextual discussion of the "language" of disability generally, and ID specifically. Following is an explanation of the critical place of communication and intersubjectivity in understanding QOL in the lives of persons with ID generally, and more severe ID specifically. The phenomenon of QOL is then explained in depth with sections on: the historical development of QOL research; conceptualization and definition; domains and indicators; theories and models; and measurement and assessment.

A more focused discussion on the literature around QOL for persons with ID then follows, with in-depth explanations about: the nature of QOL for persons with ID (and particularly subjective QOL); investigating the QOL of persons with ID; and subjective QOL for persons with more severe ID – this (probably) being the most problematic aspect of the broader discussion on QOL.

The review closes with a description and explanation of the current "state of play" with respect to the construct of QOL and its application to persons with ID (drawing substantially on the work of the Quality of Life Special Interest Research Group of the International Association for the Study of Intellectual Disabilities).

G. Lyons (✉)
The University of Newcastle
e-mail: gordon.lyons@newcastle.edu.au

R. Kober (ed.), *Enhancing the Quality of Life of People with Intellectual Disabilities*, Social Indicators Research Series 41, DOI 10.1007/978-90-481-9650-0_6,

Intellectual Disability

> Too often assumptions are made . . . that people with disabilities are a homogeneous group where in fact there is probably no other segment of the population that manifests such a broad diversity of individual problems and needs (Ferguson, 1996, p. 8).

Language reflects and influences social attitudes, especially about people with disabilities (Butow, 1993), and debates about disability language, definition, and nomenclature remain topical and contentious (Bowles, 1995; Madden, Black & Wingyan, 1995; Parmenter & Donelly, 1997; Parmenter, 2001). The World Health Organization's definitions of impairment, disability, and handicap are generally regarded as authoritative, although multiple interpretations militate against a consensus (Bowe, 1978; Fulcher, 1989; Smyer, McHale, Birkel, & Madle, 1988). A basic disagreement is whether disability is a personal tragedy, with the locus of the problem being with the individual, or a social problem arising from disabling barriers within the environment (Abberley, 1987; Bickenbach, 1993; Gleeson, 1995). Recent revisions of these definitions, as promulgated by the World Health Organization and the United Nations, refer to the complicity of impacting social and environmental factors.

Debate generally centers around three prominent groups of models of disability that have well-documented theoretical histories (Bickenbach, 1993): the medical or individual models, based on the concept of impairment; the welfare, economic, or policy models, based on the concept of disability; and the human rights or socio-political models, based on the concept of handicap (Abbott-Chapman & Easthope, 1998; Madden, Black, & Wingyan, 1995). These (groups of) models historically competed for political, social, and professional dominance, and precipitated an evolution of differing policies, practices, and outcomes for persons with disabilities (Anderson, 1988; Bickenbach, 1993; Crow, 1996; French, 1993a; Parmenter, 1995). (Roarty (1981) described an alternative model, but this is not widely discussed in the literature.) A more recent model has been posited by Low (2001), wherein he suggests that the social rights movement has gone too far by arguing for all persons with disabilities together "in a spurious solidarity" (p. 24). This view has some support among organizations that advocate for distinct groups of persons with disabilities.

Terminology in Western nations has historically distinguished less between the concepts of disability and handicap, although, for example, current Australian legislation and policy recognizes disability as a human rights and equity issue within a socio-political perspective (Butow, 1993; Einfeld, 1998; Madden, Black & Wingyan, 1993). The human rights model, as described by Bickenbach (1993) and Parmenter (1999), has current political authority in Australia arising from its adoption into legislation, although differing interpretations continue (Gleeson, 1995).

Finkelstein's (1993b) definition of disability – "the loss or limitation of opportunities that prevents people who have impairments from taking part in normal life in the community on an equal basis with others due to physical and social barriers" (p. 13) – aligns with the socio-political model, has broad international support, and reflects the contemporary usage of the term (Bigby & Ozanne, 2001;

Butow, 1993). (This author supports the positions of Bickenbach (1993), Sen (1996), and Finkelstein (1993a) wherein disability is viewed largely as a socially created phenomenon, and individuals with disabilities as a minority group constrained by disabling barriers.)

Western society generally has limited knowledge about or understanding of people with ID (Atkins, 1999). It frequently devalues those with impairments, disabilities, and handicaps, and associates these with a lower QOL (Barber, 1990; Jones, Ouellette-Kuntz, Vilela, & Brown, 2008; Wolf, 1990). In 1972, Wolfensberger warned that Cartesian dualism, a philosophy espousing the separation of the body and the mind, presented a danger to persons with ID through the discourse of deviancy (Wolfensberger & Nirje, 1972). That is, people with more severe ID could be perceived as without mind, emotion, or humanity. Given the history of discrimination, social control, and marginalization that has confronted people with ID (Barlow & Kirby, 1992), substantial contemporary opinion supporting abortion following prenatal diagnosis and euthanasia as humane courses of action is not surprising. Wolfensberger's reference to the plight of the deviant individual as a subhuman or diseased organism remains poignant and pertinent (Baily, 1986; Borthwick-Duffy, 1987; Gordon, 1984; Kuhse & Singer, 1985).

Persons with ID are referred to using a diversity of terms. This diversity reflects their origins in the fields of medicine and health care, psychology, special education, developmental disability, and habilitation (Brown, 2006; Carter, Chalmers, Clayton, & Hook, 1998; Guess, Roberts, Seigal-Causey, & Rues, 1995). Consensual definition is important because it "allows meaningful communication . . . facilitates best practice and focused research . . . and appropriate intervention and accountability" (Arthur, 1998, pp. 4–5), but debate about definition and terminology continues to be confounded by the difficulties encountered in gaining consensus about population definition (Gleason, 1993). Hogg and Sebba (1987) pointedly remarked, "The choice of a definition. . . is partly determined by the purpose for which it is required" (p. 1).

Persons with ID have been described widely (Thorley, 1993). Many of these terms, definitions, and descriptions reflect the "deficit perspective" of disability that does not acknowledge or appropriately emphasize the social place, humanity, and abilities of persons with ID. This deficit perspective precipitated out of the medical or individual models of disability (Bickenbach, 1993; Schalock, 2004b), whereas the "similarity perspective," emphasizing capability, is better reflected in the human rights or socio-political models of disability (Oliver, 1996). The author support the contention that "all persons can learn, irrespective of the degree or complexity of their disabilities" (NSW Department of Education, 1988, p. 3), and agree with Romney, Brown, and Fry (1994) and Cummins (1993) that, "even very disabled persons are capable of making choices that are meaningful and realistic" (p. 254).

Terms and classifications are generally based on medical diagnoses, psychological assessments of general cognitive ability, and developmental age. The term ID has its origins in the terms and definitions of "mental retardation" and "developmental disability" (Health Commission, 1981; Thompson & O'Quinn, 1979; Wolfe, 1992). The epidemiology of ID is generally developmental or subsequent to traumatic brain damage. Individuals may have a mild, moderate or severe ID – depending on an assessment of their cognitive ability (Arthur, 1998; Hogg & Sebba, 1987). There remains though considerable dispute about the validity of these assessments. Remarkable individuals who have discredited such assessments include Helen Keller, Annie McDonald (Crossley & McDonald, 1980), and Christy Brown (1989). Research into behavior states and arousal by Arthur (2001, 2004), Arthur, Hook and Butterfield (1995), Guess, Roberts and Behran (1998), and Guess et al. (1995) is highly pertinent, and explains how many individuals with more severe ID, who spend much of their time in apparently non-alert behavior states, are precluded from reasonable assessment.

This author has adopted the term and definition of ID put forward by the International Association for the Scientific Study of Intellectual Disabilities, the leading international professional organization in the field. The definition places an emphasis on the primacy of the individual rather than the impairment, disability, or handicap, a position widely supported in the disability and QOL literature (Blackwell, 1979; Brown, 1998a; Brown, personal communication, 1 October, 1998; 1996a, b; Guess et al., 1995; Schalock, 1994a).

Communication and Intersubjectivity

> To be labelled retarded (sic) is to have a wide range of imperfections imputed to you. One imperfection is the inability to analyse your life and your current situation. Another is the inability to express yourself – to know and say who you are and what you wish to become (Bogdan & Taylor, 1989, p. 136).

Persons with ID are most heterogeneous, particularly in terms of their abilities to communicate with others around them (Cirrin & Rowland, 1985). An understanding of the communication challenges faced by persons with ID is central to understanding them and their QOL. Communicative competence is crucial to the QOL of persons with ID (Butterfield, Arthur, & Linfoot, 1992) so establishing meaningful communication and intersubjectivity is a major challenge for families, carers, and service providers (Feil, 1993).

In simple terms, communication is the exchange of information between individuals. More specifically, intentional communication is the deliberate direction of a specific message to others that can be inferred from observable behavior, although it is important to acknowledge that "a particular function can be communicated in a wide variety of ways" (Carter & Hook, 1998, p. 44). Communication strategies are often particular to specific environments and the perceptions of the communication partners involved. Aspects of communication include: context (place, participants, and activity); generalization and application; spontaneity and dependency on prompting; and complexity, structure, and level of symbolism. People communicate to achieve a variety of goals, such as expressing needs, wants, and feelings, and to engage with others.

The importance of communication partners for persons with ID is widely recognized in the literature. Cowan (1991) referred to parents as the (first) educators of persons with ID. Fallon and Harris (1991) described parents as the experts, with professionals only facilitating the process of parents sharing their knowledge. Browne and Bramston (1996) expressed a similar view, but cautioned that mothers were the predominant parent communicator and that generalizations to fathers were unsubstantiated. Alternatively, Storey (1997) placed great emphasis on the primacy and significance of communications between teachers and students with ID in the development of social skills. Thompson and Guess (1989) also acknowledged the pivotal role of teachers in communication development, and encouraged teachers to "tune in" by considering their student's levels of alertness.

Researchers have developed some specific strategies to minimize these communication deficits. Goode and Hogg (1994) described the life sharing approach wherein (adult) clients and carers share and record life histories and biographies to enhance communication and understanding. Shaddock, Dowse, Richards, and Spinks (1998) successfully utilized the systematic gathering of information from communication partners to represent the views of adults with ID at formal legal tribunal hearings.

Persons with ID can seem difficult to "know". The nature of their inner life, life satisfaction, feelings, interests, wants, and preferences, is frequently difficult to capture, but some researchers have made creditable attempts to do so. Gustiatas and Young (1986), Goode (1984), Keenan (1992), and Sacks (1995) have all described a "knowing" that emerged after spending time with individuals with more severe ID, and this knowing seems central to the quality of relationships and understanding between persons with ID and their important others. Brudenell (1986, pp. 19–24) presented a touching and insightful description of life as a child with "profound handicaps", and refers to boundaries, adult-based childhood, physical restraints, exploration and creativity, few expectations, and the "Peter Pan Syndrome." In essence, many aspects of the lives of persons with ID are like those for all people, but their disabilities frequently impinge upon key aspects of their lives.

The literature about persons with severe ID emphasizes these challenges. Golden and Reese (1996) concluded that the quality of staff–resident interactions in residential institutions was an essential indicator of QOL, but that "lower functioning" residents received less stimulating interactions than those who were more competent. Guess, Benson and Siegel-Causey (1985) demonstrated that an improved awareness of pre-locutionary non-verbal communications among carers led to an improvement in communication and behavioral response among residents. Comparable research about elderly adults with dementia and severe communication deficits by Byrne and MacLean (1997), Parse (1996), and Bigby (2004) and about adults with mental illnesses by Mercier (1994) and Bertelli and Brown (2006), drew similar conclusions about the importance of communication (partners) to the QOL of persons with severe communication impairments.

Early research by Cirrin and Rowland (1985) into the non-verbal communications of persons with more severe communication deficits described a great diversity of types, styles, and patterns of communication. Nevertheless, the authors argued that communicative intent was evident in the frequent use of spontaneous and intentional behaviors for primary communication functions. Cirrin and Rowland believed that there could be a repertoire of communicative behaviors that might be overlooked by communication partners and professionals who are focused on more formal language behaviors. Many persons with more severe ID lack formal symbolic vocal or gestural language, and often rely on pre-symbolic, action-based, idiosyncratic communication gestures and utterances (Goode, 1990a, 1994; Hogg & Lambe, 1991). A substantial body of research describes pre-language communication in non-disabled infants, but very little research described the communicative abilities of persons with more severe ID.

Although the literature demonstrates consensus that the communicative behaviors of persons with ID are diverse and frequently difficult to interpret (Arthur, 1998; Goode, 1997), Carter and Hook (1998) concluded that contemporary research about communication training recognized the potential communicative intent of subtle, idiosyncratic, and non-symbolic behaviors, and that some learners communicated effectively without the need for conventional symbols. In a discussion paper on the ethics of communication with people with severe communication problems von Tetzchner and Jensen (1999) pointedly concluded that the most ethical approach to communicating with these persons was to take the person seriously as an authentic communicator.

Arthur and Butterfield (1996) identified three dominant issues in this area of the literature. These are socio-communicative context, partner responsivity, and the relationship between communication, social membership, and QOL. Arthur and Butterfield urged (a) communication partners to develop their communication skills to facilitate improved social membership for, and control and participation by persons with ID, (b) researchers to investigate communication across real settings, and (c) for all involved with people with ID "to be in touch to know" (p. 59). Ferguson (1994) similarly regarded communication, membership, and quality of life to be "inextricably bound". Lakin (1992), Loew and Rapin (1994), Mackay (1994), O'Brien and O'Brien (1992), and Peplau (1994) expressed comparable sentiments.

Quality of Life

> [Quality of life] ... the slipperiest creature in the conceptual zoo. (Compton, 1997, p. 120)

Quality of life (QOL) is not a phenomenon or term subject to broad consensus. Some authors have used terms such as QOL, life satisfaction, psychological wellbeing, and subjective wellbeing interchangeably (Dempsey & Foreman, 1997; Dennis, Williams, Giangreco, & Cloninger, 1993; Zhan, 1992). Others have regarded QOL as a multidimensional concept that encompasses life satisfaction and these other concepts (Abbey & Andrews, 1986; Headey & Wearing, 1992; Pavot & Diener, 1993). Still others have used the term QOL globally to subsume these concepts (Davis & Fine-Davis, 1991). Landesman (1986) suggested that life satisfaction and QOL are distinct concepts, whereas Romney et al. (1994) and Cummins (2005a) argued that QOL is more than the subjective experience of life satisfaction. The terms subjective wellbeing and subjective QOL are widely used in the literature

(Brown, Brown, & Bayer, 1994; Cummins, 2005d; Griffin, 1998; Parse, 1996; Pavot & Diener, 1993), and they refer to "the perceptions of the individual" (Andrews, 1986; Evans, 1994; Horn, 1993). Life satisfaction has been representatively defined by Evans (1994) as "the degree to which the individual's life is perceived to match some implicit or explicit internal standard or referent" (p. 53).

Subjective QOL is a personal phenomenon closely linked to the broader phenomenon of QOL. This author's view, derived from prior research (Lyons, 1999b, 1999c, 2000a, 2000b), is that an examination of the general QOL literature provides the best scaffold for investigating and understanding subjective QOL, and in accordance with the principles and assumptions underlying this review that the philosophy and ethics of QOL for persons with ID are no different from that of other persons. The following Background section provides an explanation of the history and evolution of QOL research, demonstrating the philosophical, ethical, conceptual, and paradigmatic complexity of the phenomenon.

Background

Since antiquity people have sought "the good life" (Oliver, Huxley, Bridges, & Mohamad, 1996; Reinders, 2002; Seed & Lloyd, 1997). Most notably both Aristotle and Plato reflected extensively on eudemonia, i.e., happiness and living well (Brown, 1998a; Horn, 1993; Parmenter & Donelly, 1997; Sen, 1993; Travers & Richardson, 1993). Traditional Eastern philosophies contend that a personal balance between "Yin" and "Yang" brings the best QOL (Zhan, 1992). This pursuit of goodness of life, wellbeing, life satisfaction, or QOL remains enduringly pervasive (Evans, 1994; Headey & Wearing, 1992; Keith, 1996a, 1996b; Meeberg, 1993; Romney et al., 1994). The realization of improved QOL is generally regarded to be subjectively individualistic (Davison, 1977; Dennis et al., 1993; Szalai, 1980; Zhan, 1992) notwithstanding diverse cultural interpretations and emphases (Leininger, 1994; Seed & Lloyd, 1996; Verdugo, Schalock, Keith, & Stancliffe, 2005; Wolfensberger, 1994).

In the mid-1940s, international interest in QOL research emerged following the founding of the United Nations (UN) and promulgation of the Universal Declaration of Human Rights (Einfeld, 1998). QOL subsequently developed as a political issue in the USA in the mid-1950s (Stensman, 1985) and in Europe in the 1960s (Sullivan, 1992).

QOL was identified as a field of social scientific research in the early 1960s and as a research discipline in the later 1960s (Andrews, 1986; Schuessler & Fisher, 1985). Interest in "social indicators," objective measures of social conditions normed to a population, evolved from this politicization of research (Cummins, 1996b; Dennis et al., 1993; Horn, 1993) wherein governments sought data to facilitate comparisons between population groups rather than (just) individuals (Szalai, 1980).

During the late 1950s and 1960s, the human rights movement gained popular support in western countries and research into intellectual disability and developmental disability (services) gained professional impetus (Brown, 1997c; Ferguson,

1996; Oliver et al., 1996; Parmenter, 1999; Schalock, 1990a). During this period the wider community became better informed about the (often) impoverished lives of many persons with (intellectual) disabilities who lived in institutions. A prevailing view in the community was that disability itself detracted from QOL, although this view was challenged (Edgerton, 1990).

In the 1970s and 1980s, many Western countries commissioned national research projects on QOL (Andrews & Withy, 1976; Atkinson, 1977; Blishen & Atkinson, 1980; Davis & Fine-Davis, 1991; Headey & Wearing, 1992; Headey, 1988; Vogel, Andersson, Davidsson, & Hall, 1988; Zapf et al., 1987). The United Nations Educational, Scientific and Cultural Organization (UNESCO) and the Organization for Economic Cooperation and Development (OECD) also commissioned international research projects (Parmenter & Donelly, 1997; Solomon et al., 1980; Verwayen, 1980). Strong debate about the relationship between QOL and social indicators continued. Horn (1993), for example, argued that population-based QOL research developed out of the social indicators research movement, whereas the OECD chose to enmesh QOL and social indicators research (Parmenter & Donelly, 1997). Eventually some agreement on conceptualization, definition, and application was reached, although polarized opinions about this relationship persisted (Andrews, 1980; Land, 1983; Schuessler & Fisher, 1985; Szalai, 1980).

Increasing community awareness of the poor life circumstances of many persons with ID in institutions generated popular support for Perrin and Nirje's (1985) "Normalization" and Wolfensberger's (1995) "Social Role Valorization" (Brown, 1997b; Jones et al., 2008; Kebbon, 1997). The influential disability reform movement, arising out of the human rights movement, utilized research evidence and mounting public support to bring about significant changes to human rights legislation and disability services (Parmenter, 1999, 2001; Schalock, 1997). Although the movement's primary ideology was QOL improvement for persons with disabilities (Evans, 1994; Stark & Faulkner, 1996), persons with more severe ID, who were among the most marginalized and disempowered groups of persons with disabilities, benefited least from the changes arising from this reform (Felce & Perry, 1995).

In the 1980s, QOL research proliferated across many disciplines, including philosophy, sociology, psychology, political science, economics, health sciences, and disability services (Fuhrer, 1994; Karlsson, 1992; Kolstad, 1994; Land, 1983; Renwick, Brown, & Nagler, 1996; Schuessler & Fisher, 1985; Seed & Lloyd, 1997; Solomon et al., 1980). By this time QOL was being described and explained widely using terms and concepts such as dimensions, domains, indicators, categories, components, and factors (Seed & Lloyd, 1997). Many theories and models about QOL, life satisfaction, and social indicators were published (Headey, 1993; Travers & Richardson, 1993). Social scientists investigated subjective QOL, seeking to identify relationships between objective social indicators and subjective measures (Andrews, 1991; Davis & Fine-Davis, 1991; Headey & Wearing, 1992). (Social indicators research continues as a field of research today, but is primarily concerned with comparing changes in the standard of living and QOL of cultural and/or sub-population groups (Andrews, 1991)).

In 1981, the International Year of the Disabled Person, QOL was promoted as an issue of equity. This impacted on public policy (Schalock, 1999), and QOL was linked to normalization, social role valorization, deinstitutionalization, and integration (Brown & Brown, 1996; Brown, 1997a; Cummins, 1993, 1996b; Edgerton, 1996; Goode & Hogg, 1994; Goode, 1990b; Parmenter, 1989, 1990, 1995; Renwick, 1998; Schalock, 1993, 1996b, 1999). Representatively, Dennis et al. (1993) referred to QOL as "the context for planning and evaluation of services for people with disabilities" (p. 499). By the late 1980s, prominent activists, responding to the political adoption of the human rights model of disability, identified QOL as the key research topic for the 1990s (Brown, 1999; Goode & Hogg, 1994; Hughes, Hwang, Kim, Eisenman, & Killian, 1995; Landesman, 1986; Schalock, 1990b, 1993).

Much of the subsequent research in the 1980s focused on persons with ID affected by deinstitutionalization (Hughes et al., 1995; Parmenter, Cummins, Shaddock, & Stancliffe, 1994; Richmond, 1983; Schalock, 1994a). Theorists by now had documented clear conceptual links between QOL and normalization, deinstitutionalization, integration, choice, and empowerment (Brown et al., 1994; Edgerton, 1996; Goode & Hogg, 1994; Goode, 1992; Parmenter, 1995; Romney et al., 1994; Schalock, 1994a, 1994b). Continuing impetus for research came from recognition that simplistic, objective evaluations of QOL were inadequate (Antaki & Rapley, 1996), and that consumer satisfaction and QOL improvement should be service priorities (Brown, 1999; Cheng, 1988; Conway, 1992; Fabian, 1991; Felce & Perry, 1996; Renwick, 1998).

In the 1990s, qualitative research about persons with ID that focused on specific populations and individuals became more prevalent. Cummins (1996b) and Brown (1997a) suggested that this had reinvigorated QOL research. The UN, the WHO, and the European Economic Community (EEC) investigated ways to measure life satisfaction to better inform service provision. For example, 14 of the 22 rules of the 1993 UN Standard Rules on the Equalization of Opportunities for Disabled Persons relate directly to QOL (Schalock, 1999). The Australian Government, for example, sought to develop social policy focused on the wellbeing of citizens (Everingham, 1998; McClaren, 1995; Senate Legal & Constitutional References Committee, 1996) and sought to bring together policies and services to better address citizens' QOL (Social Policy Directorate, 1994a). QOL remained a most important concern in the intellectual disability field during this period (Romney et al., 1994; Swain, Finkelstein, French, & Oliver, 1993) and QOL improvement became the major challenge facing the field (Goode & Hogg, 1994; Hughes et al., 1995; Landesman, 1986; Schalock, 1990a, 1999). Felce and Perry (1996) concluded that QOL "has emerged as a potentially unifying concept in assessing the impact of care processes on the character of people's day-to-day lives" (p. 63).

The broad emphasis in QOL research during this period was to improve population QOL (Brown, 1995; Evans, 1994). The WHO placed the study and improvement of population QOL as a primary goal (Evans, 1994). QOL researchers sought to inform decision-making for public programs and services that purported to improve QOL (Cheng, 1988; Evans, 1994; Faden & Laplege, 1992; Goodinson & Singleton, 1989; Halpern, 1993a; Hatton, 1998; Hughes & Hwang, 1996; Social

Policy Directorate, 1994b). Despite widespread agreement that improvement in QOL remained a key pursuit of governments, societies, and individuals (Bowling, 1992; Hatton, 1998; Hughes & Hwang, 1996; Nankervis, 1997; Oliver et al., 1996; Romney et al., 1994; Seed & Lloyd, 1996), there was little evidence of legislative change in the literature (Ashman, 1990).

A variety of "approaches" to QOL improvement were evident in the literature. The WHO (1986), Brown (1998a), Stokols (1992), and Tones (1986) similarly identified local, national and international top-down legislative approaches, and bottom-up approaches initiated by concerned citizens, lobbyists, and advocates. The WHO (1986) and Cowan (1991) supported a population focus based on an educational approach. More generally, Evans (1994) and Hughes and Hwang (1996) identified individual, educational, social action- or government-focused approaches. It was widely argued that normative population QOL data would enable comparisons between more specific sub-populations (Evans, 1994; Pavot & Diener, 1993; Stokols, 1992).

Schalock (1999) specifically argued that QOL research should focus on the individual, by interpreting QOL as a social construct and overriding principle for improving the perceived QOL of individuals. Schalock hoped that: countries would integrate QOL into law, policy, and service delivery systems; service providers would implement quality enhancement techniques, and individuals would pursue a life of quality, all within a QOL rubric. Similarly, Stokols (1992) and Schalock, Bontham and Marchand (2000) argued for approaches to QOL research that focused on individuals and/or their environments, and supported the implementation of environmentally and program-based enhancement techniques that responded to individual needs. Brandstadter and Baltes-Gotz (1990), Cowan (1991), Evans (1994), and Lazarus (1993) similarly argued for an individual perspective to QOL research, but they also emphasized the need to focus on personality characteristics or dispositions. Programs that aimed to develop an individual's personal skills were supported by Cowan (1991) and Lazarus (1993), as were those that sought to enhance an individual's social support milieus (Evans, 1994).

In general terms, the QOL research agenda for persons with ID has paralleled the agenda for the wider population. Additionally though, a second line of research has focused on evaluating the processes, standards, and outcomes of disability services and support programs (Brown & Bayer, 1992; Brown, Bayer, & MacFarlane, 1989; Emerson, 1985; Parmenter & Donelly, 1997; Schalock, 1990c). QOL gained popularity as a social indicator in disability services (Parmenter, 1999). Kozleski and Sands (1992), for example, promoted QOL as a more accurate yardstick of the social validity of support programs. McVilly and Rawlinson (1998) further explained why QOL process evaluations should focus on day-to-day operations and QOL outcome evaluations should focus on what services actually achieved. Schalock (1996b, 1999) similarly suggested that QOL should be interfaced with quality enhancement, assurance and management, and outcomes-based evaluation.

During this period a prevailing trend toward economic rationalism required governments and support services to rationalize and better account for resource allocations within the quality assurance and standards rubric (Brown, 1999). Unfortunately, the pressure to develop measures of QOL to help plan and evaluate these services resulted in a proliferation of instruments and techniques, many without sound theoretical or psychometric bases (Dennis et al., 1993; Goode & Hogg, 1994). This was exacerbated by continuing disagreements about conceptualization and definition (Cummins, 1996b; Fabian, 1991), and concerns about the reliability and validity of using interviews with persons with an intellectual disability as the primary data gathering technique (Antaki & Rapley, 1996).

The QOL concept is currently prominent in the disciplines of economics, medicine, and the social sciences. Each has developed a different perspective on its conceptualization and application (Bergland & Narum, 2007). With more substantial roots in the social sciences, the field of intellectual disability has adopted a more humanistic perspective facilitating engagement with key constructs of affect and cognition (Cummins, 2005a; Kahneman, Diener, & Schwartz, 1999; Russell, 2003).

Explaining QOL: Conceptualisation and Definition

Scores of concepts and hundreds of definitions of QOL are recorded in the literature (Bowling, 1992; Cummins, 1996a; Daly, Mitchell, & Jonas-Simpson, 1996; Evans, 1994; Hughes et al., 1995; Seed & Lloyd, 1997; Social Policy Directorate, 1994a). Given the continuing broad philosophical, social, and political interest in QOL research, this lack of a widely accepted concept and definition was not surprising (Andrews, 1980; Dennis et al., 1993; Fabian, 1991; Gioiella, 1994; Land, 1983; Schuessler & Fisher, 1985; Solomon et al., 1980). Felce and Perry (1995) and Romney et al. (1994) suggested that the ever-increasing range of theoretical models exacerbated this proliferation. There was strong agreement that a consensus on conceptualisation (and definition) was necessary if research was to progress collaboratively and without discipline-specific fragmentation (Borthwick-Duffy, 1996; Brown, 1997a, 1997b; Cummins, 1996b; 2005a; Felce & Perry, 1995; Ferrans & Powers, 1985; Gioiella, 1994; Romney et al., 1994).

Theorists came to some agreement about the core features of QOL (Cummins, 1996b, 1997; Daly et al., 1996; Dennis et al., 1993; Fabian, 1991; Felce & Perry, 1996; Gioiella, 1994; Parmenter, 1994). Cummins (1996b), for example, representatively explained that QOL could be measured and assessed by quantitative and qualitative methods, and objective indicators incorporated norm-referenced measures of standard of living, and subjective indicators incorporated personal measures of perceived wellbeing. Other features engendered schools of agreement, for example, that QOL was a global concept, comparable for all (Andrews, 1980; Cummins, McCabe, Romeo, Reid, & Waters, 1997); QOL was multidimensional (Felce & Perry, 1995; Loew & Rapin, 1994; Zhan, 1992); "levels" of QOL were discernible and changed over time (Schuessler & Fisher, 1985); QOL could not be measured directly, but rather through measurement and/or assessment of indicators (Andrews, 1980; Horn, 1993; Lyons, 1999b, 1999c, 2003a, 2003b, 2003c, 2003d; Solomon et al., 1980); data obtained from objective and subjective sources was often inconsistent (Borthwick-Duffy, 1992; Loew & Rapin, 1994; Schalock, 1990a); and QOL was responsive to personal judgments (Cummins et al., 1997; Daly et al., 1996; Parse, 1994, 1996; Renwick, 1998). Overall, views on conceptualization and definition generally fell into four groups, as described below.

The first group comprised the significant majority of authors who took a holistic view of QOL. Cummins's (personal communication, 21 June, 1999) definition is representative, i.e., "Quality of life is both objective and subjective, each axis being the aggregate of five domains ... objective domains comprise culturally relevant measures of objective wellbeing ... subjective domains comprise domain satisfaction weighted by their importance to the individual" (p. 2).

The second group argued that QOL was primarily a matter of personal perception (Johnstone, 1988; Schalock, 1996a; Taylor & Bogdan, 1990). Taylor and Bogdan's definition is representative "...Quality of life is satisfaction with one's lot in life and a sense of contentment with one's experiences of the world" (p. 27). Schalock (1996a, 1996b) similarly described QOL as a person's desired conditions of living and health and wellness, and suggested that a person's perceived QOL was best indicated by satisfaction.

The third group argued that agreement on conceptualization and definition was unachievable, so they opted for QOL to be regarded as a sensitizing concept (Edgerton, 1990; Goode, 1997; Neufeldt & McGinley, 1996; Taylor, 1994). Goode's remarks are representative "...Quality of life policy ... is the use of quality of life (with an emphasis on promoting general feelings of well-being, opportunities to fulfill potentials and feelings of positive social involvement) as a guide ... to decision-making in services/supports for persons. [Quality of life policy] would direct itself at minimising the discrepancies between individual's perceived and desired conditions of life" (p. 73).

The fourth group actively opposed any definition or application of the term. Sen (1993) and Taylor (1994), for example, concluded that a prescriptive definition would fail to acknowledge human diversity. Romney et al. (1994) felt that the concept of QOL was value and culture dependent and changed over time, so concluded that diversity was unavoidable. They referred to countless definitions and doubted the utility of pursuing a generic definition. This view was also shared by Hatton (1998), Luckasson et al. (1992), and Wolfensberger (1994). Goode (1992) cautioned that attempts to provide concise and clear definitions in the social sciences invariably resulted in proliferation and he argued that, "there is a kind of figure ground relationship between clarity and confusion that is necessary in social research" (p. 2). Daly et al. (1996) more contentiously stated that different disciplines required distinct definitions, and argued against meaningless global definition. Some researchers even argued that a definition was dangerous (Goode, 1994; Hatton, 1998; Wolfensberger, 1994).

In an overview of the literature, Schalock (1996b) suggested that three definitions were most representative: (1) QOL is experienced when a person's basic needs are met and he has opportunities to pursue and achieve goals (Goode, 1988); (2) QOL is a multidimensional concept involving a number of core dimensions relating to wellbeing (Felce & Perry, 1997); and (3) QOL reflects a person's desired conditions of living and health and wellness (Schalock, 1996b).

Explaining QOL: Domains and Indicators

Domains are those aspects of human existence wherein QOL may be experienced (Brown & Schalock, 2005; Lyons, 1999a; Parmenter, Briggs, & Sullivan, 1991; Schalock & Verdugo, 2002; Schalock et al., 2005; Verdugo et al., 2005). Most authors support the view that QOL is experienced across multiple domains. Cummins (personal communication, 21 June, 1999) remarked, "This convention is both intuitive and pragmatic" (p. 1). Although Michalos (1986), after conducting a comprehensive review of 10 years of QOL research, identified a complex multitude of domains used by researchers, and Van Dam, Somers, Van beck-Couzijn (1981) pointed out "almost any measure of human experience or living conditions could be co-opted as a QOL domain" (p. 1), there was some consensus about key domains. Those identified by Cummins (1996a) and Felce and Perry (1996), for example, were emotional wellbeing, health, social and family connections, material wealth or wellbeing, and work (or other forms of productive activity).

Cummins's (personal communication, 21 June, 1999) domain criteria provide valuable guidelines for identifying potentially meaningful domains, which are: (a) a set of domains must collectively encompass the totality of life experience, (b) each domain must encompass a substantial but discrete portion of the QOL construct, (c) each domain must have the potential to be measured in both objective and subjective dimensions, (d) each domain (within a generic QOL instrument) must have relevance for all people, (e) domains proposed for non-generic instruments must contribute unique variance, (f) domains must be potentially neutral, positive, or negative in their contribution, (g) domains differ from dimensions of personality, cognitive processes, and affect in that the latter cannot be measured objectively, and (h) the subjective dimension of each domain has both a cognitive and an affective component measured in terms of satisfaction.

One group of researchers (Diener, 1994; Lance, Lautenschlager, Sloan, & Varca, 1989; Pavot & Diener, 1993; Travers & Richardson, 1993) alternatively argued for the validity and utility of a single global domain. Their argument was based on the seminal research of Andrews and Withy (1976) that produced remarkably consistent data based on only one measure of QOL, and which constituted one of the few empirical benchmarks for population-based QOL research (Cummins, 1995; Cummins et al., 1997). Cummins (1995) also found that measures of global life satisfaction for large samples of the population were consistent and reliable. This global domain view has been widely criticized on four grounds. First, the approach could not explain relationships between global and domain-related QOL. Second, Michalos (1986) found that nearly half of the QOL research identified work satisfaction as a key domain, reflecting a socio-political perspective that excluded those who did not work from meaningful assessment (Kiuranov, 1980). Third, the approach implied that QOL was the same across all domains, although research has generally demonstrated a low correlation (Erikson & Uusitalo, 1987; Travers & Richardson, 1993). Fourth, critics argued that it was important to identify those who consistently scored poorly in one or more domains, in order to identify disadvantage and inequity.

More recent analyses of the international QOL literature (Schalock & Verdugo, 2002; Schalock, 2004a, 2004b) demonstrate considerable agreement on identifying key (person-referenced) QOL domains. These are, in descending order of frequency of mention in the literature: interpersonal relations, social inclusion, personal development, physical wellbeing, self-determination, material wellbeing, emotional wellbeing, rights, environment, family, recreation and leisure, and safety and security.

Indicators (as opposed to domains) are those aspects of human existence wherein QOL may be measured and/or assessed, and may be within and/or across domains (Brown & Schalock, 2005; Lyons, 2000b; Verdugo et al., 2005). Historically, QOL researchers placed different emphases on the use of subjective and objective indicators (Halpern, 1993a, 1993b). Scandinavian and Australian governments, for example, emphasized objective indicators (Erikson & Uusitalo, 1987; Travers & Richardson, 1993; Vogel et al., 1988), whereas North American researchers were oriented toward acknowledging individualism and focusing on subjective indicators (Andrews & Withy, 1976; Goode & Hogg, 1994; Romney et al., 1994).

During the 1970s, fervent debate about the validity and utility of indicators polarized views. Research at that time evidenced a poor correlation between data derived from the two types (Cheng, 1988; Fabian, 1991; Goode, 1997). By the 1980s, there was renewed recognition of the utility of both types (Andrews, 1980; Zapf, 1986), so many researchers sought to understand and describe any interrelationships. These researchers included, for example, Andrews (1980, 1986), Blishen and Atkinson (1980), Hedley, Dubin and Taveggia (1980), Horn (1993), Ingelhart and Rabier (1986); McKennell, Atkinson and Andrews (1980), Michalos (1985, 1986), Schuessler and Fisher (1985), Solomon et al. (1980), Szalai (1980), and Zapf et al. (1987).

Hankiss (1980), Land (1983), and Rapley (2003) similarly concluded, subsequent to extensive literature reviews, that significant and complicated interrelationships existed. In contrast, Brown and Shearer (1999), Ingelhart and Rabier (1986), and Zapf (1986) argued that the satisfaction paradox, wherein disadvantaged and marginalized groups of people tended to take on devalued beliefs and expectations to minimize the gap between their aspirations and circumstances, invalidated the debate. Sen (1993, 1996) supported this latter position, but emphasized the centrality of human diversity rather than the prevailing (western) philosophical view that equality could only be expressed in happiness, achievement, or materialism. Davison (1977) too, argued against hedonistic utilitarianism and the pursuit of individual happiness and wellbeing. Other theories, including Horn's (1988) gap-theoretical explanations; Michalos's (1986) multiple discrepancy theory; Ingelhart and Rabier's (1986) aspiration-adaptation model; Helson's (1964) adaptation level theory; and Cummins' (1996a) relative deprivation theory, are demonstrative of the diversity of understandings about the nature of interrelationships between objective and subjective indicators.

Evans (1994), and Olson and Schober (1993) suggested that the ascendancy of the subjective approach to QOL research had led to a dissipation of the aforementioned interest in any interrelationship. Evans, drawing on the research of Diener (1984), and Pavot and Diener (1993), argued strongly for a broader taxonomy of subjective measures. He delineated subjective measures as externally referenced to a normative sample on the basis of observation, externally referenced to a normative sample on the basis of cognitive appraisal, and internally referenced to oneself based on cognitive appraisal. Evans further argued that there were ample cognitive measures of subjective QOL, but too few based on external referents, and that most subjective indicators in the life satisfaction and affective domains were too responsive to internal changeable standards, whereas subjective measures based upon external referents and population norms were more stable.

Diener (1984), Headey (1993), and Lance et al. (1989) contended that top-down and bottom-up models explained vertical relationships between QOL indicators. Top-down models presume that personal disposition is an enduring characteristic of QOL and strongly influences outcomes in an individual's life (Peplau, 1994), whereas bottom-up models presume that environmental variables are more influential. Generally though, researchers tended to explain relationships using a combination of both models (Brief, Butcher, George, & Link, 1993; Lance et al., 1989).

In 2002, Karon and Bernard put forward representative criteria for selecting, measuring, and using indicators, i.e., indicators should have: strategic importance for maximizing wellbeing; show variation and potential for improvement when measured; be affected by the actions of supporting others; provide meaningful data that is reasonably cost effective to collect; be sensitive to cultural differences (e.g., sense of self – Triandis, 1994; perception of others – Markus & Kitayama, 1991; cultural assumptions – Keith, 1996a, 1996b; and translation of meanings – Brislin, 2000); be applicable across programs and populations; and be based on sound theory.

Explaining QOL: Theories and Models

Scores of theories and models of QOL have been proposed by many authors. The heterogeneity of these theories and models reflects the authors' diversity of approaches to the conceptualization, definition, measurement, and application of the QOL construct. The following section provides a brief overview of some of the characteristics, similarities, differences, and relationships between a selection of these theories and models. This selection emphasizes those theories and models that particularly explain subjective QOL, a concept synonymous with life satisfaction, and that aspect of global QOL most difficult to ascertain for persons with ID. From the outset, it should be noted that most theorists support holistic models, wherein objective, external, and quantifiable environmental elements are discernible from the more subjective, internal elements, and wherein these elements are combined and/or weighted by personal disposition to indicate global QOL (Borthwick-Duffy, 1992; Bowles, 1995; Brown, 1995, 1997b, 1998a; Felce & Perry, 1996, 1997; Halpern, 1993a; Seed & Lloyd 1996).

Three prevalent and widely documented perspectives on QOL, the social indicators perspective, the psychological perspective, and the goodness of fit/social policy perspective, were clearly identifiable in the literature (Campbell, Converse, & Rodgers, 1976; Halpern, 1993b; Schalock, 1990a). Other less widely promoted perspectives were notable though. For example, Bach (1994) and Mitchell and Winslade (1997) similarly described a narrative or social wellbeing approach to QOL wherein QOL correlated with the extent to which conditions and circumstances in the individual's life supported the development and realization of life plans. The involvement of all of the important others in the individual's social milieu was central to this approach. Somewhat similarly, the client-driven ecology model of Goode (1997) focused on an individual's perceived and objective environments in the context of their social relationships. Peter (1997), Schalock (1997), Stark and Faulkner (1996), and Taylor (1994) alternatively argued for a model that viewed QOL as a sensitizing concept, wherein QOL appraisal was subjective and concerned with an individual's expressed satisfaction. A primary feature of the core domains of this model was that they were experiential.

Evans (1994) categorized theorists into three groups in accordance with their views on subjective QOL. Each group supported measurement or assessment across domains, and responded to an individual's preferences and weightings of importance or relevance. The first group though supported the linear additive model, wherein global QOL was the sum of scores on a set selection of domains (e.g., Chibnall & Tait, 1990; Davis & Fine-Davis, 1991; Ouellette-Kuntz & McCreary, 1996). The second group supported the weighted sum position, wherein global QOL was the sum of scores in each domain multiplied by the individual's weighted importance in each domain. The third group supported the personal integrative model, wherein individuals included and weighted only those domains that related to their own life (e.g., Campbell et al., 1976; Diener, 1984; Pavot & Diener, 1993). (Note that these three groups do not and are not intended to correlate with the aforementioned three prevalent perspectives.)

Parmenter (1989) argued that many QOL models needed, but did not have, a sound theoretical base, and that symbolic interaction was the best theory for this purpose. Borthwick-Duffy (1992) and Felce and Perry (1995) supported this view. Parmenter and Donelly (1997) enmeshed symbolic interaction into their model of QOL wherein "quality of life represents the degree to which an individual has met their needs to create their own meanings so the individual can establish and sustain a viable self in the social world" (p. 96). Some comparisons can be drawn here with the "narrative/social wellbeing approach" of Mitchell and Winslade (1997) mentioned above. Leininger's (1994) explanation of cultural experience is also comparable.

Zapf's (1986) theory and model cogently explained four states of QOL (for any domain), which were: wellbeing, wherein a "good" perceptual evaluation and good objective life conditions prevailed; dissonance, wherein a "bad" perceptual evaluation, but good objective life conditions prevailed; adaptation, wherein a good perceptual evaluation, but bad objective life conditions prevailed; and deprivation, wherein a bad perceptual evaluation and bad life conditions prevailed. Wellbeing represented the highest QOL (for that domain). Those in the dissonant state were likely to protest or seek change. Those in the adaptation state lived the "Satisfaction Paradox" (see Zapf (1986) earlier in Domains and Indicators), and the deprived were the classic target of social policy. Zapf argued that this theory and model allowed for comparisons between domains, and had the potential to identify indicative clusters of domains and states of QOL.

Michalos's (1985) multiple discrepancies theory is a widely cited explanation for understanding subjective appraisal of QOL. Michalos claimed that subjective satisfaction was based on an individual's perceptions of discrepancies between what one (and others) had, needed, deserved, and wanted. Similarly, Renwick (1998; personal communication, August, 2003) and Raphael, Brown, Renwick, and Rootman (1996) health promotion model defined QOL as the extent to which a person enjoyed the important possibilities of life. Michalos's theory had considerable support among prominent authors (e.g., Cummins, 1996b; Fabian, 1991) although others argued that it was too complex to find useful application.

Cummins's (2000, 2005a) and Cook's (2003) theories and model posited that subjective QOL (subjective wellbeing) was moderated by a homeostasis arising from personal adaptation to environmental conditions. His extensive quantitative research suggested that QOL varied only slightly for all individuals, and that personality variables accounted for much of this variance. Key aspects of Cummins's model may be compared to Zapf's adaptation state, as abovementioned, and Cummins's model has significant implications for the validity and utility of theories and models that uphold subjective or cognitive assessments of life conditions as key determinants of QOL.

Dennis et al. (1993) described a model, based on the optimal theory of Speight, Myers, Cox, and Highlen (1991), which allowed for individual, group, and cultural perspectives to be enmeshed and compared. This model is comparable to the models of both Bergsma and Engels (1988 in Mayers, 1995, p. 148), wherein QOL can be measured at the macro-, micro-, personal-, and physical-levels, and the 3 × 3 matrix described by Heal, Borthwick-Duffy and Saunders (1994), wherein the perceiver can be the individual, an intimate acquaintance, or third party, and the focus can be on the individual, on intimate relationships, or on society at large.

Subsequent to their comprehensive review of QOL theories and models, Hughes et al. (1995) proposed a conceptual model based on a consensus of dimensions and corresponding components. This model represented a consolidation of much of the research up to that time, and is comparable to the (aforementioned) models of Felce and Perry (1997) and Brown (1997b, 1998a).

Two additional theories, although atypical and not widely adopted, are also relevant. Halpern et al.'s (1986) transition model viewed QOL from a person-referenced outcomes perspective. Halpern specifically advocated for the use of QOL as a measure of the success of the transition process. Although his model is an atypical application of the QOL concept, his views of transition and QOL as dynamic, multi-phased, lifelong processes are relevant to most theories and models. Borthwick-Duffy's (1987) model was the only one that focused specifically on assessing QOL for persons with disabilities, but was limited to measuring only the effects of changes in residential environment and community.

Evans (1994) suggested that the themes evident among prominent theories and models could be enmeshed to develop a grounded theory about QOL. For example, most theories acknowledged the importance of the individual and a subjective perspective. Satisfaction, whether overall or domain-specific, was pervasive, and closely allied to cognitive appraisal (Griffin, 1998; Lazarus, 1993; Zhan, 1992). Social context (Abbey & Andrews, 1986; Goode, 1997; Headey & Wearing, 1992; Parmenter, 1989), and personality/disposition (Costa, McCrea, & Zonderman, 1987; Cummins, 2005a; Diener, 1984; Evans, 1994) were also evident themes. The more extreme view shared by Costa et al. (1987) and Parse (1996), that personality and disposition were the only determinants of QOL, was not widely supported (Abbey & Andrews, 1986; Felce & Perry, 1996; Headey & Wearing, 1992; Peplau, 1994). There were a number of theories and models proposed specifically for persons with ID (e.g., Brown, 1997c; Raphael et al., 1996), but most prominent theories and models in the disability literature were put forward by their authors as "generic" and not specific to persons with ID (Cummins, 2005a).

There is a growing contemporary consensus about the QOL construct and its core elements, but a dearth of consensus about the ascendancy of any conceptual model or theory. Cummins (2005a) argues strongly for researchers to put current theoretical models to the test in order to "take our conceptualization of QOL to the next level." (p. 699).

Explaining QOL: Measurement and Assessment

To find out about another person's subjective QOL, researchers can generally just ask how satisfied that person is with their life. This asking is usually done in person or by means of a questionnaire, using a validated instrument or technique. Learning about another person's life satisfaction is obviously problematic when that person cannot communicate their (level of) satisfaction. Consistent with the prevailing holistic, multidimensional view of QOL (Seed & Lloyd, 1997), most researchers seek to measure and assess QOL and life satisfaction using multiple domains and indicators (Andrews, 1980; Brown et al., 1994; Cummins, 2000; Erikson & Uusitalo, 1987; Felce & Perry, 1996; Hughes et al., 1995; Parmenter, 1994, 1995; Sen, 1993; Solomon et al., 1980; Zapf et al., 1987). Nevertheless, debate continues on whether subjective QOL can or should be measured across multiple measures or whether a simple global measure is valid and achievable (Felce & Perry, 1996; Romney et al., 1994; Travers & Richardson, 1993).

The measurement and assessment of QOL has been approached using objective and subjective methods. Objective methods use observable and quantifiable indicators whereas subjective methods use an individual's perceptions and qualitative assessments of happiness or satisfaction (Land, 1983; Lyons, 2000b; Schuessler & Fisher, 1985). An early attempt to measure QOL subjectively was made by Campbell et al. (1976) who tracked the subjective feelings of a large sample of Americans using measures of satisfaction, affect, and stress. Schalock (1999) and Lyons (2000b) put the view that objective aspects of QOL relating to standard of living are measurable but that subjective aspects of life satisfaction can and should only be assessed.

The use of subjective methods for ascertaining people's perceptions attracted polarized views. Although strongly supported (by, e.g., Dale, 1995; Diener, 1994; Headey & Wearing, 1992; McKennell et al., 1980; Pavot & Diener, 1993; Zapf et al., 1987), the approach was also criticized for a variety of reasons (see Andrews & Withy, 1976; Ingelhart & Rabier, 1986; Land, 1983). Cummins (personal communication, 21 June, 1999), Diener (1994), Headey and Wearing (1992), Pavot and Diener (1993), Schuessler and Fisher (1985), for example, all argued that, as indicators, happiness and affect were too labile and emotive, and life satisfaction overly stable. Andrew and Whitny (1976), Diener (1994), and Headey (1993) argued that positive and negative feelings were independent, and thus both necessary for assessment. Subjective wellbeing was also often interpreted as inclusive of life satisfaction, positive affect, and negative affect. Land (1983) particularly criticized the use of happiness and life satisfaction as major measures, and argued for the use of measures like expectations, aspirations, attitudes, and values. Andrew and Whitny (1976), Ingelhart and Rabier (1986), Schalock and Keith (1993), and Seed and Lloyd (1996) held similar views.

The use of objective methods alone was also criticized (Abberley, 1986; Andrews, 1980; Horn, 1993; Oliver, 1990) even though there was wide support for the use of objective instruments (Cummins, personal communication, 21 June, 1999; Schalock & Keith, 1993). Browne and Bramston (1996) explained two major criticisms of using objective methods alone. First, that it was ethnocentric to assume that one set of objective standards could apply to all people (Edgerton, 1990), and second, that environmental factors played only a small role in subjective wellbeing (Abbey & Andrews, 1986; Costa et al., 1987).

A further issue of interest is the question of the stability of QOL over time. Although there was comparatively little research on this issue, the consensus in the literature was that time was a variable in any judgment about QOL (Parmenter, 1992; Schipper, Clinch, & Powell, 1990, Szalai, 1980). There was little longitudinal research focusing on measures which were trait or state-related, whereas cognitive measures have been demonstrated to be very responsive to life events (Cheng, 1988; Goodinson & Singleton, 1989). Nevertheless, Costa et al. (1987), in a seminal longitudinal study, found QOL to be very stable over time, and concluded that future QOL was best predicted by past QOL. This study, and others conducted by Brandstadter and Baltes-Gotz (1990), supported the contention that an individual's QOL remained relatively stable over time, despite the impact of life events and conditions. Edgerton pointedly remarked, "The current body of research tells little about changes in quality of life or subjective well-being" (p. 153). Halpern's (1993a, 1993b) aforementioned research on QOL and transition is relevant here. Cummins' seminal (continuing) longitudinal study on population wellbeing (in Australia), provides arguably indisputable evidence for the validity and rigor of his homeostasis theory and model (Cummins et al., 2004).

Given the now widely accepted view that QOL consists of (some combination) both objective and subjective measures that neither is more "valid" than the other, and that there is a weak relationship between them, one strong agreement is that a comprehensive global assessment of QOL must include both measures (Cummins, 2000, 2005a; International Wellbeing Group, 2005).

QOL and Persons with ID

> The logic and relationships of QOL for persons with disabilities are no different from that of those without (Goode, 1992, p. 5).

A strong consensus in the literature supports the view that the conceptualization and assessment of QOL should be the same for persons with or without ID (Borthwick-Duffy, 1992, 1996; Brown, 1998a; Brown, 1999; Cummins, 2005a; Felce, 1997; Goode, 1994; Holm, Holst, & Perit, 1994; Hughes & Hwang, 1996; Keith, 1996a; Lyons, 2000b; Renwick, 1998; Schalock, 1996b, 2002; Seed & Lloyd, 1996; Woodill, Renwick, Brown, & Raphael, 1994). Turnbull and Brunk (1990) and Ashman (1990), for example, argued cogently for this position on the basis of values, morality, and social policy arguments. Cummins (1995) concluded, subsequent to his literature review of life satisfaction studies that results for persons with ID showed values in the normal range. Kozleski and Sands (1992) also compared QOL assessments for adults with and without ID and found a moderate correlation.

One exceptional position was put by Rosen, Simon, and McKinsey (19895) who argued that QOL should be defined differently for persons with ID on the basis of what could be "appreciated, responded to, integrated and utilized by that individual [and] that comparisons of QOL should be made within relatively homogeneous groups of mental disability" (p. 365). This position was widely opposed. Cummins (1997), for example, expressed the concern that "there is a great danger in any conception of quality of life that is restricted to some minority group . . . It is imperative that all definitions and models of life quality be referenced to the general population both in their conception and in their operational measurement" (p. 127). Brown and Brown (1996) also explained that, as most minority groups had a lower standard of living than the general population, a definition that might seem appropriate for minority groups might well be unacceptable to the general population. Such definitions, they argued, were "shaped by the deficits of the groups to which they refer and, as a consequence, have been downgraded to reflect the assumption of a lower life quality than normal" (p. 123).

The literature on the concept of QOL for persons with ID does though show some different emphases to that in the general QOL literature. First, conceptualizations tended to reflect the social justice, individual rights, and equity origins of the research (Brown, 1998a). Schalock's (1999) core dimensions of QOL for persons with ID were indicative of these different emphases, and included emotional wellbeing, personal development, physical wellbeing, self-determination, social inclusion, and rights. Second, there was an emphasis on individual rather than population QOL improvement (Brown, 1998a; Cummins, 1996b; Zapf et al., 1987) that impacted upon policy development, service planning, delivery and evaluation, and quality assurance and enhancement programs in (intellectual) disability services (Brown, Bayer, & MacFarlane, 1988, 1989; Cummins, 1993; Emerson, 1985; Goode, 1992; Parmenter, 1989, 1995; Schalock, 1990c, 1994b; Schalock et al., 2000). This second emphasis reflected the abovementioned recognition that consumer satisfaction and QOL improvement should be service priorities (Brown, 1999; Cheng, 1988; Conway, 1992; Fabian, 1991; Felce & Perry, 1996; Renwick, personal communication, August, 2003). Third, and synchronous with the focus on the individual, Brown, 1995; Brown, McLinden, & Porter, 1998, Goode and Hogg (1994), Nankervis (1997), Schalock (2002), and Schalock and Verdugo (2002) argued that persons with ID should be more involved in decision-making about policies and programs aimed at improving their QOL.

Other different emphases were put forward by Halpern (1993a), who representatively identified the individual perceptions of satisfaction, wellbeing, and connections between the individual and important others as core concepts, and Schalock (1994a), who identified three key concepts in the disability literature, i.e., general feelings of wellbeing, opportunities to fulfill one's potential, and feelings of positive social involvement.

An extensive literature review conducted by the American National Institute on Disability and Rehabilitation Research (Goode, 1992) found four types of definitions to be prevalent in the disability field. Implicit definitions were those that assumed normalization led to a better QOL. Operational definitions were research methodology driven. Rational definitions reflected authors' values or beliefs. Unintentional definitions reflected unstated beliefs or values. Goode (1992) and Dempsey and Foreman (1997) noted that QOL could be defined at international, national, local, and individual levels, although the majority of definitions in the disability field were individually oriented.

Although general conceptualizations of QOL prevail in the intellectual disability literature, many definitions of QOL specific to intellectual disability have been recorded (Brown et al., 1994; Evans, 1994; Goode & Hogg, 1994; Hatton, 1998; Heal et al., 1994; McVilly & Rawlinson, 1998; Nankervis, 1997; Schalock, 1994a; Taylor, 1994). Schalock (1997), for example, referred to perceived QOL as satisfaction with the main areas of one's life. Brown et al. (1994) suggested that QOL enhancement was related to a reduction in the discrepancy between an individual's achieved and unmet needs, and included perceived and objective assessments across domains. Brown (1998a) referred to QOL as the extent to which individuals have increasing control of their environments. Heal et al. (1994) described QOL in terms of global satisfaction with one's lifestyle and control over resources that produced satisfactions.

A broadly held concern was that QOL (and disability) research was drawing on a proliferating base of concepts and definitions (Heal & Sigelman, 1996) and measurement instruments (Cummins, 2003, 2007). Hughes et al. (1995), for example, identified 1243 measures of QOL. Similarly, Cummins (2007) has catalogued over 1000 instruments for measuring QOL. Goode (1992) warned that, unless there was substantive progress in defining and confining terms, the QOL concept would lose utility.

Investigating the QOL of Persons with ID

> We know all too little about the quality of (the lives of persons with intellectual disabilities), and next to nothing about their satisfaction with those lives (Edgerton, 1990, p. 153).

The general debate about relationships between subjective and objective methods and indicators in mainstream literature (see, e.g., Rapley, 2003) was similarly evident in the disability literature (Brown, Bayer, & Brown, 1992; Emerson et al., 2005; Goode, 1990b; Parmenter et al., 1994; Schalock & Felce, 2004; Schalock, 1990a; Verdugo et al., 2005). Schalock (1994a) argued that QOL research for persons with ID requires a holistic approach using interactional indicators based on both types. Goode and Hogg (1994) noted that the indicators debate was the source of continuing tension in the disability literature. Ingelhart and Rabier (1986) and Brown et al. (1994), for example, refuted any meaningful interrelationship between the two types of indicators and argued that the satisfaction paradox confounds any definitive analysis. The satisfaction paradox is particularly pertinent to persons with ID, as it can provide one explanation as to why persons with ID tend to take on devalued beliefs and expectations.

The use of indicators in the disability/QOL research does differ from that in mainstream research, in that disability/QOL theorists tried to account for atypical needs and circumstances. Antaki and Rapley (1996) and Hughes et al. (1995), for example, criticized the earlier and prevailing use of objective QOL measures and argued that they were only used to indicate changes in functional and/or adaptive skills. Objective indicators were widely criticized as susceptible to value bias and inadequately responsive to individual needs (French, 1993b; Oliver, 1993). Many authors (e.g., Branson & Miller, 1992; Fullagher & Hardaker, 1993; Goode, 1994; Holm et al., 1994; Kuehn & McClainm, 1994; Parmenter, 1992; Schalock, 1994a) warned against "the tyranny of the normal," wherein diversity was challenged as inappropriate. Nevertheless, Kozleski and Sands (1992) were able to explain how general community values could be taken positively into account to avoid potential value bias.

Subjective indicators found wide support in the disability field because they were regarded to be more reflective of individual needs, perceptions, and diversity (see Brown et al., 1992; Brown et al., 1989; Cummins, 1993; Ferrans & Powers, 1985; Goode & Hogg, 1994; Parmenter, 1989; Parmenter et al., 1994; Rosen, Simon, & McKinsey, 1995; Schalock, 1994a; Taylor & Bogdan, 1990). More specifically, subjective indicators were widely used as QOL measures for individuals with intellectual disabilities (Cummins et al., 1997). Brown (1998, personal communication, 1 October, 1998), however, criticized the term "subjective" as implying imprecision, and suggested the term "perceived" as preferable. Antaki and Rapley (1996) and Brown et al. (1994) concluded that subjective indicators were facilitative because they provided opportunities for researchers to use both qualitative and quantitative research approaches in investigating QOL and life satisfaction.

Some of the more widely supported subjective indicators in the disability research included control and choice (Brown & Bayer, 1992; Brown, Bayer, & McFarlane, 1989; Schalock, 1994a), beliefs, goals, values, empowerment, happiness and control (Antaki & Rapley, 1996; Parmenter, 1992), self esteem, satisfaction, independence and responsibility (Brown et al., 1989; Rosen et al., 1995), friendship, intimacy, understanding and security (Cummins, 1993; McVilly, 2004), and mastery and social networks (Holm et al., 1994). Seed and Lloyd (1996) preferred degree of reciprocity to independence as a key indicator, and Rosen et al. (1995) regarded perceived stress, affect, loneliness, and dissatisfaction to be the most relevant criteria.

Despite this widespread support, Felce and Perry (1996) argued that subjective evaluations of emotional wellbeing have been neglected in the intellectual disability literature because of the difficulties these persons have in communicating the nuances and complexities of abstract feelings and emotions. Emerson (1985) similarly identified resident satisfaction as significantly under-researched. Antaki and Rapley (1996), Matikka and Vesala (1997), and McVilly and Rawlinson (1998) agreed that these difficulties render data obtained from interviews with persons with ID to be of questionable validity. Despite this criticism, Brown et al. (1988) were able to demonstrate measurements of perceived QOL obtained directly from adults with mild to moderate ID to have reliabilities of greater than 0.45.

In 1991, Fabian, on the basis of an extensive review of 10 years of the QOL/disability literature, identified three approaches to measuring QOL. The first two, viewing QOL as an objective social indicator for specific groups, and viewing QOL as a broad subjective measure of life satisfaction, have been discussed earlier in this chapter. The third, viewing QOL as a measure of adaptive functioning, was identified as one alternative for those individuals who were unable to self-report or whose life experiences were inequitably limited. However, Antaki and Rapley (1996) argued that behavioral data provides only dubious inference for how persons with ID felt about their life. Further still, Fabian, although conceding that adaptive functioning had some value in a comprehensive assessment, concluded that it was inadequate as a sole measure or indicator. Conversely, Barlow and Kirby (1992), Brown and Bayer (1992), and McVilly and Rawlinson (1998) similarly concluded that patterns of engagement in daily activities are potentially valid indicators for persons with more severe ID.

This review of the QOL/disability literature identified two principal schools of thought among theorists about QOL measurement and assessment (DisAbility Services Division, 2000). The first most widely supported school of thought, represented by, for example, Bowling (1992); Felce (1997) Felce and Perry (1996), Goode (1997), Goode and Hogg (1994), Oliver et al. (1996), Schalock (1993) and Seed and Lloyd (1996), upheld a holistic approach, inclusive of both qualitative and quantitative approaches. Romney et al. (1994) concluded, "There seems to be a remarkable degree of agreement on this point, at least among researchers in the field of developmental disabilities" (p. 248).

At the same time, though, there was considerable criticism of this holistic approach. Felce and Perry (1996) argued that it lacked an empirical basis, although they accepted the reasonable evidence of its face validity. Bowling (1992) and Hatton (1998) criticized attempts to measure subjective indicators, and concluded that self-reporting lacked validity and reliability. Bowling (1992) went so far as to suggest, "... most studies of quality of life are hampered by poor design and inadequate assessment methods." (p. 9). Similar research by Dagnan (1996), and Dagnan, Look, Ruddick, and Jones (1995) pointed to methodological inadequacies in many studies that purportedly assessed QOL for persons with ID. Edgerton (1996) argued that objective measures must be separated from subjective reports of wellbeing. Some researchers (e.g., Antaki & Rapley, 1996; Stensman, 1985; Taylor & Bogdan, 1990) argued that the radical subjectivity of QOL presented a serious obstacle to the use of QOL in policy and programs for persons with ID.

Conversely, Raphael et al. (1996) suggested that differences in reports between persons with ID and their proxy reporters were not problematic, but simply reflected real differences in perceptions and worldviews. Goode (1997) also put an alternative position, and argued that a third relational or social factor should be included, wherein data sourced from proxy reporters should be regarded as a valued subset of subjective data.

The second major school of thought, represented by, for example, Edgerton (1996), Keith (1996a, 1996b), Taylor (1994), and Taylor and Bogdan (1990), argued that QOL could be described but not measured, lacks definitive characteristics and benchmarks, and should only be conceived as a sensitizing concept to guide thinking. Authors upholding this position supported qualitative research that reflected cultural and personal diversity. Edgerton pertinently remarked, "Judging whether a reasonable level of quality of life exists is a separate issue to its measurement" (p. 59).

This review generated four themes about measurement and assessment in the QOL/disability literature. First, the subjective nature of QOL was prominent. Second, the centrality of the individual's perspective was widely emphasized (Brown et al., 1998; Goode & Hogg, 1994; McVilly & Rawlinson, 1998). Third, there was a focus on responding to an individual's expressed wants (Brown et al., 1992; Edgerton, 1990; Taylor, 1994). Fourth, there was a consensus that QOL could and should be applied in (disability services) policy development, quality assurance, and enhancement (Brown, 1995; Hughes & Hwang, 1996; Knoll, 1990; Newton, Ard, Horner, & Toews, 1996; Oliver et al., 1996; Parmenter, 1994; Roth & Morse, 1996; Schalock, 1993, 1999). Collectively, the research of Abbott-Chapman and Easthope (1998), Brown et al. (1992) Cummins (1993), Hughes et al. (1995), Parmenter et al. (1994), and Schalock et al. (2000) all showed that better outcomes were achieved when people with disabilities were encouraged to pursue their own goals.

QOL assessment and measurement for individuals with more severe ID brings about specific and complex challenges for researchers, decision-makers, and practitioners (Cummins, 2005d). First, accounting for the subjective nature of assessment at the individual level is highly problematic (Goode & Hogg, 1994; Goode, 1994; Heal & Sigelman, 1996). Second, it is problematic to involve the individual in the process of conceptualizing and assessing QOL (Brown, 1995; Hughes et al., 1995; Romney et al., 1994), meaning the cognitive impairments of persons with ID clearly limit their levels of understanding, life experiences, communicative capacities, and perceptions of QOL (Evans, 1994; McVilly & Rawlinson, 1998; Oliver et al., 1996; Seed & Lloyd, 1997). Third, the experiences and perceptions of persons conducting these assessments are significant (Antaki & Rapley, 1996; Neufeldt & McGinley, 1996), and if these persons do not have shared experiences or culture, and cannot assume a reciprocity of perspectives or intersubjectivity (Goode, 1997; Keith, 1996a; Leininger, 1994; Luckasson et al., 1992), then communication and understanding may be unreliable and/or invalid (Heal & Sigelman, 1996). While this need for mutual understanding was widely discussed in the literature, little research has been published in this area (Golden & Reese, 1996). Fourth, attempts to use reputational data from proxy reporters for persons with ID have been demonstrated to be of dubious validity and reliability (Borthwick-Duffy, 1992; Cummins et al., 1997; Heal & Sigelman, 1990; Holm et al., 1994; Oliver et al., 1996; Schalock, 1994a), as there is a strong likelihood of misreading the other's thoughts or feelings (Dale, 1995; Goode, 1997). Prominent authors further criticized proxy reporting for distancing the subject person (Bannerman, Sheldon, Sherman, & Harchick, 1990; Brown, 1997a; Verdugo et al., 2005), and Goode (1997) noted that proxy interviews placed adults with severe ID in a passive role.

Direct interviewing approaches, using contemporary assessment instruments designed specifically for persons with mild or moderate ID, include the MLSS (Harner & Heal, 1993), the Com QOL-ID (Cummins et al., 1997), the Lifestyle Satisfaction Scale (Heal & Chadsey-Rusch, 1985), the QOL questionnaire (Schalock & Keith, 1993), PALS (Rosen et al., 1995), and an instrument designed by Renwick et al. (1996). Direct interviewing is inappropriate for use with people with more severe ID (Brown et al., 1992, 1998; Fabian, 1991). Even for persons with some verbal skills, acquiescence, inconsistency, and last-option responding impinge upon the validity and reliability of these assessments (Baroff, 1986; Felce & Perry, 1996; Heal & Sigelman, 1992; Matikka & Vesala, 1997). These problems are exacerbated when an individual has atypical expression, lacks formal communication skills, or tends to acquiesce (Matikka & Vesala, 1997). Dale (1995) noted that similar problems were widely reported in the medical and nursing literature.

Alternatively, the QOL questionnaire (Schalock & Keith, 1993) and the Lifestyle Satisfaction Scale (Harner & Heal, 1993) are widely used instruments designed for proxy reporters who know the subject person well. The QOL questionnaire is rigorous for objective items but remains problematic for subjective issues (Campo, Sharpton, Thompson, & Sexton, 1997). Stancliffe (1995) and Heal and Sigelman (1992) suggested that the validity and reliability of surrogate reporting could be enhanced by discussions and detailed behavioral observation. Similarly, Heal and Sigelman (1992) suggested that the validity of interview techniques could be enhanced if data from multiple interviews with familiar others was included. Brown

(1997c), holding a different view, suggested that differences between proxy and consumer responses, if appreciated as verbalized perceptions, were critical to furthering an understanding of the true individuality of perceptions about QOL. (More recently, researchers have successfully trained adults with ID to interview others about their QOL (Schalock, Bontham, & Marchand, 2000). This has reduced the need for proxy reporting and given persons with moderate ID the opportunity to self-report in a meaningful way.)

Schalock and Felce (2004) suggest that the measurement of QOL for persons with ID should depend on its use, i.e., if one wants to find out whether people with ID are as satisfied with their lives as others they should asses their level of satisfaction on the same measures and compare. If one wants to evaluate the support services/environment, objective indicators of life experiences and circumstances within an agreed QOL framework should be investigated.

Given the now widely supported view that the construct of QOL is the same for all people, it follows that it should be possible to develop a valid "generic" instrument to assess QOL for all people – regardless of disability, economic status, or culture. The proliferation of specific QOL assessment instruments in recent years is problematic, particularly when these are not generally comparable to any "gold standard" generic instrument (Cummins & Lau, 2005; Cummins, 2005a). While these instruments may inform diagnosis or therapeutic intervention they may have little value for measuring global QOL (Cummins et al., 2004).

Subjective QOL for Persons with More Severe ID

> One of the field's greatest needs is the development and application of strategies that evaluate subjective or idiosyncratic dimensions of quality of life to supplement, and in some cases replace, more traditional objective indices. However, particularly difficult measurement challenges are presented by the many individuals with severe or profound mental retardation who cannot understand or respond meaningfully to questions designed to gauge subjective perspectives on their quality of life. (Campo et al., 1997, p. 335)

The connections between theory, ideology, and methodology are subject to continuing debate. Baum (1995) explains ideology as a stable system of beliefs that is resistant to change, and theory as subject to constant development and modification. Mosby's Dictionary of Medical, Nursing and Allied Health (1990) defined methodology as a system of principles or methods of procedure, and method as a technique or procedure for producing a desired effect. Oliver (1993) explained the relationship between theory, research, policy, and practice as complex, and highlighted the need for researchers to explicate their understanding of the relationships between their theoretical paradigms and research activities (Johnson, 1998). Research in disability studies has a history of "a lack of transparency" in this regard (Parmenter, 1989), which has contributed to difficulties in comparison, analysis, and validation (Landesman & Butterfield, 1987). Consequently, theories with wider contemporary support have gained predominance in the literature (Oliver, 1993). This review sought to account for competing approaches to disability and to undertake an investigation that was directly relevant to improving the lives of people with

ID (Bickenbach, 1993; Emerson, Hatton, Thomson, & Parmenter, 2004; Oliver & Barnes, 1993; Parmenter et al., 1991).

Theoretical approaches to, and the selection of research methods for, investigating the subjective QOL of persons with ID have to respond to the nature of the topic, the purpose and goals of the research, and the researchers' world views (Guba & Lincoln, 1994). There are several methods of inquiry that aim to develop knowledge, each with its own theoretical perspectives based on ontological, epistemological, and methodological differences (Denzin & Lincoln, 2000). It is this author's view that investigations into the subjective QOL of persons with ID are best conducted using interpretism as an inquiry paradigm, symbolic interactionism as a guiding theory of inquiry, and a grounded theory methodology and methods. Participant observation and semi-structured interviewing are facilitative as the primary means of field data collection.

Evidence and support for a qualitative/ethnographic approach, and symbolic interactionism as a guiding theory of inquiry, was evident in prior research that had comparable research questions and methodologies. For example, Atkins (1999) investigated nurses' perceptions of QOL for persons with severe and multiple impairments; Goode (1994) explored the communicative milieu surrounding children born deaf, blind, and alingual, and their parents and teachers; Clements, Copeland and Loftus (1990) studied parents' perceptions of caring for critically ill children; Hutchinson (1984) researched nurses' understandings about their work in a neonatal intensive care unit; Kearney (1996) investigated parents' feelings about caring for children with developmental disabilities; and Byrne and MacLean (1997) utilized grounded theory methodology to develop a QOL instrument for aged persons with dementia. Further strong evidence and support was also evident in the disability literature, particularly with respect to investigations into the nature of feelings about satisfaction and wellbeing expressed by persons with ID. A summary of this evidence follows.

Daly et al. (1996), Edgerton (1996), Goode (1994, 1995, 1997), and Romney et al. (1994) all strongly supported qualitative research methods as part of a holistic approach to understanding and assessing QOL. Dennis et al. (1993) supported the use of participatory research methods to increase the validity of current QOL assessment techniques, and noted that this has become the preferred approach for the American National Institute on Disability and Rehabilitation. Hughes et al. (1995) recommended triangulation of methods and multiple sources of information for future research into QOL for persons with ID.

Brown et al. (1989) and Brown (1990, 1995) argued that understanding the emotions of individuals required an appraisal of the individual within the context of his or her environment, and supported the ecological model of Bronfenbrenner (1979). Brown (1995) suggested that the adoption of a QOL model required researchers to conduct qualitative and ethnographic studies, given that the primary purpose of QOL assessment was to seek the perceptions of the individual. Similarly, Brown (1997b) and Christiansen (1993) concluded that qualitative methods were most appropriate for investigating the changing patterns of an individual's life. To quote Brown (1997b), "Insofar as such personal views can be presented orally or registered non-verbally, they represent an externalization of external and internal processes in forms that are measurable and replaceable. . .To ignore these data is to restrict scientific investigation" (p. 2).

Edgerton (1990) concluded, subsequent to his seminal 10-year ethnographic study, that the only viable means of assessing the QOL of an individual was to use an ethnographic approach. He also suggested that research into life satisfaction and intellectual disability should address the need for refinement of measurement technologies for gaining subjective appraisals of personal satisfaction and the importance a person places on various lifestyle issues. Johnson (1998) similarly identified qualitative action research, using an ethnographic approach, as the best means of establishing some form of reciprocity with participants.

Goode's (1994) seminal study into the lives of children born deaf–blind and with severe ID explored the social construction of children and their communications with their parents, paid carers and teachers using qualitative, ethnographic, participant–observer, and action research approaches. Goode uncovered a complex, contextual, and intersubjective communicative milieu surrounding these individuals and their communication partners, and suggested that "Establishing an understanding (intersubjectivity) with the children in their 'own terms' would be significant not only for our understanding of them but for our efforts at teaching and socializing" (p. 17). He argued that the more traditional quantitative methodologies were incompatible with this task, and could obfuscate potential understandings of these persons, and of the milieu of communicative intersubjectivity surrounding them.

Haring (1996) criticized much of the quantitative research as being irrelevant to current practice, and urged researchers to link qualitative and quantitative methods to include participants as active collaborators in research, and to pursue and support meaningful research that could improve people's lives. Miller and Davey (1993) similarly demonstrated that quantitative approaches were unable to capture the essential nuances of subjective QOL for individuals with severe ID. They argued that qualitative approaches demonstrated a potential to interpret communicative intent with respect to an individual's inner state and their feelings about their environment.

Mitchell and Winslade (1997), O'Brien and Mount (1998), and Romney et al. (1994) all supported a narrative approach when working with families of persons with ID, based on the developmental systems approach of Bronfenbrenner (1979), as did Brown et al. (1989), Brown (1990, 1995), Bach (1994), and Miller and Davey (1993). Pare (1995) similarly viewed families as "interpretive communities or storying cultures" (p. 16), wherein making meaning from the family communicative milieu predominated over clinical explanations of formal observations. Peter (1997) representatively concluded that qualitative research into QOL for persons with ID produced rich descriptive data about the complexities and ambiguities of QOL from that person's and other's views, reflected the holistic nature of a person's life, contextualized data within the individual's social/cultural milieu, and had strong internal validity.

Despite comprehensive literature reviews conducted by Marinoble and Hegenauer (1988), Borthwick-Duffy (1992), and Mayers (1995), there was no research identified until 1995 that focused on the QOL of people with more severe

ID. Since then, Brown (1997c) noted that most of the pertinent research had focused on adults with mild to moderate ID and that very little research, other than that of Halpern (1993a, 1993b) and Timmons and Brown (1997), focuses on children (or the elderly). This reflected the strong government, professional and community interest in the deinstitutionalization of adults at that time (Atkins, 1999). Consequently, research by Atkins (1999), Borthwick-Duffy (1990), Campo, Sharpton, Thompson, and Sexton (1996, 1997), and Goode (1994) emerged as the only basic research specifically examining QOL for persons with more severe ID, although Green and Reid (1996) had conducted research on happiness among adults. Campo et al. (1997) concluded that there was a clear unmet need for the development of ways to evaluate QOL for persons with more severe ID. Atkins (1999), Baroff (1986), Dennis et al. (1993), Edgerton (1996), Fabian (1991), Goode (1994), Halpern (1993a), Lyons (2000a, 2000b, 2003a, 2003b, 2003c, 2003d, 2005), Newton et al. (1996), and Rosen et al. (1995) have expressed similar views.

Both Goode (1997) and Hogg (1992), after having referred to the well-documented disjunction between objective and subjective approaches to measurement and assessment, suggested that a holistic and comprehensive approach was preferable. "Direct and detailed observation of the lives of persons with profound disabilities should be resonant with qualitative assessments of these lives" (Goode, 1997, p. 87). Goode strongly advocated qualitative methods as "uniquely suited to discover the subjective viewpoints of actors under study . . . These methods produce relatively valid reputational data about how subjects view their own quality of life" (p. 78).

Goode (1997), consistent with the earlier work of Fabian (1991), identified two qualitative approaches to investigating QOL for persons with more severe ID. First, through behavioral observation and evaluation of disposition based on reputational data, and second, by describing the lives of persons with more severe ID and producing data that was both reputational and sociological (relational). Goode argued that this second approach produced valid subjective data, as it allowed the researcher to get close to the individual. Parents and carers of persons with more severe ID have expressed considerable disenfranchisement with the evolution of QOL assessment and measurement (see Crutcher, 1990; Turnbull & Brunk (1990)), so Goode's call to get close to these individuals clearly responds to these concerns. More specifically, Goode and Hogg (1994) and Schalock and Keith (1993) argued that expressions of positive affect are central to assessing subjective QOL. Parmenter et al. (1991) and Zhan (1992) similarly expressed enthusiasm for the development of a QOL model wherein satisfaction (and happiness) were key measures for persons with more severe ID. Green, Gardner and Reid (1997) and Ivancic and Barrett (1997) alternatively preferred a behavior-analytic approach and argued that their research results supported the efficacy of this approach to increasing indices of QOL for people with more severe ID.

Although the general literature on persons with ID and QOL per se provided limited and conflicting direction for research into the nature of life satisfaction for persons with ID, the specific literature on severe ID that focuses on individual happiness and satisfaction provides some direction and insight into the world views of these individuals. Edgerton (1996) pointedly described satisfaction with life as "a separate and ultimately more important criterion of individual welfare" (p. 55), and concluded that expressions of satisfaction are "a datum that most commentators agree lies somewhere near the heart of quality of life" (p. 57). Edgerton believed that the judging of a reasonable QOL is a separate issue to its measurement, and that gaining insight into an individual's feelings, concerns, and values is far more important than providing only a limited assessment of QOL using objective indicators. Felce and Perry (1995) similarly described life satisfaction as a personal assessment wherein "the frame of reference is personal and affected by experience and the judgment of what is possible and typical for a person in one's situation" (pp. 56–7). Leininger (1994) and Romney et al. (1994) referred similarly to the importance of "cultural synchronicity" when judging QOL for persons with narrow life experiences and communication difficulties.

Green and Reid's (1996) research into happiness for persons with more severe ID was closely related. Although happiness per se is generally viewed by theorists as more transient and emotional than life satisfaction, a body of researchers and theorists acknowledged a considerable correlation between the two phenomena (e.g., Edgerton, 1990; Halpern, 1993a; Taylor & Bogdan, 1990). Byrne and MacLean (1997) suggested, "Satisfaction may be a more appropriate term than happiness because it suggests cognitive appraisal and evaluation, which has a greater degree of permanence than happiness" (p. 22). Halpern (1993a) preferred the explanation that happiness, life satisfaction, and wellbeing were encapsulated within the notion of personal fulfillment. Despite the fact that people with more severe ID generally demonstrated limited affect (Ivancic & Barrett, 1997), a confluence of anecdotal evidence derived from this review and discussions with colleagues, parents, and carers supported this author's contention that intellectual functioning is not simply related to judgments of or feelings about satisfaction (Diener, 1984; Harner & Heal, 1993).

This literature review identified only one reference (Timmons & Brown, 1997) that focused on QOL for children with less severe ID, though it was essentially a philosophical chapter discussing the scarcity of basic research on this topic. No basic research specifically investigated the subjective QOL of persons with ID.

Overall, the case for blending qualitative and quantitative research methods to promote a holistic QOL assessment for persons with more severe ID is strongly supported by prominent authors (e.g., Cummins, 2005a; Dennis et al., 1993; Dossa, 1989; Edgerton, 1990; Fabian, 1991; Goode, 1997; Schalock, 1994a).

Contemporary Best Practice in QOL Research for Persons with ID

(This final section of the review draws substantially on the more recent work of members of the Quality of Life Special Interest Research Group (QOL SIRG) of the International Association for the Scientific Study of Intellectual Disabilities. The SIRG's mission is to "further work that enhances the QOL of individuals with ID and their families.")

The previous 10 years have seen a fundamental movement from a "quality of care" toward a QOL emphasis in programs and services for persons with ID (De Waele & Van Hove, 2005; De Waele, van Loon, Van Hove, & Schalock, 2005; Schalock, 2005b). This shift has placed an increasing demand on researchers, policy makers, and practitioners to clarify and apply the QOL construct in "real" settings – to enhance personal outcomes for these persons.

Brown and Schalock (2005) have suggested that five international socio-political trends have driven this movement, i.e., an increased concern for the social and psychological aspects of the subjective wellbeing of people with ID; increasing awareness of the need for more supports for these persons to realize their potentials through self-determination; recognition of the true challenges and value of meaningful participation in society; a widening acceptance of a more ecological model of disability and associated policy imperatives; and a shift in prevailing scientific conceptions of disability toward the environmental and rights-outcome models.

The IASSID QOL SIRG put forward six criteria for best practice in QOL research for persons with ID. These are best practice research should: embrace a multidimensional construct; be guided by operational principles; adopt methodological pluralism; incorporate a systems perspective; use the QOL concept as a change agent; and focus on both the individual with ID and their family.

1. Multidimensionality

The construct of QOL (both individual and family-centered) encompasses multiple factors (Schalock & Verdugo, 2002; Turnbull, Brown & Turnbull, 2004). Although the specific factors (domains or dimensions) vary somewhat across investigators, most QOL researchers generally support the stance that: the number of domains is less important than the recognition; any proposed QOL construct must recognize the need to employ a multi-element framework; individuals and families know what is important to them, and any set of domains must cover all aspects of the construct.

The importance of identifying these domains which should have (as far as possible) cross-culturally validity is that it allows the field to move from a general to a specific, multidimensional construct with measurable properties and attributes. (For a representative contemporary taxonomy of core QOL domains and indicators, see particularly Schalock, Verdugo, Bontham, Fantova, & Van Loon, 2008, but also, e.g., Cummins, 1997; Felce & Perry, 1996; Gardner & Carran, 2005; Renwick, Brown, & Raphael, 2000.)

2. Guiding operational principles

The SIRG nominate 12 principles to guide future research (Schalock et al., 2002), which are based upon their social validity in terms of desirability, feasibility, and effectiveness. The premise upon which these principles were developed is "that QOL provides an ongoing framework to promote well-being at the personal, family, service delivery, community, national, and international levels." The principles are ... (In regard to conceptualization) QOL: is multidimensional and influenced by personal and environmental factors and the interaction of these factors; has the same components for all people; has both subjective and objective components; and is enhanced by self-determination, resources, purpose in life, and a sense of belonging. (In regard to measurement) QOL: reflects the degree to which people have life experiences that they value; embraces the domains that contribute to a full and interconnected life; considers the contexts of important physical, social, and cultural environments; and includes measures of experiences both common to all humans and those unique to individuals. (In regard to application) QOL: should be evidence-based and enhance well-being within cultural contexts; should be the basis for interventions and supports; and take a prominent place in professional education and training (Brown & Brown, 2005; Brown & Shearer, 2004).

3. Methodological pluralism

Best practice QOL research is based on a well-delineated model, clearly articulated domains and indicators, and reliable and valid assessment instruments, and should use methodological pluralism with respect to its focus, design, and methodology. It should employ both subjective and objective measures to assess quality indicators. Subjective measures assess perceptual issues and typically use dependent variables such as importance or satisfaction (in regard to the persons with ID). Objective measures assess personal experiences and circumstances and typically use dependent variables such as frequency or quantity.

Researchers should use both between- and within-group designs for the assessment of subjective and objective quality indicators. Between-group designs are prevalent in cross-cultural studies and serve as a basis to understand and verify the etic and emic properties of the QOL domains and indicators. Within-group designs are being used to understand better the predictors (or causal factors) of quality outcomes, and the role that life events and circumstances play in a life of quality. Good QOL research is also characterized by a balance of qualitative and quantitative research methods. The importance of this balance is that it allows for the assessment of both the subjective and objective properties and attributes of a life of quality, and the triangulation/comparison of results across research designs and methods.

4. A systems perspective

Conceptualization, measurement, and application of the construct are best facilitated when a systems perspective – that integrates the micro-, meso-, and macro-systems in which individuals with ID and their families live – is adopted. The importance of this is that it allows researchers to understand better the predictors of and causal factors in a life of quality that extend beyond the individual with ID to his/her family/carers, associated support organizations and service delivery systems, and society.

Considerable current research focuses on the micro-system ostensibly because impact upon the other systems will be greater when research is based on a clear understanding of the personal and family QOL domains and their indicators. However, the QOL concept is now being increasingly applied at the organizational level and service delivery system (Schalock et al., 2008), and cross-cultural studies are indicating the value of the construct at the macro-systemic level. In this regard, the use of valid QOL domains and indicators has permitted significant progress in the cross-cultural validation of the construct's etic and emic properties.

5. QOL as a change agent

Historically, the QOL concept was used primarily as a sensitizing notion that gave a sense of reference to what was valued and desired from the individual's perspective. During the last decade, its role has broadened to include a conceptual framework for assessing quality outcomes, a social construct to guide quality enhancement strategies, and a criterion for assessing the effectiveness of those strategies. It has become an agent for social change that encourages others to think differently about people with ID, and how change might be brought about in policy and practice to enhance quality outcomes related to objective life conditions (Schalock & Felce, 2004) and reduced social inequalities (Emerson et al., 2005).

6. Individual and family foci

Best practice QOL research should take into account both individual and family-centered QOL. (Note that this chapter does focus on individual QOL, but the principles discussed are relevant to both. Comprehensive discussions about family-referenced QOL can be found in Park et al. (2003), Poston et al. (2003) and Turnbull et al. (2004)). This approach necessitates: the definition of quality in terms of individual and family-centered outcomes; the active involvement of individuals with ID and their families in the design, implementation, and evaluation of QOL-related research; and the development of individual or family-centered supports to enhance these outcomes. This is most apparent at the micro-systemic (individual/family) level, but can be applied productively at the meso-systemic and macro-systemic levels as well.

Contemporary Best Practice in QOL Policy and Support Service Development for Persons with ID

An increasing diversity of authorities and organizations have been making major changes to policies about services and supports for persons with ID – particularly by moving toward a QOL rationale and a "systems" perspective (see, e.g., Bronfenbrenner, 1979; Gardner, 1985 Senge, 2006). Similarly, an increasing number of education, residential, rehabilitation, and other service providers have adopted evidence-based best practices focusing more on improving personal outcomes (Schalock et al., 2008). These changes have been variously "top-down" and "bottom-up" initiatives but regardless are resulting in real and positive changes for people with ID (and their families). (Schalock et al. (2008) provide an excellent overview of these best practices.)

Good practice seems to be aligning with good policy and good research. These good practices, as so cogently described and explained by Schalock et al. (2008), include: individual supports as "vehicles" for an enhanced QOL; the community as the context for a life of quality; organizations operating as "bridges" to the community; service delivery practices such as person-centered planning, individualized supports, and consumer (and family) involvement in service delivery planning and evaluation; and evidence-based practices involving assessing personal QOL-related outcomes for quality improvement. (See also, e.g., Fantova, 2005a, 2005b; Schalock, Gardner, & Bradley, 2007; Verdugo et al., 2005; Walsh et al., 2006.) In seeking to adopt this QOL rationale and systems perspective, and to improve personal outcomes through evidence-based best practice, organizations are developing and implementing facilitative and efficacious guidelines and strategies. They include the following:

Schalock et al. (2008) describe facilitative strategies for implementing a QOL approach. The first set of strategies are about changing inhibiting "mental models," i.e., organizations identify, challenge, and change mental models that inhibit change. These include mental models: of disablement – that regard disability is internalized and unchangeable; that emphasize quality of care over QOL; and that regard organizations as fixed systems with inbuilt obstacles to change – incapable of self-reorganization. (See also, Jones et al., 2008; Senge, 2006.) Organizations that: embrace and act upon the principles of QOL (especially relating to conceptualization around core domains, indicators, measurement, and application); adopt a progressive and flexible "learning organization" position; and act upon a rigorous and valid code of ethics (see, e.g., Schalock & Luckasson, 2005) are well positioned to implement a QOL approach.

The second set of strategies is about designing assessments to focus on improving (valued) personal outcomes using the QOL approach. Schalock et al. (2007) and Walsh et al. (2006) identify some criteria that have a wide acceptance in the literature, i.e., outcome measures should: resonate with what individuals want/prefer; are based on a validated QOL model; facilitate organizational quality improvement; are psychometrically sound; meaningfully engage the individual; and are synchronous with policy imperatives. Best practice assessment and measurement is about improved practices, programs and policies, and ultimately of course about an improved QOL for the persons with ID (Schalock et al., 2007).

Valid, formal support needs assessments (see, e.g., the "Supports Intensity Scale" explained by Thompson et al., 2004) are a preferred approach to assessment, as they can be applied at the personal (individual support plan) and organizational (service/resource planning/distribution) levels. Organizations can then select meaningful performance indicators, based on collective individual data, to inform a systemic approach to organizational (self) evaluation and development.

The third set of strategies is about service delivery. Progressive service delivery systems for persons with ID are increasingly adopting personal outcomes improvement and quality improvement as core service goals (Fantova, 2005a, 2005b; ISO, 2003; MTAS, 2005; Nabaskues, 2003). To bring about this change, successful organizations delegate top-down authority to local management units to enable them to self-monitor, implement, evaluate, and report on service improvements. This allows for better planning of and use of human and other resources. Furthermore they delegate to well-trained support staff, particularly about QOL issues and person-centered planning principles, bringing about more informed and responsive QOL-based and individualized planning.

Providing opportunities for management staff to take initiatives that improve organizational culture, encourage participatory management practices, and implement action research initiatives is similarly effective. This can involve offering more choices to support workers and consumers to encourage greater self-responsibility and autonomy. Consequently, this encourages workers to take initiatives with planning and services at the individual consumer level.

Services that actively seek out and engage with their local communities gain the benefits of their communities "social capital." By building links with local support groups, businesses, and similar agencies, organizations can establish "self-perpetuating" collaborations between consumers, workers, and communities members. These initiatives are (of course) about "normalization" and providing opportunities to engage in the "ebb and flow" of daily domestic and community living.

Finally, and arguably most importantly, organizations that develop their service delivery practices around the principle of maximizing consumer participation in decision-making (in both day-to-day activities and particularly in the ISP process) demonstrate the benefits of developing self-advocacy among their consumers. Service delivery, simply put, is about delivering valued quality outcomes for consumers. Ethical ISP processes are person-centered, responsive, data-based, and flexible across the life span.

The fourth set of strategies is about quality improvement (QI). QI involves good leadership, the adoption of learning teams as part of a "learning organization" (see, e.g., Orthner, Cook, Sabah, & Rosenfeld, 2006 & Senge, 2006), evidence-based practices and reflective self-evaluation.

Schalock et al. (2008, 281–282) suggest that these organizational strategies are best implemented in accordance with the following guidelines: that "systems thinking" should provide the lens for seeing and responding to the interrelationship at the individual, organizational, and system levels; that public policy reflects QOL principles and valued personal outcomes; that all stakeholders are actively engaged in the processes of planning, implementation, assessment, and evaluations – in order to nurture a collective commitment to this process of change; and that quality improvement is the "mechanism" for change.

Conclusion

For the QOL construct to be a more effective facilitator of social change and improved personal outcomes for persons with ID (and their families) attention must be focused toward meeting a number of critical needs. These include: the need to develop public policies based on valued QOL principles and practices; the need to base the provision of services and supports on key predictors of a life of quality such as self-determination, empowerment, equity; the need to focus on individual experiences and circumstances; the need to incorporate QOL operational principles and methodological pluralism into professional training and ongoing human resource development; the need to rethink what we measure – particularly by going beyond subjective measures to include objective measures of personal experiences and circumstances; and the need to apply and evaluate the QOL construct in less developed countries.

The ultimate benchmark is – "Does the QOL construct make a difference in the lives of individuals with ID (and their families)?" As we address these needs, we go beyond (just) models, concepts, and ideals toward the development of a comprehensive use of the QOL construct which will embrace the criteria for best practice research and synchronize this research with QOL policy and practice development.

In thinking about synchronizing our future work, we need to pursue: research that describes and explains the QOL construct and how QOL is best assessed to provide a framework for application and evaluation; practices that incorporates quality enhancement strategies, and bring about valued outcomes that reflect personal experiences and circumstances; and policies that reduce social inequalities and improve the overall level of "good" (Emerson 2005).

This synchronicity is both necessary and possible. It requires, however, that we build on what we know and move our thinking forward. This includes moving from: models to theories; descriptive to explanatory and evaluative levels of theory construction; a general to a specific, multidimensional construct with measurable properties and attributes; and processes to outcomes. Research must be more theory-based and have greater "explanatory power." This movement will allow research to better meet the criteria of evaluability, precision, and certainty (Schalock, 2005a, p. 698).

The last two decades have provided a sound foundation for future QOL research, and policy and practice development for persons with intellectual disabilities. We now have a good understanding of the operational procedures that will guide our future endeavors: a clearer understanding of the multidimensionality of QOL and its etic and emic properties; and increasingly valid strategies for its measurement, application, and evaluation.

Eudemonia (the "good life") for persons with intellectual disabilities engaged in a support milieu is at least in part in our hands.

References

Abberley, P. (1986). Modeling the psychological determinants of life quality. In F. M. Andrews (Ed.), *Research on the quality of life*. Ann Arbor, MI: Institute for Social Research, University of Michigan.

Abberley, P. (1987). The concept of oppression and the development of a social theory of disability. *Disability, Handicap and Society*, 2(1), 5–19.

Abbey, A., & Andrews, F. M. (1986). Modeling the psychological determinants of life quality. In F. M. Andrews (Ed.), *Research on the quality of life*. Ann Arbor, MI: Institute for Social Research, University of Michigan.

Abbott-Chapman, J., & Easthope, G. (1998). Participation and inclusion: A discourse of welfare or a discourse of rights? *Australian Journal of Social Issues, 33*(2), 99–118.

Anderson, R. (1988). The quality of life of stroke patients and their carers. In R. Anderson & M. Bury (Eds.), *Living with chronic illness: The experience of patients and their families*. London: Unwin Hyman.

Andrews, F. M. (1980). Comparative studies of life quality: Comments on the current state of the art and some issues for future research. In *The quality of life: Comparative studies* (pp. 273–285). Beverly Hills, CA: Sage Publications.

Andrews, F. M. (1986). Introduction. In F. M. Andrews (Ed.), *Research on the quality of life*. Ann Arbor, MI: Institute for Social Research, University of Michigan.

Andrews, F. M. (1991). Stability and change in levels and structure of subjective well-being. *Journal of Health and Social Behaviour, 32*, 238–253.

Andrews, F. M., & Withy, S. B. (1976). *Social indicators of well-being: Americans' perceptions of life quality*. New York: Plenum Press.

Antaki, C., & Rapley, M. (1996). Questions and answers to psychological assessment schedules: Hidden troubles in 'quality of life' interviews. *Journal of Intellectual Disability Research, 40*(5), 421–437.

Arthur, M. (1998). *Socio-communicative variables and behaviour states in students with the most severe and multiple disabilities: An observational study*. Unpublished PhD dissertation, Macquarie University, Sydney.

Arthur, M. (2001). *Educational implications of socio-communicative variables and behavior states in students with profound and multiple disabilities*. Unpublished manuscript, University of Newcastle.

Arthur, M. (2004). Patterns amongst behaviour states, socio-communicative and activyt variables in education programs for students with profound and multiple disabilities. *Journal of Developmental and Physical Disabilities, 16*, 125–149.

Arthur, M., & Butterfield, N. (1996). Parental perspectives on communication processes involving students with high support needs: A pilot study. *Special Education Perspectives, 5*(2), 59–63.

Arthur, M., Hook, J., & Butterfield, N. (1995). Behaviour state: Exploring issues in best practice for students with the most severe and multiple disabilities. *Australasian Journal of Special Education, 19*(1), 37–44.

Ashman, A. F. (1990). Sterilization and training for normal sexual development: Human rights and obligations. *Australia and New Zealand Journal of Developmental Disabilities, 16*(3), 359–368.

Atkins, C. (1999). *Just little things: Nurses' perceptions of quality of life for people with severe multiple impairments*. Unpublished PhD dissertation, University of Sydney, Sydney.

Atkinson, T. (1977, August). *Is satisfaction a good measure of the perceived quality of life?* Paper presented at the 10th Meeting of the American Statistical Association, Toronto, ON.

Bach, M. (1994). Quality of life: Questioning the vantage points for research. In M. H. Rioux & M. Bach (Eds.), *Disability is not measles: New research paradigms in disability* (pp. 127–152). North York, ON: Roeher Institute.

Baily, C. F. (1986). Withholding or withdrawing treatment on handicapped newborns. *Pediatric Nursing, 12*(6), 413–416.

Bannerman, D. J., Sheldon, J. B., Sherman, J. A., & Harchick, A. E. (1990). Balancing the right to habilitation with the right to personal liberties: The rights of people with developmental disabilities to eat too many donuts and take a nap. *Journal of Applied Behavior Analysis, 23*(1), 79–89.

Barber, P. (1990). *Literature review: Medical decision-making for newborns with disabilities. Quality of life as a criterion*. Lawrence, KS: The University of Kansas/Beach Center on Family and Disability.

Barlow, J., & Kirby, N. (1992). Residential satisfaction of persons with an intellectual disability living in an institution or in the community. *Australian and New Zealand Journal of Developmental Disabilities, 17*(1), 7–24.

Baroff, G. S. (1986, December). Maximal adaptive competency. *Mental Retardation, 24*, 367–368.
Baum, F. (1995). Researching public health: Behind the qualitative-quantitative methodological debate. *Social Science and Medicine, 40*(4), 459–468.
Bergland, A., & Narum, I. (2007). Quality of life: Diversity in context and meaning. *Critical Reviews in Physical and Rehabilitation Medicine, 19*(2), 115–139.
Bertelli, M., & Brown, I. (2006). Quality of life for people with intellectual disabilities. *Current Opinion in Psychiatry, 19*(5), 508–513.
Bickenbach, J. E. (1993). *Physical disability and social policy*. Toronto, ON: University of Toronto Press.
Bigby, C. (2004). *Ageing with a lifelong disability: A guide to practice, program and policy issues for human services professionals*. London: Jessica Kingsley.
Bigby, C., & Ozanne, E. (2001). Shifts in the model of service delivery in intellectual disability in Australia. *Journal of Intellectual and Developmental Disability, 26*(2), 177–190.
Blackwell, M. W. (1979). *Care of the mentally retarded*. Boston: Little Brown.
Blishen, B., & Atkinson, T. (1980). Anglophone and Francophone differences in perceptions of the quality of life in Canada. In A. Szalai & F. M. Andrews (Eds.), *The quality of life: Comparative studies*. Beverly Hills, CA: Sage Publications.
Bogdan, R. C., & Taylor, S. J. (1989). Relationships with severely disabled people: The social construction of humanness. *Social Problems, 36*(2), 135–148.
Borthwick-Duffy, S. A. (1987). *Quality of life of mentally retarded people: Development of a model*. Unpublished PhD dissertation, University of California, Riverside, CA.
Borthwick-Duffy, S. A. (1990). Quality of life of persons with severe or profound mental retardation. In R. L. Schalock & M. J. Begab (Eds.), *Quality of life: International perspectives and issues* (pp. 177–190). Washington, DC: American Association on Mental Retardation.
Borthwick-Duffy, S. A. (1992). Quality of life and quality of care in mental retardation. In L. Rowitz (Ed.), *Mental retardation in the year 2000* (pp. 52–56). New York: Springer.
Borthwick-Duffy, S. A. (1996). Evaluation and measurement of quality of life: Special considerations for persons with mental retardation. In R. L. Schalock (Ed.), *Quality of life: Volume 1: Conceptualization and measurement* (pp. 105–119). Washington, DC: American Association on Mental Retardation.
Bowe, F. (1978). *Handicapping America: Barriers to Disabled People*. New York: Harper and Row.
Bowles, W. (1995). *Quality of life of adults with spina bifida: An issue of equality*. Unpublished PhD dissertation, Macquarie University, Sydney, Australia.
Bowling, A. (1992). *Measuring health*. Milton Keynes: Open University Press.
Brandtstadter, J., & Baltes-Gotz, B. (1990). Personal control over development and quality of life perspectives in adulthood. In P. B. Baltes & M. M. Baltes (Eds.), *Successful aging: Perspectives from the behavioral sciences*. Cambridge: Cambridge University Press.
Branson, J., & Miller, D. (1992). Normalisation, community care and the politics of difference. *Australian Disability Review, 92*(4), 17–28.
Brief, A. P., Butcher, A. H., George, J. M., & Link, K. E. (1993). Integrating bottom-up and top-down theories of subjective well-being: The case of health. *Journal of Personality and Social Psychology, 64*(4), 646–653.
Brislin, R. (2000). *Understanding culture's influence on behaviour* (2nd ed.). Fort Worth, TX: Harcourt College Publishers.
Bronfenbrenner, U. (1979). *The ecology of human development*. Cambridge, MA: Harvard University Press.
Brown, C. (1989). *My left foot*. London: Mandarin.
Brown, F., Davis, R., Richards, M., & Kelly, K. (1989). Residential services for adults with profound disabilities. In F. Brown & D. H. Lehr (Eds.), *Persons with profound disabilities: Issues and practices* (pp. 295–331). Baltimore, MD: Paul H. Brookes.

Brown, I. (1999). Embracing quality of life in times of spending restraint. *Journal of Intellectual and Developmental Disability, 24*(4), 299–308.

Brown, N., McLinden, M., & Porter, J. (1998). Sensory needs. In P. Lacey & C. Ouvry (Eds.), *People with profound and multiple learning disabilities: A collaborative approach to meeting complex needs* (pp. 29–38). London: David Fulton.

Brown, P. M., & Brown, R. I. (1996). *Developmental handicaps and gender differences in quality of life*. Ottawa, ON: Health and Welfare.

Brown, R. I. (1990). Quality of life for people with learning difficulties: The challenge for behavioural and emotional disturbance. *International Review of Psychiatry, 2*, 23–32.

Brown, R. I. (1995). Measuring new dimensions through quality of life: The personal equation. *Evaluation Journal of Australasia, 7*(1), 14–23.

Brown, R. I. (1997a). Quality of life: Challenges and dilemmas. *Journal on Developmental Disabilities, 5*(2), 22–33.

Brown, R. I. (1997b). Quality of life: The development of an idea. In R. I. Brown (Ed.), *Quality of life for people with disabilities: Models, research and practice* (2nd ed, pp. 1–10). Cheltenham: Stanley Thornes.

Brown, R. I. (Ed.). (1997c). *Quality of life for people with disabilities: Models, research and practice*. Cheltenham: Stanley Thornes.

Brown, R. I. (1998a, October). *Conceptualisation of quality of life: An overview*. Paper presented at the 1998 Australian Society for the Study of Intellectual Disability (ASSID) Conference: Conceptualisation of quality of life workshop, Flinders University of South Australia, Adelaide, Australia.

Brown, R. I. (2006). Professional development: Education and practice. In I. Brown, & M. Percy (Eds.), *Intellectual and developmental disabilities*. Baltimore, MD: Paul H. Brookes.

Brown, R. I., & Bayer, M. B. (1992). Rehabilitation Programmes Study. In R. I. Brown (Ed.), *Empowerment and developmental handicaps: Choices and quality of Life* (pp. 7–20). London: Chapman and Hall.

Brown, R. I., Bayer, M. B., & Brown, P. M. (1992). *Empowerment and developmental disabilities*. Toronto, ON: Captus Press.

Brown, R. I., Bayer, M. B., & MacFarlane, C. (1988). Quality of life amongst handicapped adults. In R. I. Brown (Ed.), *Quality of life for handicapped people* (pp. 111–140). London: Croom Helm.

Brown, R. I., Bayer, M. B., & MacFarlane, C. (1989). *Rehabilitation programmes: The performance and quality of life of adults with developmental handicaps (Vol. 1)*. Toronto, ON: Lugus Productions.

Brown, R. I., & Brown, I. (2005). The application of quality of life. *Journal of Intellectual Disability Research, 49(10)*, 718–733.

Brown, R. I., Brown, P. M., & Bayer, M. B. (1994). A quality of life model: New challenges resulting from a six year study. In D. Goode (Ed.), *Quality of life for persons with disabilities: International perspectives and issues*. Cambridge, MA: Brookline Books.

Brown, R. I., & Schalock, R. I. (2005). *The concept of quality of life and its application to persons with intellectual disabilities*. Unpublished manuscript.

Brown, R. I., & Shearer, J. (1999). Challenges for inclusion within a quality of life model for the 21st century. *Australasian Journal of Special Education, 22*(3), 180–194.

Brown, R. I., & Shearer, J. (2004). Challenges for inclusion within a quality of life model for the 21st century. In D. Mitchell (Ed.), *Special educational needs and inclusive education: Major themes in education* (*Vol.* 2, pp139–pp156). London: Routledge Falmer.

Browne, G., & Bramston, P. (1996). Quality of life in the families of young people with intellectual disabilities. *Australian and New Zealand Journal of Mental Health Nursing, 5*, 120–130.

Brudenell, P. (1986). *The other side of profound handicap*. Hampshire: Macmillan.

Butow, H. (1993). Australian disability strategy. *Australian Disability Review, 93*(4), 5–11.

Butterfield, N., Arthur, M., & Linfoot, K. (1992). Meeting communication needs in communication programming for students with severe intellectual disability: The creating communicative contexts manual. *Special Education Perspectives, 1*(1), 35–43.

Byrne, H., & MacLean, D. (1997). Quality of life: Perceptions of residential care. *International Journal of Nursing Practice, 3*, 21–28.

Campbell, A., Converse, P. E., & Rodgers, W. L. (1976). *The quality of American life: Perceptions, evaluations and satisfactions*. New York: Sage Publications.

Campo, S. F., Sharpton, W. R., Thompson, B., & Sexton, D. (1996). Measurement characteristics of the Quality of Life Index when used with adults who have severe mental retardation. *American Journal on Mental Retardation, 100*(5), 546–550.

Campo, S. F., Sharpton, W. R., Thompson, B., & Sexton, D. (1997). Correlates of the quality of life of adults with severe or profound mental disabilities. *Mental Retardation, 35*(5), 329–337.

Carter, M., Chalmers, S. E., Clayton, M., & Hook, J. (1998). Teachers' perceptions of possible best practices, reported implementation and training needs for students with high support needs: Comparisons across qualification status and teacher location. *Australasian Journal of Special Education, 22*(1), 50–70.

Carter, M., & Hook, J. (1998). Communication programming for students with high support needs: A model for deciding what to teach. *Special Education Perspectives, 7*(1), 42–55.

Cheng, S. (1988). Subjective quality of life in the programming and evaluation of programs. *Evaluation and Program Planning, 11*, 123–134.

Chibnall, J. T., & Tait, R. C. (1990). The quality-of-life scale: A preliminary study with chronic pain patients. *Evaluation and Health Professions, 10*, 186–200.

Christiansen, C. (1993). Continuing challenges of functional assessment in rehabilitation: Recommended changes. *American Journal of Occupational Therapy, 47*(3), 258–259.

Cirrin, F. M., & Rowland, C. M. (1985). Communicative assessment of non-verbal youths with severe/profound mental retardation. *Mental Retardation, 23*(2), 52–62.

Clements, D. B., Copeland, L. G., & Loftus, M. (1990). Critical times for families with a chronically ill child. *Pediatric Nursing, 16*(2), 157–161.

Compton, D. A. (1997). (Ed.). *Issues in therapeutic recreation: a profession in transition.* Champaign: Sagamore Press.

Conway, R. N. F. (1992). Disability and legislation: The relationship between changing policy and changing practices. *Australia and New Zealand Journal of Developmental Disabilities, 18*(2), 65–73.

Cook, V. (2003). *Subjective wellbeing: An integration of depression, stress, and Homeostasis Theory*. Unpublished PhD Thesis, Deakin University, Melbourne, Australia.

Costa, P. T., McCrea, R. R., & Zonderman, A. B. (1987). Environmental and dispositional influences on well-being: Longitudinal follow-up of an American national sample. *British Journal of Psychology, 78*, 299–306.

Cowan, E. L. (1991). In pursuit of wellness. *American Psychologist, 46*(4), 404–408.

Crossley, R., & McDonald, A. (1980). *Annie's coming out*. Ringwood, NJ: Penguin.

Crow, L. (1996). Including all of our lives: Renewing the social model of disability. In C. Barnes & G. Mercer (Eds.), *Exploring the divide: Illness and disability* (pp. 55–73). Leeds: The Disability Press.

Crutcher, D. M. (1990). Quality of life verses quality of life judgements: A parent's perspective. In R. L. Schalock & M. J. Begab (Eds.), *Quality of life: Perspectives and issues* (pp. 17–22). Washington, DC: American Association on Mental Retardation.

Cummins, R. (2007). Subjective wellbeing and quality of life: a cross-cultural perspective. In K. Rao, I. J. Prakash, K. Srinivasan, & NIMHANS (Institute) (Eds.), *Mindscapes: Global perspectives on psychology in mental health*, pp. 21–31.

Cummins, R. (2003). Normative life satisfaction: measurement issues and a homeostatic model, *Social indicators research, 64*(2), 225–256.

Cummins, R. A. (1993). On being returned to the community: Imposed ideology verses quality of life. *Australian Disability Review, 93*(2), 64–72.

Cummins, R. A. (1995). On the trail of the golden standard for subjective well-being. *Social Indicators Research, 35*, 179–200.

Cummins, R. A. (1996a). *Bibliography on quality of life and cognate areas of study* (5th ed.). Melbourne: School of Psychology, Deakin University.

Cummins, R. A. (1996b). Assessing quality of life. In R. L. Schalock (Ed.), *Quality of life. Volume I: Conceptualization and measurement*. Washington, DC: American Association on Mental Retardation.

Cummins, R. A. (1997). Assessing quality of life. In R. I. Brown (Ed.), *Quality of life for people with disabilities: Models, research and practice* (2nd ed, pp. 116–150). Cheltenham: Stanley Thornes.

Cummins, R. A. (2000). Objective and subjective quality of life: An interactive model. *Social Indicators Research, 52*, 55–72.

Cummins, R. A. (2005a). Moving from the quality of life concept to a theory. *Journal of Intellectual Disability Research, 49(10)*, 698–706.

Cummins, R. A. (Ed.). (2005d). *Issues in the systemic assessment of quality of life*. Malden, MA: Blackwell Publishing.

Cummins, R. A., Eckersley, R., Lo, S. K., Okerstrom., E., Hunter, B., & Davern, M. (2004). *Australian unity wellbeing index: Cumulative psychometric record*. Melbourne: Australian Centre of Quality of Life, School of Psychology, Deakin University.

Cummins, R. A., & Lau, A. L. D. (2005). Quality of life measurement. In R. Norman & D. Currow (Eds.), *Supportive care of the urology patient*. Oxford: Oxford University Press.

Cummins, R. A., McCabe, M., Romeo, Y., Reid, S., & Waters, L. (1997). An initial evaluation of the Comprehensive quality of life scale: Intellectual disability. *International Journal of Disability, Development and Education, 44*(1), 7–19.

Dagnan, D. (1996). Levels of engagement in hospital and community-based homes for people with learning disabilities: Can individual characteristics account for differences? *International Journal of Rehabilitation Research, 19*, 313–319.

Dagnan, D., Look, R., Ruddick, L., & Jones, J. (1995). Changes in the quality of life of people with learning disabilities who moved from hospital to live in community-based homes. *International Journal of Rehabilitation Research, 18*(2), 115–122.

Dale, A. E. (1995). A research study exploring the patient's view of quality of life using the case study method. *Journal of Advanced Nursing, 22*, 1128–1134.

Daly, J., Mitchell, G. J., & Jonas-Simpson, C. M. (1996). Quality of life and the human becoming theory: Exploring discipline-specific contributions. *Nursing Science Quarterly, 9*(4), 170–174.

Davis, E., & Fine-Davis, M. (1991). Social indicators of living conditions in Ireland with European comparison. *Social Indicators Research, 25*(2–4), 318–353.

Davison, I. (1977). *Values, ends and society*. St. Lucia: University of Queensland Press.

Dempsey, I., & Foreman, P. (1997). Towards a clarification of empowerment as an outcome of disability service provision. *International Journal of Disability, 44*(4), 287–303.

Dennis, R. E., Williams, W., Giangreco, M. F., & Cloninger, C. J. (1993). Quality of life as a context for planning and evaluation of services for people with disabilities. *Exceptional Children, 59*(6), 499–512.

Denzin, N. K., & Lincoln, Y. S. (Eds.). (2000). *Handbook of qualitative research*. Thousand Oaks, CA: Sage Publications.

De Waele, I., & Van Hove, G. (2005). Modern times: An ethnographic study on the quality of life of peole with a high support need in a Flemish residence. *Disability & Society, 20*, 6.

De Waele, I., van Loon, J., Van Hove, G., & Schalock, R. L. (2005). Quality of life versus quality of care: Implications for people and programs. *Journal of Policy and Practice in Intellectual Disabilities, 2*(3/4), 229–239.

Diener, E. (1984). Subjective well-being. *Psychological Bulletin, 95*(3), 542–575.

Diener, E. (1994). Assessing subjective well-being: Progress and opportunities. *Social Indicators Research, 31*, 103–157.

DisAbility Services Division. (2000). *Quality of life assessment for people with a disability*. Melbourne: Victorian Government Department of Human Services.
Dossa, P. A. (1989). Quality of life: Individualism or holism? A critical review of the literature. *International Journal of Rehabilitation Research, 12*(2), 121–136.
Edgerton, R. B. (1990). Quality of life from a longitudinal research perspective. In R. L. Schalock & M. J. Begab (Eds.), *Quality of life: Perspectives and issues* (pp. 149–160). Washington, DC: American Association on Mental Retardation.
Edgerton, R. B. (1996). A longitudinal-ethnographic research perspective on quality of life. In R. L. Schalock (Ed.), *Quality of life: Volume 1: Conceptualization and measurement* (pp. 53–90). Washington, DC: American Association on Mental Retardation.
Einfeld, M. (1998, November/December). Rights, obligations, responsibilities: The human dimension: 1998 Kenneth Jenkins Oration. *ACROD Newsletter* [Australian Council for Rehabilitation of Disabled], 8–17.
Emerson, E. (1985). Evaluating the impact of deinstitutionalisation on the lives of mentally retarded people. *American Journal on Mental Deficiency, 90*, 277–288.
Emerson, E., Hatton, C., Thomson, T., & Parmenter, T. (2004). *The international handbook of applied research in intellectual disability*. Chichester: Wiley.
Emerson, E., Robertson, J., Hatton, C., Knapp, M., Walsh, P. N., & Hallam, A. (2005). Costs and outcomes of community residential supports in England. In R. Stancliffe & C. Lakin (Eds.), *Cost and outcomes of community services for peole with intellectual disabilities*. Baltimore: P. H. Brookes.
Erikson, R., & Uusitalo, H. (1987). The Scandinavian approach to welfare research. *International Journal of Sociology, 15*(3–4), 176–193.
Evans, D. R. (1994). Enhancing quality of life in the population at large. *Social Indicators Research, 33*, 47–88.
Everingham, C. (1998). The imagined community of access and equity. *Australian Journal of Social Issues, 33*(1), 1–16.
Fabian, E. S. (1991). Using quality-of-life indicators in rehabilitation program evaluation. *Rehabilitation Counselling Bulletin, 34*(4), 344–356.
Faden, R., & Laplege, A. (1992). Assessing quality of life: Moral implication for clinical practice. *Medical Care, 30*, 166–175.
Fallon, M., & Harris, M. (1991). Training parents to interact with their young children with handicaps: Professional -directed or parent-oriented approaches. *Infant-Toddler Intervention, 1*, 297–313.
Fantova, F. (2005a). *Manual para la gestion de la intervencion social (manual for social intervention management)*. Madrid: CCS.
Fantova, F. (2005b). *Tercer sector e intervencion social (Third sector and social intervention)*. Madrid: PPC.
Feil, N. (1993). *The validation breakthrough*. Sydney: McLennan & Petty.
Felce, D. (1997). Defining and applying the concept of quality of life. *Journal of Intellectual Disability Research, 41*(2), 126–135.
Felce, D., & Perry, J. (1995). Quality of life: Its definition and measurement. *Research in Developmental Disabilities, 16*(1), 51–74.
Felce, D., & Perry, J. (1996). Assessment of quality of life. In R. L. Schalock (Ed.), *Quality of life: Volume 1: Conceptualization and measurement* (pp. 63–72). Washington, DC: American Association on Mental Retardation.
Felce, D., & Perry, J. (1997). Quality of life: The scope of the term and its breadth of measurement. In R. I. Brown (Ed.), *Quality of life for people with disabilities: Models, research and practice* (2nd ed, pp. 56–71). Cheltenham: Stanley Thornes.
Ferguson, D. L. (1994). Is communication really the point? Some thoughts on intervention and membership. *Mental Retardation, 32*(1), 7–18.
Ferguson, R. V. (1996). Environmental design and quality of life. In R. I. Brown (Ed.), *Quality of life for people with disabilities: Models, research and practice*. Cheltenham: Stanley Thornes.

Ferrans, C., & Powers, M. (1985). Quality of Life Index: Development and psychometric properties. *Advances in Nursing Science, 8*, 15–24.

Finkelstein, V. (1993a). Disability: A social challenge or an administrative responsibility? In J. Swain, V. Finkelstein, S. French & M. Oliver (Eds.), *Disabling barriers – enabling environments* (pp. 34–43). London: Sage.

Finkelstein, V. (1993b). The commonality of disability. In J. Swain, V. Finkelstein, S. French & M. Oliver (Eds.), *Disabling barriers – enabling environments* (pp. 13–16). London: Sage.

French, S. (1993a). Disability, impairment or something in between? In J. Swain, V. Finkelstein, S. French & M. Oliver (Eds.), *Disabling barriers – enabling environments* (pp. 17–25). London: Sage.

French, S. (1993b). What's so great about independence? In J. Swain, V. Finkelstein, S. French & M. Oliver (Eds.), *Disabling barriers – enabling environments* (pp. 44–48). London: Sage.

Fuhrer, M. J. (1994). Subjective well-being: Implications for medical rehabilitation outcomes and models of disablement. *American Journal of Physical Medicine and Rehabilitation, 73*(5), 358–364.

Fulcher, G. (1989). Disability: A social construction. In G. Lupton & J. Najman (Eds.), *Sociology of health and illness: Australian readings*. Melbourne: Macmillan.

Fullagher, S., & Hardaker, K. (1993). Debating disability: A critical review of current issues in service provision for people with intellectual disability. *Australian Disability Review, 93*(4), 36–46.

Gardner, H. (1985). *The mind's new science*. New York: Basic Books.

Gardner, J. E., & Carran, D. (2005). Attainment of personal outcomes by people with developmental disabilities. *Mental Retardation, 43*, 157–174.

Gioiella, E. C. (1994). Guest editorial – Quality of life: An international commitment. *Nursing Science Quarterly, 7*(1), 1.

Gleason, J. J. (1993). The creation of meaning: What persons with severe or profound multiple disabilities do in context. *Australia and New Zealand Journal of Developmental Disabilities, 18*(3), 157–167.

Gleeson, B. (1995). Disability: A state of mind? *Australian Journal of Social Issues, 30*(1), 10–23.

Golden, J., & Reese, M. (1996). Focus on communication: Improving interaction between staff and residents who have severe or profound mental retardation. *Research in Developmental Disabilities, 17*(5), 363–382.

Goode, D. A. (1984). Socially produced identities, intimacy and the problem of competence among the retarded. In L. Barton & S. Tomlinson (Eds.), *Special education and social interests* (pp. 228–248). London: Croom Helm.

Goode, D. A. (1988). *Quality of life for persons with disabilities: A review and synthesis of the literature*. New York: Mental Retardation Institute.

Goode, D. A. (1990a). On understanding without words: Communication between a deaf-blind child and her parents. *Human Studies, 13*, 1–37.

Goode, D. A. (1990b). Thinking about and discussing quality of life. In R. L. Schalock & M. J. Begab (Eds.), *Quality of life: Perspectives and issues* (pp. 41–57). Washington, DC: American Association on Mental Retardation.

Goode, D. A. (1992, May). *Quality of life policy: Some issues and implications of a generic social policy concept for people with developmental disabilities*. Paper presented at the Annual Meeting of the American Association on Mental Retardation, New Orleans, LA.

Goode, D. A. (1994). *A world without words: The social construction of children born deaf and blind*. Philadelphia, PA: Temple University Press.

Goode, D. A. (1995). *Self-determination and choice by people with severe intellectual disability*. New York: College of Staten Island.

Goode, D. A. (1997). Assessing the quality of life of adults with profound disabilities. In R. I. Brown (Ed.), *Quality of life for people with disabilities: Models, research and practice* (2nd ed., pp. 72–90). Cheltenam: Stanley Thornes.

Goode, D. A., & Hogg, J. (1994). Towards an understanding of holistic quality of life in people with profound intellectual and multiple disabilities. In D. Goode (Ed.), *Quality of life for persons with disabilities: International perspectives and issues* (pp. 197–207). Cambridge, MA: Brookline Books.

Goodinson, S. M., & Singleton, J. (1989). Quality of life: A critical review of current concepts, measures and their clinical implications. *International Journal of Nursing Studies, 26*, 327–341.

Gordon, A. K. (1984). Reaction to Gibson. *Mental Retardation, 22*(4), 164–166.

Green, C. W., Gardner, S. M., & Reid, D. H. (1997). Increasing indices of happiness among people with profound multiple disabilities: A program replication and component analysis. *Journal of Applied Behavior Analysis, 30*(2), 217–228.

Green, C. W., & Reid, D. H. (1996). Defining, validating, and increasing indices of happiness among people with profound multiple disabilities. *Journal of Applied Behavior Analysis, 29*(1), 67–78.

Griffin, T. (1998, May). *Quality in action or quality inaction: Reflections on quality. Keynote address*. Paper presented at the Australian Society for the Study of Intellectual Disability (ASSID; NSW): 4th Annual State Conference, University of Sydney, Sydney, Australia.

Guba, E. G., & Lincoln, Y. S. (1994). Competing paradigms in qualitative research. In N. K. Denzin & Y. S. Lincoln (Eds.), *Handbook of qualitative research*. Thousand Oaks, CA: Sage Publications.

Guess, D., Benson, H. A., & Siegal-Causey, E. (1985). Concepts and issues related to choice-making and autonomy among persons with severe disabilities. *The Journal of the Association for People with Severe Handicaps, 10*, 79–86.

Guess, D., Roberts, S., & Behrens, G. A. (1998). Response to Mudford, Hogg, and Roberts on continuous recording of behavior state. *American Journal on Mental Retardation, 103*(1), 75–79.

Guess, D., Roberts, S., Seigal-Causey, E., & Rues, J. (1995). Replication and extended analysis of behaviour state, environmental events, and related variables among individuals with profound disabilities. *American Journal on Mental Retardation, 100*(1), 36–51.

Gustiatas, R., & Young, E. W. D. (1986). *A time to be born, a time to die: Conflicts and ethics in an intensive care nursery*. Reading, MA: Addison-Wesley.

Halpern, A. S. (1993a). Quality of life as a conceptual framework for evaluating transition outcomes. *Exceptional Children, 59*(6), 486–498.

Halpern, A. S. (1993b, July). *Evaluation of the transition process from a qualitative process*. Paper presented at the Second International Transition Conference, Sydney, Australia.

Halpern, A. S., Nave, G., Close, D. W., & Nelson, D. (1986). An empirical analysis of the dimensions of community adjustments for adults with mental retardation in semi-independent living situations. *Australian and New Zealand Journal of Developmental Disabilities, 12*(3), 147–157.

Hankiss, E. (1980). Structural variables in cross-cultural research on the quality of life. In A. Szalai & F. M. Andrews (Eds.), *The quality of life: Comparative studies*. Thousand Oaks, CA: Sage Publications.

Haring, T. G. (1996). The role of research in the continuing development of the field of severe disabilities. *Journal of the Association for Persons with Severe Handicaps, 21*(1), 6–8.

Harner, C. J., & Heal, L. W. (1993). The multifaceted lifestyle satisfaction scale (MLSS): Psychometric properties of an interview schedule for assessing personal satisfaction of adults with limited intelligence. *Research in Developmental Disabilities, 14*, 221–236.

Hatton, C. (1998). Whose quality of life is it anyway? Some emerging problems with the quality of life consensus. *Mental Retardation, 36*(2), 104–115.

Headey, B. (1988). The life satisfactions and priorities of Australians. In J. Kelly & C. Gean (Eds.), *Australian attitudes: Social and political analyses from the national social science survey* (pp. 163–175). Sydney: Allen and Unwin.

Headey, B. (1993). An economic model of subjective well-being: Integrating subjective and sociological theories. *Social Indicators Research, 28*, 97–116.

Headey, B., & Wearing, A. (1992). *Understanding happiness: A theory of subjective well-being*. Melbourne: Longman Cheshire.

Heal, L. W., Borthwick-Duffy, S. A., & Saunders, R. R. (1994). Assessment of quality of life. In D. A. Goode (Ed.), *Quality of life for persons with disabilities: International perspectives and issues* (pp. 199–209). Cambridge, MA: Brookline Books.

Heal, L. W., & Chadsey-Rusch, J. (1985). The lifestyle satisfaction scale (LSS): Assessing individuals satisfaction with residence, community setting and associated services. *Applied Research in Mental Retardation, 6*, 475–490.

Heal, L. W., & Sigelman, C. K. (1990). Methodological issues in measuring the quality of life of individuals with mental retardation. In R. L. Schalock & M. J. Begab (Eds.), *Quality of life: Perspectives and issues* (pp. 161–176). Washington, DC: American Association on Mental Retardation.

Heal, L. W., & Sigelman, C. K. I. (1992). *Interviewing respondents who have limited mental ability.* Paper presented at the International Symposium on the Assessment of Exceptional Children, Changhua, Taiwan.

Heal, L. W., & Sigelman, C. K. (1996). Methodological issues in quality of life measurement. In R. L. Schalock (Ed.), *Quality of life: Volume 1: Conceptualization and measurement* (pp. 91–104). Washington, DC: American Association on Mental Retardation.

Health Commission of New South Wales. (1981). *Circular 81/8.* Sydney: Health Commission of New South Wales.

Hedley, R. A., Dubin, R., & Traveggia, T. C. (1980). The quality of working life, gender and occupational status: A cross-national comparison. In A. Szalai & F. M. Andrews (Eds.), *The quality of life: Comparative studies.* Beverly Hills, CA: Sage Publications.

Hogg, J. (1992). *Behavioural state and affective communication in people with profound intellectual and multiple disabilities as indicators of their response to service provision: Grant Application to the Scottish Home Office and Health Department.* Dundee: White Tops Research Unit, Dundee University.

Hogg, J. A., & Lambe, L. (1991). People with profound and multiple disabilities: Retrospect and prospects. In S. Segal & V. Varma (Eds.), *Prospects for people with learning difficulties* (pp. 61–71). London: David Fulton.

Hogg, J., & Sebba, J. (1987). *Profound retardation and multiple impairment: Volume 1: Development and learning.* Rockville, MD: Aspen Publishers.

Holm, P., Holst, J., & Perit, B. (1994). Co-write your own life: Quality of life as discussed in a Danish context. In D. A. Goode (Ed.), *Quality of life for persons with disabilities: International perspectives and issues.* Cambridge, MA: Brookline Books.

Horn, R. V. (1993). *Statistical indicators for the economic and social sciences.* Port Melbourne: Cambridge University Press.

Hughes, C., & Hwang, B. (1996). Attempts to conceptualize and measure quality of life. In R. L. Schalock (Ed.), *Quality of life: Volume 1: Conceptualization and measurement* (pp. 51–61). Washington, DC: American Association of Mental Retardation.

Hughes, C., Hwang, B., Kim, J. -H., Eisenman, L. T., & Killian, D. J. (1995). Quality of life in applied research: A review and analysis of empirical measures. *American Journal on Mental Retardation, 99*(6), 623–641.

Hutchinson, S. A. (1984). Creating meaning: A grounded theory of NICU nurses. *Nursing Outlook, 32*, 86–90.

Ingelhart, R., & Rabier, J. R. (1986). Aspirations adapt to situations – But why are the Bavarians so much happier than the French? In F. M. Andrews (Ed.), *Research on the quality of life.* Ann Arbor, MI: University of Michigan.

International Organisation for Stanndardization (ISO). (2003). *ISO 9000 quality management: ISO Standards compendium.* New York: American Standards Institute.

International Wellbeing Group. (2005). *Normative data – International.* Melbourne: Deakin University.

Ivancic, M., & Barrett, G. T. (1997). A replication to increase happiness indices among some people with profound multiple disabilities. *Research in Developmental Disabilities, 18*(1), 77–92.

Johnson, K. (1998). *Deinstitutionalising women. An ethnographic study of institutional closure*. Cambridge: Cambridge University Press.

Johnstone, M. J. (1988). Quality versus quality of life: Who should decide? *Australian Journal of Advanced Nursing, 6*(1), 30–37.

Jones, J., Ouellette-Kuntz, H., Vilela, T., & Brown, H. (2008). Attitudes of community developmental services agency staff towards issues of inclusion for individuals with intellectual disabilities. *Journal of Policy and Practice in Intellectual Disabilties, 5(4)*, 219–226.

Kahneman, D., Diener, E., & Schwartz, N. (Eds.) (1999). *Well-being: The foundations of hedonic psychology*. New York: Russell Sage Foundation.

Karlsson, G. (1992). The health economist's point of view concerning quality of life. *Nordic Journal of Psychiatry, 46*, 95–99.

Karon, S. L., & Bernard, S. (2002). *Development of operational definitions of quality indicators for Medicaid Services for people with disabilities*. Washington, DC: Centres for Medicare and Medical Services.

Kearney, P. M. (1996). *Between joy and sorrow: Being the parent of a child with a developmental disability*. Unpublished Master's thesis, University of Western Sydney, Penrith South, Australia.

Kebbon, L. (1997). Nordic contributions to disability policies. *Journal of Intellectual Disability Research, 41*(2), 120–125.

Keenan, B. (1992). *An evil cradling*. London: Vintage Press.

Keith, K. D. (1996a). Measuring quality of life across cultures: Issues and challenges. In R. L. Schalock (Ed.), *Quality of life: Volume 1: Conceptualization and measurement* (pp. 73–82). Washington, DC: American Association on Mental Retardation.

Keith, K. D. (1996b). Cross-cultural measurement of critical quality of life concepts. *Journal of Intellectual and Developmental Disability, 21*(4), 273–293.

Kiuranov, C. (1980). An integral indicator of the quality of work and the quality of life. In A. Szali, & F. M. Andrews (Eds.), *The quality of life: Comparative studies*. Beverly Hills, CA: Sage Publications.

Knoll, J. A. (1990). *Defining quality in residential services*. Baltimore, MD: Paul A. Brookes.

Kolstad, A. (1994). *Quality of life: The concept and how to measure it*. Paper presented at the Social Research and the Quality of Life, Inaugural Conference of the Australian Association for Social Research, University of Tasmania, Launceston, Australia.

Kozleski, E. B., & Sands, D. J. (1992). The yardstick of social validity: Evaluating quality of life as perceived by adults without disabilities. *Education and Training in Mental Retardation, 27*(2), 119–131.

Kuehn, M. L., & McClainm, J. W. (1994). Quality of life in the United States: A multicultural context. In D. A. Goode (Ed.), *Quality of life for persons with disabilities. International perspectives and issues*. Cambridge, MA: Brookline Books.

Kuhse, H., & Singer, P. (1985). *Should the baby live? The problem of handicapped infants*. Oxford: Oxford University Press.

Lakin, K. C. (1992, Fall). Improving the quality of community living to empower people with mental retardation. *OSERS News*, 30–35.

Lance, C. E., Lautenschlager, G. J., Sloan, C. E., & Varca, P. E. (1989). A comparison between bottom-up, top-down, and bi-directional models of relationships between global and life facet satisfaction. *Journal of Personality, 57*(3), 601–623.

Land, K. C. (1983). Social indicators. *Annual Review Sociology, 9*, 1–26.

Landesman, S. (1986). Quality of life and personal satisfaction: Definition and measurement issues. *Mental Retardation, 24*(3), 141–143.

Landesman, S., & Butterfield, E. C. (1987). Normalization and deinstitutionalisation of mentally retarded individuals: Controversy and facts. *American Psychologist, 42*, 809–816.

Lazarus, R. S. (1993). Coping theory and research: Past, present and future. *Psychosomatic Medicine, 55*, 234–247.

Legal, S., & Constitutional References Committee (1996). *National well-being: A system of national citizenship indicators and benchmarks*. Canberra: Senate Legal & Constitutional References Committee, Parliament of the Commonwealth of Australia.

Leininger, M. (1994). Quality of life from a trans-cultural perspective. *Nursing Science Quarterly*, *7*(1), 22.

Loew, F., & Rapin, C. H. (1994). The paradoxes of quality of life and its phenomenological approach. *Journal of Palliative Care*, *10*(1), 37–41.

Low, C. (2001). *Have disability rights gone too far? City Insights Lecture, 3rd April 2001*. Retrieved 15 June, 2001, from http://www.city.ac.uk/whatson/low.htm.

Luckasson, R., Coulter, D. L., Polloway, E. A., Reiss, S., Schalock, R. L., Snell, M. E., et al. (1992). *Mental retardation: Definition, classification and systems of support*. Washington, DC: American Association of Mental Retardation.

Lyons, G. S. (1999a, October). *Quality of life and substitute decision-making: Rhetoric or reality?* Paper presented at the 7th National Guardianship and Administration Conference, Sydney, Australia.

Lyons, G. S. (1999b, September). *Quality of life for students with profound intellectual and multiple disabilities*. Paper presented at the 1999 Australian Association of Special Educators National Conference, Sydney, Australia.

Lyons, G. S. (1999c, September). *Assessing/measuring quality of life for individuals with the most severe intellectual disabilities: Unearthing eudaemonia*. Paper presented at the 35th Annual Australian Society for the Study of Intellectual Disability (ASSID) National Conference, Sydney, Australia.

Lyons, G. S. (2000a, December). *Individuals with the most severe intellectual disabilities, quality of life and decision-making: Unearthing eudaemonia*. Paper presented at the 2000 Annual Conference of Psychologists in Developmental Disability Services, University of Western Sydney, Australia.

Lyons, G. S. (2000b). *Embracing eudaemonia: Quality of life for individuals with intellectual disabilities*. Unpublished MEd thesis, University of Newcastle, Australia.

Lyons, G. S. (2003a, 20–22). *Life satisfaction for children with profound and multiple disabilities*. Paper presented at the Australian Group on Severe Communication Impairment 2003 National Conference, Sydney, Australia.

Lyons, G. S. (2003b, July 10–11). *Life satisfaction for children with profound and multiple disabilities: What is it? A research report*. Paper presented at the Australian Society for the Study of Intellectual Disability (ASSID; NSW) Annual Conference, Charles Sturt University, Albury, NSW, Australia.

Lyons, G. S. (2003c, July 10–11). *The Life Satisfaction Matrix: A (preliminary) instrument/procedure for assessing and improving the life satisfaction of individuals with profound and multiple disabilities*. Paper presented at the Australian Society for the Study of Intellectual Disability (ASSID; NSW) Annual Conference, Charles Sturt University, Albury, NSW, Australia.

Lyons, G. S. (2003d, September 17–20). *Life satisfaction for children with profound and multiple disabilities*. Paper presented at the 4th European Conference: SIRM 3rd National Conference 'Mental Health and Mental Retardation: A Lifespan Multidisciplinary Approach', Rome.

Lyons, G. S. (2005). The life satisfaction matrix: An instrument and procedure for assessing the subjective quality of life of individuals with profound multiple disabilities. *Journal of Intellectual Disability Research*, *49(10)*, 766–769.

Mackay, H. (1994, July). *Values, relationships and community: Where do our values spring from?* Paper presented at the Office on Social Policy, Social Policy Directorate: Seminar, Sydney.

Madden, R., Black, K., & Wingyan, W. (1995). *The Definition and categorisation of disability in Australia*. Canberra: Australian Government Publishing Service.

Marinoble, R., & Hegenauer, J. (1988). *Quality of life for individuals with disabilities: A conceptual framework*. Eric Document 302–015.

Markus, H., & Kitayama, S. (1991). Culture and the self: Implications for cognition, emotion, and motivation. *Psychological Review*, *98*, 224–253.

Matikka, L. M., & Vesala, H. T. (1997). Acquiescence in quality-of-life interviews with adults who have mental retardation. *American Journal on Mental Retardation, 35*, 75–82.

Mayers, C. A. (1995). Defining and assessing quality of life. *British Journal of Occupational Therapy, 58*(4), 146–150.

McClaren, P. (1995). Critical pedagogy in the age of global capitalism: Some challenges for the educational left. *Australian Journal of Education, 39*(1), 5–21.

McKennell, A., Atkinson, T., & Andrews, F. M. (1980). Structural constancy's in surveys of perceived well-being. In A. Szalai & F. M. Andrews (Eds.), *The quality of life: Comparative studies*. Beverly Hills, CA: Sage.

McVilly, K. R. (2004). *'I get by with a little help from my friends': Adults with intellectual disability discuss friendship*. Unpublished PhD Thesis. Sydney, Australia: The University of Sydney.

McVilly, K. R., & Rawlinson, R. B. (1998). Quality of life issues in the development and evaluation of services for people with intellectual disability. *Journal of Intellectual and Developmental Disability, 23*(3), 199–218.

Meeberg, G. A. (1993). Quality of life: A conceptual analysis. *Journal of Advanced Nursing, 18*, 32–38.

Mercier, C. (1994). Improving the quality of life of people with chronic mental disorders. *Social Indicators Research, 33*, 165–192.

Michalos, A. C. (1985). Multiple discrepancies theory (MDT). *Social Indicators Research, 16*, 347–443.

Michalos, A. C. (1986). Job satisfaction, marital satisfaction and the quality of life: A review and a preview. In F. M. Andrews (Ed.), *Research on the quality of life*. Ann Arbor, MI: Institute for Social Research, University of Michigan.

Miller, L., & Davey, R. (1993, November). *"There are fairies at the bottom of the garden..." A description and evaluation of Barkuma's Linkwater Service*. Paper presented at the 29th Australian Society for the Study of Intellectual Disability (ASSID) National Conference, Newcastle University, Australia.

Mitchell, D., & Winslade, J. (1997). Developmental systems and narrative approaches to working with families of persons with disabilities. In R. I. Brown (Ed.), *Quality of life for people with disabilities: Models, research and practice* (2nd ed, pp. 151–182). Cheltenham: Stanley Thornes.

MTAS (Ministerio de Trabajo Asuntos Sociales). (2005). *Preliminary plan of the law of promotion of personal autonomy and attention to people in dependency situations*. Madrid: Author.

Nabaskues, I. (2003). *Globalization and new politics*. Victoria-Gasteiz: IVAP.

Nankervis, K. (1997). *Keynote Address*. Paper presented at the Annual Conference, Australian Society for the Study of Intellectual Disability [ASSID], Hobart, Australia.

Neufeldt, A. H., & McGinley, P. (1996). Human spirituality in relation to quality of life. In R. I. Brown (Ed.), *Quality of life for people with disabilities: Models, research and practice* (2nd ed., pp. 292–309). Cheltenham: Stanley Thornes.

New South Wales Department of Education. (1988). *Curriculum statement for the education of students with severe intellectual disability*. Sydney: Author.

Newton, J. S., Ard, W. R., Horner, R. H., & Toews, J. D. (1996). Focusing on values and lifestyle outcomes in an effort to improve the quality of residential services in Oregon. *American Journal on Mental Retardation, 34*, 1–12.

O'Brien, J., & Mount, B. (1998, June). Telling new stories: The search for capacity among people with severe handicaps. *Newsletter of the Citizen Advocacy NSW Association*, 3–6.

O'Brien, J., & O'Brien, C. L. (1992). Members of each other: Perspectives on social support for people with severe disabilities. In J. Nisbet (Ed.), *Natural supports in school, at work, and in the community for people with severe disabilities* (pp. 17–63). Baltimore, MD: Paul H. Brookes.

Oliver, J., Huxley, P., Bridges, K., & Mohamad, H. (1996). *Quality of life and mental health services*. London: Routledge.

Oliver, M. (1990). *The politics of disablement*. London: Macmillan.

Oliver, M. (1993). Redefining disability: A challenge to research. In J. Swain, V. Finkelstein, S. French & M. Oliver (Eds.), *Disabling barriers – enabling environments* (pp. 61–67). London: Sage.

Oliver, M. (1996). *Understanding disability: From theory to practice*. London: Macmillan Press.

Oliver, M., & Barnes, C. (1993). Discrimination, disability and welfare: From needs to rights. In J. Swain, V. Finkelstein, S. French & M. Oliver (Eds.), *Disabling barriers – enabling environments* (pp. 267–277). London: Sage.

Olson, G. I., & Schober, B. I. (1993). The satisfied poor: Development of an intervention-oriented theoretical framework to explain satisfaction with a life in poverty. *Social Indicators Research, 28*, 173–193.

Orthner, D. K., Cook, P., Sabah, Y., & Rosenfeld, J. (2006). Organization learning: A cross-sectional pilot test of effectiveness in children's services. *Evaluation and Programming, 29*, 71–78.

Ouellette-Kuntz, H., & McCreary, B. (1996). Applying quality of life to assessment and intervention. In R. Renwick, I. Brown & M. Nagler (Eds.), *Quality of life in health promotion and rehabilitation: Conceptual approaches, issues, and applications* (pp. 268–278). Thousand Oaks, CA: Sage.

Pare, D. (1995). Of families and other cultures: the shifting paradigm of family therapy. *Family Process, 34*, 1–19.

Park, J., Hoffman, L., Marquis, J., Turnbull, A. P., Poston, D., Mannan, H., et al. (2003). Towards assessing family outcomes of service delivery: Validation of a family quality of life survey. *Journal of Intellectual Disability Research, 47*, 367–384.

Parmenter, T. R. (1989). An International Perspective: The Australian Experience. In R. I. Brown, M. B. Bayer & C. MacFarlane (Eds.), *Rehabilitation Programmes: Performance and the quality of life of adults with developmental handicaps* (pp. 209–225). Toronto, ON: Lugus Productions.

Parmenter, T. R. (1990). Evaluation and service delivery research in the area of severe intellectual disability in Australia. *Australian & New Zealand Journal of Developmental Disability, 16*(3), 187–193.

Parmenter, T. R. (1992). Quality of life of persons with developmental disabilities. *International Review of Research in Mental Retardation, 18*, 246–287.

Parmenter, T. R. (1994). Quality of life as a concept and measurable entity. *Social Indicators Research, 33*, 9–46.

Parmenter, T. R. (1995). The utility of quality of life as a construct for social and health policy development. In R. Renwick, I. Brown & M. Nagler (Eds.), *Quality of life in health promotion and rehabilitation: Conceptual approaches, issues and applications*. Thousand Oaks, CA: Sage.

Parmenter, T. R. (1999). Implications of social policy for service delivery: The promise and the reality, "Are we getting real?". *Journal of Intellectual and Developmental Disabilities, 24*(4), 321–331.

Parmenter, T. R. (2001, September). *Disability into the 21st century: Where are we heading?* Paper presented at the 3rd International Respite Care Conference, Sydney, Australia.

Parmenter, T. R., Briggs, L., & Sullivan, R. (1991). Quality of life: Intellectual disabilities and community living. *Evaluation Journal of Australia, 3*(1), 12–25.

Parmenter, T. R., Cummins, R., Shaddock, A. J., & Stancliffe, R. (1994). In D. A. Goode (Ed.), *Quality of life for persons with disabilities: International perspectives and issues* (pp. 75–102). Cambridge, MA: Brookline Books.

Parmenter, T. R., & Donelly, M. (1997). An analysis of the dimensions of quality of life. In R. I. Brown (Ed.), *Quality of life for people with disabilities: Models, research and practice* (2nd ed, pp. 91–115). Cheltenham: Stanley Thornes.

Parse, R. R. (1994). Quality of life: Sciencing and living the art of human becoming. *Nursing Science Quarterly, 7*(1), 16–21.

Parse, R. R. (1996). Quality of life for persons living with Alzheimer's Disease: The human becoming perspective. *Nursing Science Quarterly, 9*(3), 126–133.

Pavot, W., & Diener, E. (1993). The affective and cognitive context of self-reported measures of subjective well-being. *Social Indicators Research, 28*, 1–20.

Peplau, H. E. (1994). Quality of life: An interpersonal perspective. *Nursing Science Quarterly, 7*(1), 10–15.

Perrin, B., & Nirje, B. (1985). Setting the record straight: A critique of some frequent misconceptions of the normalization principle. *Australia and New Zealand Journal of Developmental Disabilities, 11*(2), 69–74.

Peter, D. (1997). A focus on the individual, theory and reality: Making the connection through the lives of individuals. In R. I. Brown (Ed.), *Quality of life for people with disabilities: Models, research and practice* (2nd ed, pp. 27–55). Cheltenham: Stanley Thornes.

Poston, D., Turnbull, A. P., Park, J., Mannan, H., Marquis, J., & Wang, M. (2003). Family quality of life: A qualitative inquiry. *Mental Retardation, 41*, 313–328.

Raphael, D., Brown, I., Renwick, R., & Rootman, I. (1996). Assessing the quality of life of persons with developmental disabilities: Description of a new model, measuring instruments, and initial findings. *International Journal of Disability, Development, and Education, 43*(1), 25–42.

Rapley, M. (2003). *Quality of life research: A critical introduction*. London: Sage Publications.

Reinders, J. S. (2002). The good life for citizens with intellectual disability. *Journal of Intellectual Disabilities Research, 46*(1), 1–5.

Renwick, R. (1998). Quality of life: A guiding framework for practice with adults who have developmental disabilities. In S. Bachner & M. Ross (Eds.), *Adults with developmental disabilities: Current approaches in occupational therapy*. Bethesda, MD: American Occupational Therapy Association.

Renwick, R., Brown, I., & Nagler, M. (Eds.). (1996). *Quality of life in health promotion and rehabilitation*. Thousand Oaks, CA: Sage Publications.

Renwick, R., Brown, I., & Raphael, D. (2000). Person-centered quality of life. Contribution from Canada to an international understanding. In K. D. Keith & R. L. Schalock (Eds.), *Cross-cultural perspectives on quality of life* (pp. 5–22). Washington, DC: AAMR.

Richmond, D. (1983). *Inquiry into health services for the psychiatrically ill and developmentally disabled*. Sydney: New South Wales State Health Department.

Roarty, J. (1981). *Captives of care*. Sydney: Hodder and Stoughton.

Romney, D. M., Brown, R. I., & Fry, P. S. (1994). *Improving the quality of life: Recommendations for people with and without disabilities*. Dordrecht: Kluwer Academic.

Rosen, M., Simon, E. W., & McKinsey, L. (1995). Subjective measures of quality of life. *American Journal on Mental Retardation, 33*, 31–34.

Roth, S. P., & Morse, J. S. (1996). *A life-span approach to nursing care for individuals with developmental disabilities*. Sydney: Paul A. Brookes.

Russell, J. A. (2003). Core affect and the psychological construction of emotion. *Psychological Review, 110*, 145–172.

Sacks, O. (1995). *An anthropologist on Mars*. Sydney: Pan Macmillan Australia.

Schalock, R. L. (1990a). Attempts to conceptualize and measure quality of life. In R. L. Schalock & M. J. Begab (Eds.), *Quality of life: Perspectives and issues* (pp. 141–148). Washington, DC: American Association on Mental Retardation.

Schalock, R. L. (1990b). Where do we go from here? In R. L. Schalock & M. J. Begab (Eds.), *Quality of life perspectives and issues* (pp. 235–240). Washington, DC: American Association on Mental Retardation.

Schalock, R. L. (1990c). Preface. In R. L. Schalock (Ed.), *Quality of life: Perspectives and issues*. Washington, DC: American Association on Mental Retardation.

Schalock, R. L. (1993). Viewing quality of life in the larger context. *Australia and New Zealand Journal of Developmental Disabilities, 18*(4), 201–208.

Schalock, R. L. (1994a). The concept of quality of life and its current application in the field of mental retardation/developmental disabilities. In D. Goode (Ed.), *Quality of life for persons with disabilities: International perspectives and issues*. Cambridge, MA: Brookline Books.

Schalock, R. L. (1994b). Quality of life, quality enhancement and quality assurance: Implications for program planning and evaluation in the field of mental retardation and developmental disabilities. *Evaluation and Program Planning, 17*(2), 121–131.

Schalock, R. L. (1996a). Preface. In R. L. Schalock (Ed.), *Quality of life: Volume 1: Conceptualization and measurement* (pp. vii–xi). Washington, DC: American Association on Mental Retardation.

Schalock, R. L. (1996b). Reconsidering the conceptualization and measurement of quality of life. In R. L. Schalock (Ed.), *Quality of life: Volume 1: Conceptualization and measurement* (pp. 123–139). Washington, DC: American Association on Mental Retardation.

Schalock, R. L. (1997). The concept of quality of life in 21st century disability programmes. In R. I. Brown (Ed.), *Quality of life for people with disabilities: Models, research and practice* (2nd ed, pp. 327–340). Cheltenham: Stanley Thornes.

Schalock, R. L. (1999, September). *The application of the concept of quality of life: IASSID Quality of Life Consensus Document: Discussion draft.* Paper presented at the 35th National Conference of the Australian Society for the Study of Intellectual Disabilities [ASSID], Sydney.

Schalock, R. L. (2002, June). *The concept of quality of life: What we know and do not know.* Paper presented at the Inaugural IASSID [International Association for the Scientific Study of Intellectual Disabilities] Europe Quadrennial Conference, University College, Dublin, Ireland.

Schalock, R. L. (2004a). Quality of life: What we know and what we don't know. *Journal of Intellectual Disability Research, 48*, 203–216.

Schalock, R. L. (2004b). The emerging disability paradigm and its implications for policy and practice. *Journal of Disability Policy Studies, 14*(4), 204–215.

Schalock, R. L. (2005a). Introduction and overview. *Journal of Intellectual Disability Research, 49(10)*, 695–698.

Schalock, R. L. (2005b). *Moving from a quality of care to a quality of life program emphasis.* Paper presented at the international congress about quality of life of persons with disability, Quito, Ecuador, 17–21 October.

Schalock, R. L., Bontham, G. S., & Marchand, C. B. (2000). Consumer based quality of life assessment: A path model of perceived satisfaction. *Evaluation and Program Planning, 23*(1), 77–87.

Schalock, R. L., Brown, I., Brown, R., Cummins, R. A., Felce, D., Matikka, L., et al. (2002). Quality of life: Its conceptualization, measurement, and application: Results of an international consensus process. *Mental Retardation, 40*, 457–470.

Schalock, R. L., & Felce, D. (2004). Quality of life and subjective well-being: Conceptual and measurement issues. In E. Emerson, C. Hatton, T. Thompson & T. Parmenter (Eds.), *Handbook of applied research in intellectual disabilities* (pp. 261–279). Chichester: Wiley.

Schalock, R. L., Gardner, J. F., & Bradley, V. J. (2007). *Quality of life of persons with intellectual and other disabilities: Applications across individuals, organizations, systems, and communities.* Washington, DC: American Association on Intellectual and Developmental Disabilities.

Schalock, R. L., & Keith, K. D. (1993). Quality of life questionnaire. In R. L. Schalock (Ed.), *Quality of life. Volume I: Conceptualization and measurement.* Washington, DC: American Association of Mental Retardation.

Schalock, R. L., & Luckasson, R. (2005). *Clinical judgement.* Washington, DC: AAMR.

Schalock, R. L., & Verdugo, M. A. (2002). *Handbook on quality of life for human services practitioners.* Washington, DC: American Association on Mental Retardation.

Schalock, R. L., Verdugo, M. A., Bontham, G. S., Fantova, F., & Van Loon, J. (2008). Enhancing personal outcomes: Organizational strategies, guidelines, and example. *Journal of Policy and Practice in Intellectual Disabilities, 5(4)*, 276–285.

Schalock, R. L., Verdugo, M. A., Jenaro, C., Wang, M., Wehmeyer, M., Xu, J., et al. (2005). A cross cultural study of quality of life indicators. *American Journal on Mental retardation, 110*, 298–311.

Schipper, H., Clinch, J., & Powell, V. (1990). Definitions and conceptual issues. In B. Spilker (Ed.), *Quality of life assessments in clinical trials* (pp. 11–24). New York: Raven.

Schuessler, K. F., & Fisher, G. A. (1985). Quality of life research and sociology. *Annual Review of Sociology, 11*, 129–149.

Seed, P., & Lloyd, G. (1997). *Quality of life*. London: Jessica Langley.

Sen, A. (1993). Capability and well-being. In M. Mussbaum & A. Sen (Eds.), *The quality of life*. Oxford: Clarendon Press.

Sen, A. (1996). *Inequality re-examined*. Boston: Harvard University Press.

Senge, P. M. (2006). *The fifth discipline: The art and practice of the learning organization* (Rev. Ed.). New York: Doubleday.

Shaddock, A. J., Dowse, L., Richards, H., & Spinks, A. T. (1998). Communicating with people with an intellectual disability in Guardianship Board hearings: An exploratory study. *Journal of Intellectual and Developmental Disability, 23*(4), 278–293.

Smyer, M. A., McHale, S. M., Birkel, R., & Madle, R. A. (1988). Impairments, handicapping environments, and disability: A life-span perspective. In P. S. Van Hasselt, P. S. Dtrain & M. Herson (Eds.), *Handbook of developmental and physical disabilities* (pp. 9–20). New York: Permagon.

Social Policy Directorate. (1994a). *Quality of life: A social policy approach*. Sydney: New South Wales Office on Social Policy, Office on Social Policy.

Social Policy Directorate. (1994b, July). *Quality of life: Our values our future*. Paper presented at the New South Wales Office on Social Policy Seminar, Sydney, Australia.

Solomon, E. S., Bouchouchi, N., Denisov, V., Hankiss, E., Mallman, C. A., & Milbrath, L. W. (1980). UNESCO's policy-relevant quality of life research program. In A. Szalai & F. M. Andrews (Eds.), *The quality of life: Comparative studies*. Beverly Hills, CA: Sage.

Speight, S., Myers, L., Cox, C., & Highlen, P. (1991). A redefinition of multicultural counseling. *Journal of Counseling and Development, 70*, 29–36.

Stancliffe, R. J. (1995). Assessing opportunities for choice making: A comparison of self and staff reports. *American Journal on Mental Retardation, 99*(4), 418–429.

Stark, J., & Faulkner, E. (1996). Quality of life across the life span. In R. L. Schalock (Ed.), *Quality of life: Volume 1: Conceptualization and measurement* (pp. 23–32). Washington, DC: American Association on Mental Retardation.

Stensman, R. (1985). Severely mobility-disabled people assess the quality of their lives. *Scandinavian Journal of Rehabilitation, 17*(2), 87–89.

Stokols, D. (1992). Establishing and maintaining health environments: Towards a social ecology of health promotion. *American Psychologist, 47*, 6–22.

Storey, K. (1997). Quality of life issues in social skills assessment of persons with disabilities. *Education and Training in Mental Retardation and Developmental Disabilities, 32*, 197–200.

Strauss, A., & Corbin, J. (1994). Grounded theory methodology: An overview. In N. K. Denzin & Y. S. Lincoln (Eds.), *Handbook of qualitative research* (pp. 273–285). Thousand Oaks, CA: Sage.

Sullivan, M. (1992). Quality of life assessment in medicine: Concepts, definitions, purposes and basic tools. *Nordic Journal of Psychiatry, 46*, 79–83.

Swain, J., Finkelstein, V., French, S., & Oliver, M. (Eds.). (1993). *Disabling barriers – Enabling environments*. London: Sage.

Szalai, A. (1980). Prologue. In A. Szalai & F. M. Andrews (Eds.), *The quality of life: Comparative studies* (pp. 7–24). Beverly Hills, CA: Sage Publications.

Taylor, S. J. (1994). In support of research on quality of life, but against QOL. In D. A. Goode (Ed.), *Quality of life for persons with disabilities: International perspectives and issues*. Cambridge, MA: Brookline Books.

Taylor, S. J., & Bogdan, R. C. (1990). Quality of life and the individual's perspective. In R. L. Schalock & M. J. Begab (Eds.), *Quality of life: Perspectives and issues* (pp. 27–40). Washington, DC: American Association on Mental Retardation.

Thompson, J. T., Bryant, B. R., Campbell, E. M., Craig, E. M., Hughes, C. M., Rotholz, D. A., et al. (2004). *Support intensity scale manual*. Washington, DC: AAMR.

Thompson, B., & Guess, D. (1989). Students who experience the most profound disabilities: Teacher perspectives. In F. Brown & D. H. Lehr (Eds.), *Persons with profound disabilities: Issues and practices* (pp. 3–41). Baltimore, MD: Paul H. Brookes.

Thompson, R. J., & O'Quinn, A. N. (1979). *Developmental disabilities: Etiologies, manifestations, diagnoses, and treatments*. New York: Oxford.

Thorley, B. (1993). Servicing students with special needs: More categories plus more specialist equals more problems. *Special Education Perspectives, 2*(1), 17–21.

Timmons, V., & Brown, R. I. (1997). Quality of life: Issues for children with handicaps. In R. Brown (Ed.), *Quality of life for people with disabilities: Models, research and practice* (2nd ed.). Cheltenham: Stanley Thornes.

Tones, B. K. (1986). Health education and the ideology of health promotion: A review of alternative approaches. *Health Education Research, 1*, 3–12.

Travers, P., & Richardson, S. (1993). *Living decently: Material well-being in Australia*. Melbourne: Oxford University Press.

Triandis, H. C. (1994). Culture and social behaviour. In W. J. Lonner & R. Malpass (Eds.), *Psychology and culture*. Boston: Allyn & Bacon.

Turnbull, A., Brown, I., & Turnbull, H. R. (2004). *Families and people with mental retardation and quality of life: international perspectives*. Washington, DC: American Association on Mental Retardation.

Turnbull, R., & Brunk, G. L. (1990). Quality of life and public policy: Quality of Life: Perspectives and Issues. In R. L. Schalock (Ed.), *Mental retardation monograph series*. Washington, DC: American Association on Mental Retardation.

Van Dam, F. S. A. M., Somers, R., & Van Beck-Couzijn, A. L. (1981). Quality of life: Some theoretical issues. *Journal of Clinical Pharmacology, 21*, 1665–1685.

Verdugo, M. A., Schalock, R. L., Keith, K. D., & Stancliffe, R. J. (2005). Quality of life and its measurement: Important principles and guidelines. *Journal of Intellectual Disability Research, 49(10)*, 707–717.

Verwayen, H. (1980). The specification and measurement of the quality of life in OECD countries. In A. Szalai & F. M. Andrews (Eds.), *The quality of life: Comparative studies*. Beverly Hills, CA: Sage.

Vogel, J., Andersson, L., Davidsson, U., & Hall, L. (1988). *Living conditions report No. 58: Inequality in Sweden, trends and current situation, statistics*. Stockholm: SCB Statistics Sweden.

von Tetzchner, S., & Jensen, K. (1999). Interacting with people who have severe communication problems: Ethical considerations. *International Journal of Disability, Development and Education, 46*(4), 453–462.

Walsh, P. N., Emerson, E., Bradley, V. J., Schalock, R. L., Hatton, C., & Moseley, C. (2006). *The outcomes and costs of supported accommodation for people with intellectual disabilities*. Dublin: National Disability Authority.

Wolf, N. (1990). *The beauty myth*. London: Vintage.

Wolfe, P. S. (1992). Challenges for service providers. In P. J. McLaughlin & P. Wejman (Eds.), *Developmental disabilities: A handbook for best practice* (pp. 124–141). Boston: Andover Medical.

Wolfensberger, W. (1994). Let's hang up "quality of life" as a hopeless term. In D. Goode (Ed.), *Quality of life for persons with disabilities: International perspectives and issues*. Cambridge, MA: Brookline Books.

Wolfensberger, W. (1995). Social role valorization is too conservative. No, it's too radical. *Disability and Society, 10*(3), 365–367.

Wolfensberger, W., & Nirje, B. (1972). *Normalization: The principle of normalization in human services*. Toronto, ON: National Institute on Mental Retardation.

Woodill, G., Renwick, R., Brown, I., & Raphael, D. (1994). Being, belonging and becoming: An approach to the quality of life of persons with developmental disabilities. In D. A. Goode (Ed.), *Quality of life for persons with disabilities: International perspectives and issues*. Cambridge, MA: Brookline Books.

World Health Organisation. (1986). A discussion document on the concept and principles of health promotion. *Health Promotion, 1*, 73–76.

Zapf, W. (1986). Development, structure and prospects of the German social state. In R. Rose & R. Shiratori (Eds.), *The welfare state: East and west*. Oxford: Oxford University Press.

Zapf, W., Glatzer, W., Noll, H. H., Habich, R., Berger-Schmitt, R., Breuer, S., et al. (1987). German social report: Living conditions and subjective well-being, 1978–1984. *Social Indicators Research, 19*, 1.

Zhan, L. (1992). Quality of life: Conceptual and measurement issues. *Journal of Advanced Nursing, 17*(1), 795–800.

Chapter 7
The Effect of Employment on the Quality of Life of People with Intellectual Disabilities: A Review of the Literature

Ralph Kober

There have been numerous studies using quality of life measures to investigate the outcomes achieved by different methods of accommodation services for people with an intellectual disability (for example, Conroy, 1996; Heal & Chadsey-Rusch, 1985; Hemming, Lavender, & Pill, 1981; Schalock & Genung, 1993; Schalock & Lilley, 1986). However, there has been surprisingly little research investigating whether different methods of employment result in different quality of life outcomes. As such, this chapter first summarizes the literature on whether employment affects the quality of life of people with intellectual disabilities, and then reports those papers that investigate whether differences exist in the quality of life of people with intellectual disabilities employed in sheltered employment[1] compared with open employment.[2]

Does Employment Make a Difference?

Schalock and Lilley (1986) developed a quality of life questionnaire to evaluate the successfulness, in living and work, of individuals 8–10 years after being deinstitutionalized. In relation to work, they found that those individuals who had successful work placements had a higher quality of life than those who have unsuccessful work placements. Schalock and Lilley (1986) found that living success appears to be independent of work success, but the converse does not hold. However, they also found

R. Kober (✉)
Department of Accounting and Finance, Monash University, Caulfield East, VIC 3145, Australia
e-mail: ralph.kober@monash.edu

[1] *Sheltered employment* refers to the situation where people with intellectual disabilities work alongside other people with a disability in a segregated, specially tailored setting. Typically, in this setting, the only people without disabilities in the workplace with whom people with intellectual disabilities would interact would be their supervisors.

[2] *Open employment* is where people with intellectual disabilities work alongside people without disabilities in integrated, meaningful employment in a community setting, supported by their employment agency. The alternative terms of *competitive employment* or *supported employment* are also often used.

R. Kober (ed.), *Enhancing the Quality of Life of People with Intellectual Disabilities*, Social Indicators Research Series 41, DOI 10.1007/978-90-481-9650-0_7,

that individuals who retained their jobs are generally higher functioning and have fewer disabilities. Thus, it is not clear whether it is the employment or the level of disability that is impacting on their results.

Fabian (1991) used the Lehman (1988) Quality of Life Interview to assess whether people with severe intellectual disabilities in open employment report higher quality of life scores compared with people with intellectual disabilities seeking employment. Fabian (1991) found that people in open employment reported statistically significantly higher scores than job seekers in two of the eight areas of the Quality of Life Interview; the two areas being *work* and *finance*. Neither of these findings is surprising. First, it could be expected that people in work would be more satisfied with their work situation than those unemployed. Second, it could be expected that those earning a wage would be more satisfied with their finances than those not earning a regular income. It is interesting to note that employment does not lead to higher scores in the other six areas of the Quality of Life Interview. The results of Fabian (1991) suggest that employment does not impact on quality of life, thus contradicting the findings of Schalock and Lilley (1986).

Does Type of Employment Make a Difference?

Relatively few studies compare the quality of life of people participating in open employment compared with those in sheltered employment (Eggleton, Robertson, Ryan, & Kober, 1999; Inge, Banks, Wehman, Hill, & Shafer, 1988; Kober & Eggleton, 2005; Pedlar, Lord, & Loon, 1990; Sinnott-Oswald, Gliner, & Spencer, 1991; Verdugo, Jordán de Urríes, Jenaro, Caballo, & Crespo, 2006). Pedlar et al. (1990) conducted a qualitative study of 12 people placed in open employment. Based on content analysis of the interviews they concluded that open employment considerably enhanced participants' quality of life. However, exactly how this conclusion was drawn is not clear, as no established link between the content of the interviews and quality of life was made. Additionally, given that no statistical analysis was conducted, it is not possible to determine whether the enhancement in quality of life is statistically significant.

Inge et al. (1988) and Sinnott-Oswald et al. (1991) both conducted quantitative analysis and found that people participating in open employment experienced a higher quality of life than those employed in a sheltered environment. Inge et al. (1988) identified 20 people employed in sheltered employment and matched them to people in open employment based on gender, age, physical and sensory involvement, parental support, and functioning level. They assessed participants' quality of life using three proxy measures: first, the AAMD Adaptive Behavior Scale (Nihira, Foster, Shellhaas, & Leland, 1974); second, a parent/guardian survey that measured participants' community participation, social vocational skills, fiscal responsibility, financial activity, and weekly work income; and finally, five physical health measures, including weight, resting pulse, blood pressure, hand strength, and body fat.

Inge et al. (1988) found that participants in open employment had statistically significantly higher scores for three of the five sub-scales of the adaptive behavior scale (economic activity, language development, and numbers and time) as well as all five aspects of the parent/guardian survey. No significant differences were found in terms of the health of the two samples. Though not explicitly stated, they assumed that the higher scores for the adaptive behavior scale and parent/guardian survey meant that participants in open employment had a higher quality of life. However, whether such a conclusion can be drawn is questionable. In the absence of theoretical underpinning, a person's assessment of the quality of life he/she experiences can neither be assumed to be related to his/her adaptive behavior nor necessarily others' opinions on his/her level of community participation, social vocational skills, fiscal responsibility, financial activity, and weekly work income.

Sinnott-Oswald et al. (1991) compared the quality of life of ten people employed in open employment with ten people employed in sheltered employment who were matched based on age, gender, and degree of intellectual disability. Quality of life was assessed using a questionnaire the authors developed, based on Schalock and Lilley's (1986) quality of life questionnaire. Sinnott-Oswald et al. (1991) found participants in open employment reported statistically significantly higher scores for ten of the 18 questions contained in their questionnaire (ability to make independent decisions, self-esteem, use of public transport, frequency of use of public transport, participation in leisure/recreation activities, with whom they eat out, use of leisure time in the past year, changes in mobility during the past year, changes in job skills during the past year, changes in income during the past year). Based on these statistically significant differences Sinnott-Oswald et al. (1991) concluded that people with intellectual disabilities placed in open employment had a higher quality of life than those people placed in sheltered employment. Whether such a conclusion can be drawn is questionable, given that the quality of life questionnaire did not undergo any form of psychometric validation, the non-significant changes in eight of the questions, and the fact that their questionnaire does not allow the calculation of a total quality of life score.

Both Inge et al. (1988) and Sinnott-Oswald et al. (1991) had small sample sizes, and neither used a psychometrically validated quality of life questionnaire. As such, it is not clear whether their findings can be generalized. Overcoming these problems, Eggleton et al. (1999) used the Schalock and Keith (1993) QOL.Q to investigate the impact of open employment on people with intellectual disabilities.

The QOL.Q has 40 questions, each relating to an aspect of a person's life. For each question the interviewer provides the interviewee with three possible responses, and the interviewee selects the response most appropriate to their life situation. These responses are scored from 1 (low) to 3 (high), thus giving the overall quality of life score a theoretical range of 40–120. In addition to being able to compute an overall quality of life score, the QOL.Q is designed to allow the computation of four sub-dimensions (factors), which measure the following different domains of quality of life: (1) personal life satisfaction, (2) individual competence and productivity at work, (3) feelings of empowerment and independence in the living environment, and (4) feelings of belonging and community integration (Schalock &

Keith, 1993). As each factor comprises ten questions, each factor has a theoretical range of 10–30.

The QOL.Q has successfully undergone more psychometric assessment than any other quality of life questionnaire developed for people with intellectual disabilities. The factor structure of the QOL.Q has been broadly confirmed by Rapley and Lobley (1995), Kober and Eggleton (2002), and Caballo, Crespo, Jenaro, Verdugo, and Martinez (2005). Also, past studies have confirmed that the QOL.Q and its four factors have acceptable internal reliability in terms of reported Cronbach alpha scores (Caballo et al., 2005; Eggleton et al., 1999; Kober & Eggleton, 2005; Rapley & Lobley, 1995; Schalock & Keith, 1993).

Eggleton et al. (1999) interviewed 25 people who were in open employment, and a matched sample of 25 people who were seeking open employment. As in Fabian (1991), Eggleton et al. (1999) found that people with intellectual disabilities in open employment reported statistically significantly higher quality of life scores than job seekers. Further, Eggleton et al. (1999) also compared a subset of their sample who were working in open employment, but had previously worked in a sheltered employment setting, with those people still working in a sheltered employment setting (sheltered employment participants were included in their job seekers sample). Eggleton et al. (1999) found that those in open employment reported statistically significantly higher quality of life scores than their sheltered employment counterparts.

However, what drives the result of Eggleton et al. (1999) is not entirely clear. Given that Eggleton et al. (1999) noted all participants in their research were drawn from the list of an open employment agency, this means those people who were in sheltered employment were probably not satisfied with their employment situation, otherwise they would not have been on the list of an open employment agency, and seeking open employment. As such, it is not clear whether the results of Eggleton et al. (1999) are driven by the differences in the nature of the two methods of employment (open employment versus sheltered employment), or due to the fact that participants in sheltered employment were seeking open employment.

From the abovementioned research, it is not entirely clear whether open employment and sheltered employment produce different outcomes in terms of quality of life. As such, Kober and Eggleton (2005) specifically investigate this question.[3] They interviewed 117 people with intellectual disabilities participating in either open employment (64 people) or sheltered employment (53 people), using the Schalock and Keith (1993) QOL.Q.

Kober and Eggleton (2005) found that when the entire sample was considered, participants working in open employment reported statistically significantly higher scores compared with those working in sheltered employment for overall quality of life as well as the QOL.Q factors of *empowerment/independence* and *social*

[3]The discussion of Kober and Eggleton (2005) is based on the discussion from Kober and Eggleton(2006). I am grateful to Springer for granting permission to incorporate this discussion into this chapter.

belonging/community integration. However, when the authors conducted separate analyses for participants with high levels of functional work ability[4] and those with low levels of functional work ability, the above results of statistically significant differences between open employment and sheltered employment in terms of *empowerment/independence*, *social belonging/community integration*, and *quality of life* are found only for people with high levels of functional work ability, and not for people with low levels of functional work ability.

The results of Kober and Eggleton (2005) therefore indicate that for people with low functional work ability, there is no difference in relation to the quality of life of participants in open employment compared with sheltered employment. However, participants with high functional work ability reported higher quality of life scores in open employment compared with sheltered employment.

Given that the results of Kober and Eggleton (2005) revealed statistically significantly higher scores for *empowerment/independence, social belonging/community integration*, and *total quality of life* for people with high level of functional work ability the results appear to support the placement of people with intellectual disabilities with a high level of functional work ability in open employment rather than in sheltered employment. Conversely, given that there was no statistically significant difference between methods of employment for people with low levels of functional work ability it appears that it does not matter where people with intellectual disabilities with low levels of functional work ability are placed. The results of Kober and Eggleton (2005) combined with the results of research showing that from a societal point of view the benefits of open employment compared with supported employment (e.g., increased tax revenues, decreased service expenditure, decreased government pensions) outweigh the associated costs (e.g., employment agency funding, subsidies paid to employers) (e.g., Conley, Rusch, McCaughrin, & Tines, 1989; Hill & Wehman, 1983; Hill et al., 1987; McCaughrin, Ellis, Rusch, & Heal, 1993; Noble, Conley, & Banerjee, 1991; Rusch, Conley, & McCaughrin, 1993; Shearn, Beyer, & Felce, 2000; Tines, Rusch, McCaughrin, & Conley, 1990; Tuckerman, Smith, & Borland, 1999) could be taken to support the closure of sheltered employment options for people with intellectual disabilities. However, I would strongly caution against any such course of action, as it would only serve to limit the options available to people with intellectual disabilities. However, what I would encourage is the dissemination of the results of Kober and Eggleton (2005) to people with intellectual disabilities and their parents/guardians to aid their decision-making processes when deciding upon what type of employment they believe best suits their needs. I would also encourage an exploration of what are the underlying factors

---

[4]Functional work ability was measured by the Functional Assessment Inventory (FAI) (Crewe & Athelstan, 1984). The FAI consists of 30 behaviourally anchored rating items, ranging from 0 (no significant impairment) to 3 (severe impairment), which assess a person's work capabilities and deficiencies, thus giving a theoretical range of 0–90; the higher the score, the lower the person's functional work ability. Low functional work ability was defined as a score of equal to or greater than 26, with high functional work ability defined as a score of 20 or less. These cut-off scores were selected as they represented approximately the top and bottom 40% of the sample, respectively.

that cause these statistically significant differences between the open employment and sheltered employment. Is it the employment method per se, or some other factor, such as the lower level of wages received in sheltered employment compared with open employment? As noted by Cummins (2000), income can act as an external buffer that can protect a person from negative input from the surrounding environment.

The argument that the income level could be driving the results of Kober and Eggleton (2005) is supported by the results of Verdugo et al. (2006). Verdugo et al. (2006) also used the Schalock and Keith's (1993) QOL.Q in comparing the quality of life of people with intellectual disabilities placed in open employment ($n = 160$) compared with sheltered employment ($n = 72$) in Spain. In contrast to the results of Kober and Eggleton (2005), they found no difference in the quality of life of the two samples. Verdugo et al. (2006) note that unlike most other countries (and prior research) in Spain people placed in sheltered employment receive at least the minimum wage as well as benefits such as over-time and medical benefits and that this may explain the differences in their results compared with prior research. Given the differing results of Verdugo et al. (2006), further research is definitely warranted as to the effect of income on the quality of life of people with intellectual disabilities. It will be interesting to determine if it is the typical income disparity between sheltered employment and open employment, which does not afford the person in sheltered employment the opportunity to buffer themselves from their external environment, that is driving the differences in reported quality of life between the two methods of employment.

In addition to assessing the outcomes of one method of employment relative to another method of employment, Kober and Eggleton (2005) also showed how performance can also be evaluated based on the percentage of scale maximum score. Percentage of scale maximum involves the conversion of a scale into a standard form that ranges from 0 to 100% (Cummins, 2000). As the QOL.Q has a theoretical range of 40–120, the QOL.Q score can be converted to a percentage of scale maximum using the following formula: [(QOL.Q score – 40) $\div$ 80] $\times$ 100. To convert the four sub-domain QOL.Q scores, which have a theoretical range of 10–30, to a percentage of scale maximum, the following formula can be used: [(QOL.Q sub-domain score – 10) $\div$ 20] $\times$ 100. Cummins (2000, p. 136) notes that "the average level of life satisfaction [quality of life] can be described by 75 $\pm$ 2.5" percent scale maximum. Using two standard deviations around the mean to determine a normative range, Cummins (2000) notes that population quality of life can be predicted to range between 70 and 80% of scale maximum. He argues that in a western population the value of 70% of scale maximum holds significance in that values below this level indicate that homeostasis[5] has been defeated. That is, the environment experienced by that population "has become so aversive that, on average, it exceeds the average person's adaptational capacity" (Cummins, 2000, p. 137).

[5]For an explanation of homeostasis and homeostatic theory of subjective well-being, see Cummins (1995, 1998, 2000).

Kober and Eggleton (2005) found that in relation to *social belonging/community integration*, irrespective of the method of employment, on all occasions the percent of scale maximum score was below 70% of scale maximum. Their results highlight that people with intellectual disabilities are not integrating to a satisfactory level with their communities for both forms of employment. As noted in Kober and Eggleton (2005), addressing this issue may be beyond the scope of individual employment agencies and may require initiatives at governmental level. Nonetheless, the results are still informative in highlighting that both open employment and sheltered employment methods are not performing well on this aspect of quality of life.

Kober and Eggleton (2005) also found that in all instances for participants in sheltered employment, their percentage of scale maximum scores for *empowerment/independence* and *quality of life* were below 70%. This indicates that in relation to *empowerment/independence* and *quality of life* sheltered employment is not performing to a satisfactory level in that the environment provided by this method of employment resulted in participants' homeostasis being defeated. A similar observation in relation to *empowerment/independence* can be made for participants with low functional work ability in open employment, as the mean percentage scale maximum score for these participants was also found by Kober and Eggleton (2005) to be below 70%. This suggests that irrespective of method of employment, disability employment agencies need to consider methods to improve the performance of their services to people with low functional work ability in terms of their feelings of *empowerment/independence*.

Kober and Eggleton (2005) found that participants with high functional work ability reported mean scores below 70% of scale maximum for the *satisfaction* factor of the QOL.Q. Again, it appears that homeostasis was defeated in relation to this domain of quality of life irrespective of method of employment. For participants with high functional work ability in sheltered employment it is likely that this reflects that they compare their employment situation to people without a disability. For those participants with high functional work ability in open employment, it is probable defeat of homeostatic on this factor reflects they are not interacting on a socially meaningful level with their co-workers, and as such do not feel part of their work community. If this is the case, disability employment agencies may need to educate/train the co-workers without disabilities as to how to interact meaningfully and socially involve people with intellectual disabilities. It is clear that disability employment agencies need to ameliorate those aspects of their services to people with high functional work ability that impacts on this quality of life domain.

Conclusion and Future Research Opportunities

The review of literature undertaken in this chapter has shown there still exists a dearth of literature relating to the effect of different methods of employment on quality of life, with most research being conducted using small sample sizes and/or non-psychometrically validated questionnaires. The exception to this being Kober and Eggleton (2005), who found that for participants with high functional work ability, open employment results in a higher quality of life. While, for people with low functional work ability, there appears to be no difference in quality of life between sheltered employment and open employment.

Given that Kober and Eggleton (2005) was the first study to comprehensively explore the question of the effect of method of employment on quality of life it is important that other studies continue with this vein of research. One particularly fruitful area for future research would be to investigate the effect of income levels on the quality of life of people with intellectual disabilities. Given the disparity in the wages paid to participants in open employment compared with those in sheltered employment Kober and Eggleton (2005) were unable to control for the differences between the two methods of employment with regards to this demographic variable. As such it is not clear whether it is the type of employment per se, or possibly the differences in income levels between participants in open employment and sheltered employment that are driving their results. This is all the more pertinent given that the findings of Cummins (2000) suggest that people with low socio-economic status (as may be expected of people with intellectual disabilities) report higher quality of life with higher levels of wealth; as the additional income can be used to help buffer themselves from their external environment. As such it would be interesting to survey people with intellectual disabilities placed in sheltered employment who received considerably higher wages than those in the Kober and Eggleton's (2005) sample. This would allow for a determination of whether it is the method of employment or income levels that are driving Kober and Eggleton's (2005) results.

There are many other fruitful avenues for further research into the effect employment has on the quality of life experienced by people with intellectual disabilities. It would be interesting to conduct further research to investigate whether within a method of employment (open employment or sheltered employment) the nature of the occupation (that is, laboring positions versus non-laboring positions) has a bearing on quality of life. It would also be interesting to know whether within sheltered employment, the extent of opportunities for interaction with people without disabilities has a bearing on participants' quality of life. For example, people employed in a mobile gardening crew have greater opportunities to interact with people without a disability, compared with those people employed in a sheltered workshop. This degree of interaction may impact on their quality of life. Additionally, it would be worth investigating the effect the length of employment has on a participant's quality of life. Anecdotal evidence would suggest that people with intellectual disabilities placed in either open employment or sheltered employment tend to have limited opportunities for promotion and consequently remain in the same position for extended periods of time. It would be interesting to investigate the effect this has on the person's quality of life as a basis for formulating appropriate career plans for people with disabilities

References

Caballo, C., Crespo, M., Jenaro, C., Verdugo, M. A., & Martinez, J. L. (2005). Factor structure of the Schalock and Keith quality of life questionnaire (QOL-Q): Validation on Mexican and Spanish samples. *Journal of Intellectual Disability Research, 49*, 773–776.

Conley, R. W., Rusch, F. R., McCaughrin, W. B., & Tines, J. (1989). Benefits and costs of supported employment: An analysis of the Illinois supported employment project. *Journal of Applied Behavior Analysis, 22*, 441–447.

Conroy, J. W. (1996). The small ICF/MR program: Dimensions of quality and cost. *Mental Retardation, 34*, 13–26.

Crewe, N. M., & Athelstan, G. T. (1984). *Functional assessment inventory manual*. Menomonie, WI: Stout Vocational Rehabilitation Institute, University of Wisconsin-Stout.

Cummins, R. A. (1995). On the trail of the gold standard for life satisfaction. *Social Indicators Research, 35*, 179–200.

Cummins, R. A. (1998). The second approximation to an international standard for life satisfaction. *Social Indicators Research, 43*, 307–334.

Cummins, R. A. (2000). Personal income and subjective well-being: A review. *Journal of Happiness Studies, 1*, 133–158.

Eggleton, I., Robertson, S., Ryan, J., & Kober, R. (1999). The impact of employment on the quality of life of people with an intellectual disability. *Journal of Vocational Rehabilitation, 13*, 95–107.

Fabian, E. S. (1991). Using quality-of-life indicators in rehabilitation program evaluation. *Rehabilitation Counseling Bulletin, 34*, 344–356.

Heal, L. W., & Chadsey-Rusch, J. (1985). The lifestyle satisfaction scale (LSS): Assessing individuals' satisfaction with residence, community setting, and associated services. *Applied Research in Mental Retardation, 6*, 475–490.

Hemming, H., Lavender, T., & Pill, R. (1981). Quality of life of mentally retarded adults transferred from large institutions to new small units. *American Journal of Mental Deficiency, 86*, 157–169.

Hill, M., & Wehman, P. (1983). Cost benefit analysis of placing moderately and severely handicapped individuals into competitive employment. *TASH Journal, 8*, 30–38.

Hill, M. L., Banks, P. D., Handrich, R. R., Wehman, P. H., Hill, J. W., & Shafer, M. S. (1987). Benefit-cost analysis of supported competitive employment for persons with mental retardation. *Research in Developmental Disabilities, 8*, 71–89.

Inge, K. J., Banks, P. D., Wehman, P., Hill, J. W., & Shafer, M. S. (1988). Quality of life for individuals who are labelled mentally retarded: Evaluating competitive employment versus sheltered workshop employment. *Education and Training in Mental Retardation, 6*, 97–104.

Kober, R., & Eggleton, I. R. C. (2002). The factor stability of the Schalock and Keith (1993) quality of life questionnaire. *Mental Retardation, 40*, 157–165.

Kober, R., & Eggleton, I. (2005). The effects of different types of employment on quality of life. *Journal of Intellectual Disability Research, 49*, 756–760.

Kober, R., & Eggleton, I. R. C. (2006). Using quality of life to assess performance in the disability services sector. *Applied Research in Quality of Life, 1*, 63–77.

Lehman, A. F. (1988). A quality of life interview for the chronically mentally ill. *Evaluation and Program Planning, 11*, 51–62.

McCaughrin, W. B., Ellis, W. K., Rusch, F. R., & Heal, L. W. (1993). Cost-effectiveness of supported employment. *Mental Retardation, 31*, 41–48.

Nihira, K., Foster, R., Shellhaas, M., & Leland, H. (1974). *AAMD adaptive behavior scale*. Washington, DC: American Association on Mental Deficiency.

Noble, J. H., Conley, R. W., & Banerjee, S. (1991). Supported employment in New York State: A comparison of benefits and costs. *Journal of Disability Policy Studies, 2*, 39–71.

Pedlar, A., Lord, J., & Loon, M. V. (1990). Quality of life outcomes of supported employment. *Canadian Journal of Community Mental Health, 9*, 79–96.

Rapley, M., & Lobley, J. (1995). Factor analysis of the Schalock and Keith (1993) quality of life questionnaire: A replication. *Mental Handicap Research, 8*, 194–202.
Rusch, F. R., Conley, R. W., & McCaughrin, W. B. (1993). Benefit-cost analysis of supported employment in Illinois. *Journal of Rehabilitation, 59*, 31–36.
Schalock, R. L., & Genung, L. T. (1993). Placement from a community-based mental retardation program: A 15-year follow-up. *American Journal of Mental Retardation, 98*, 400–407.
Schalock, R. L., & Keith, K. D. (1993). *Quality of life manual*. Hastings, NE: Self Published.
Schalock, R. L., & Lilley, M. A. (1986). Placement from community-based mental retardation programs: How well do clients do after 8 to 10 years. *American Journal of Mental Deficiency, 90*, 669–676.
Shearn, J., Beyer, S., & Felce, D. (2000). The cost-effectiveness of supported employment for people with severe intellectual disabilities and high support needs: A pilot study. *Journal of Applied Research in Intellectual Disabilities, 13*, 29–37.
Sinnott-Oswald, M., Gliner, J. A., & Spencer, K. C. (1991). Supported and sheltered employment: Quality of life issues among workers with disabilities. *Education and Training in Mental Retardation, 26*, 388–397.
Tines, J., Rusch, F. R., McCaughrin, W., & Conley, R. W. (1990). Benefit-cost analysis of supported employment in Illinois: A statewide evaluation. *American Journal on Mental Retardation, 95*, 44–54.
Tuckerman, P., Smith, R., & Borland, J. (1999). The relative cost of employment for people with a significant intellectual disability: The Australian experience. *Journal of Vocational Rehabilitation, 13*, 109–116.
Verdugo, M. A., Jordán de Urríes, F. B., Jenaro, C., Caballo, C., & Crespo, M. (2006). Quality of life of workers with an intellectual disability in supported employment. *Journal of Applied Research in Intellectual Disabilities, 19*, 309–316.

Part III
International Perspectives

Chapter 8
Quality of Life in the Polder: About Dutch and EU Policies and Practices in Quality of Life for People with Intellectual Disabilities

Alice Schippers

Introduction

Typical Dutch: Polder model

The Netherlands is probably best known for clogs, tulips, bikes and above all taming the water. Many parts of the Netherlands are below sea level, and with a dense population in a small country (17 million people on 41.500 km^2), land was gained from the sea: the polders. These facts influenced the Dutch culture. For centuries the Dutch have had to fight the water. Landlords have had to negotiate with each other to build and maintain dikes around the polders. When in the 1990s the Dutch economy had better results than other EU countries, the explanation was found in the so-called 'polder model'. In the political field no left or right wing were dominant, but a 'third way' of consensus after elaborate negotiating between parties was found (Wikipedia, 2008).

When describing Dutch policy and practice in the intellectual disabilities field, and more specifically in relation to quality of life (QoL), one should keep this so-called polder model in mind. In striving for QoL in the disabilities field, the Dutch stakeholders negotiated about what and how QoL should have a place in the debate. In the following sections these developments will be described and discussed.

We will continue with a description of QoL as a sensitizing, organizing and reflecting concept. In the second section the Dutch health-care system and relevant legislation is described, highlighting changing paradigms, changing roles of stakeholders, and at national level the QoL framework. We will briefly refer to EU developments in this respect. How QoL is put into practice is described in the third section. We will give examples from perspectives of several stakeholders in the disabilities field. In the last section we conclude with the discussion.

A. Schippers (✉)
Disability Studies in the Netherlands, Utrecht, The Netherlands; Policy and Quality Affairs, Amsterdam, The Netherlands
e-mail: alice.schippers@tiscali.nl

R. Kober (ed.), *Enhancing the Quality of Life of People with Intellectual Disabilities*, Social Indicators Research Series 41, DOI 10.1007/978-90-481-9650-0_8,

Quality of Life

Aristotle defined quality of life or 'eudaimonia' as the meaning and the purpose of life, the whole aim and end of human existence. Quality of life is a universal concept, of all places and times. As Aristotle stated, it is even the meaning of life. Searching the internet for QoL, you come up with millions of hits, indicating the widespread use of the concept.

Over the past decades, in the field of care and disabilities, the concept of QoL has received an international or global perspective, and been applied in several ways; as a *sensitizing, organizing* and *reflecting* concept (Brown & Schalock, 2006; WHO, 1993). Quality of life can be considered as a sensitizing concept that gives a general idea of what is important in life. The concept gives sense to several stakeholders in the disabilities field to be aware of 'what it is all about': people with and without disabilities want to live a quality life. As an organizing concept QoL (operationalized in dimensions and/or domains) provides a framework at several levels. For example, at a macro level, the WHO uses the concept in describing poverty around the world (WHO, 1993). At a meso and micro level, domains of QoL are used in similar ways, as highlighted in the third section relating to the Dutch situation. QoL as a reflecting or evaluating concept gives a reference for evaluating performance, e.g. legislation or care provision. QoL has influenced Dutch policy on intellectual disabilities as a sensitizing, organizing and reflecting concept.

Policy

In the past few decades, mostly after deliberate debates and 'poldering', the Dutch health-care system has changed. We will first provide a general overview of the Dutch health-care system and the associated changes followed by a more specific discussion in relation to the disabilities field.

Health-Care System

The Dutch health-care system has significantly changed over the past decade. The *cost* system changed the *structure* and reflects the changing paradigm.

In the Netherlands we have an insurance-based *cost system* in health care, similar to other European countries such as Germany, Austria and Belgium. Other EU countries, like the UK and Sweden have a national health-care system. In the Netherlands, the government does not participate directly in the actual provision of care. This is a task principally for private care providers: individual practitioners and care institutions.

In 2006 a new insurance system was introduced, following decades of debate about the escalating cost of the health-care system. The Netherlands spends almost 10% of GDP on health care; the highest of any EU country (Ministry of HWS, 2006). With the expected change in demographics caused by an aging population it was feared the old health system would become unaffordable. Compared with the old system of standard insurance for all citizens, the new system is more market-driven. It gives citizens the possibility to change insurance company, and for insurers and care providers to compete on cost and performance (Ministry of HWS, 2006). Chronic illness and disabilities are insured via the so-called AWBZ, the General Act for Special Health Care Costs. The aforementioned principles apply to this act as well.

The new cost system changed the *structure* of Dutch health care, amongst other things, it meant changing roles for the stakeholders such as government, the insurance companies, the care providers and, of course, the citizens (as well care consumers as/or insurance payers). Citizens have more choice between insurance companies and care providers.

Other legislation defines more or less the roles of the different stakeholders and their relationships in the care system. Those acts apply in the disabilities field as well. The Quality Act obliges care providers to provide care that is at a high standard, effective, efficient and client-centred. The care provider has to maintain a quality system. The Act on Individual Professions in Health Care aims for good professional practice through a process of registration, education and disciplinary rules. The Act on the Medical Intervention Agreement defines the relationship between the client and the care provider by means of a formal agreement and informed consent. In the Act on Complaints of Clients in the Care Sector, clients have means of complaining about interventions or omissions of the (individual) care provider. Recently, the Community Support Act was adopted, followed by the introduction of a number of essential changes in the distribution of responsibility in respect of participation by vulnerable citizens. These acts all came into practice in the last decade, reflecting the *changing visions* in health care. Before elaborating on these changes we will first describe the disabilities field in the Netherlands.

People with Intellectual Disabilities: Some Facts and Figures

The number of people with intellectual disabilities (IQ<80) in the Netherlands is approximately 112,000. This number is estimated to remain stable until 2020 (SCP, Social and Cultural Planning Office of the Netherlands, 2005).

The majority of people with intellectual disabilities need support to contribute to their quality of life. Support varies in intensity, complexity, continuity and labour-intensity and can change over time, depending on the individual's own development and changes in their social context. Informal and formal support can be distinguished. Informal support is provided by the social network such as family, relatives and neighbours. Whereas, formal support is provided by general and specific service providers (Schippers, 2003). Professional support is provided to approximately 88,000 persons with intellectual disabilities (VGN, 2007). The above described General Act on Special Health Care Costs (AWBZ) and the Community Support Act entitle individuals to professional support, if required. In every region a person can choose from several professional care providers. These agencies, or sometimes individual professionals, provide all common types of support such as living and vocational support, respite care and 24-h care. Allocation of resources differs at local level, but most people can choose from different providers, despite some waiting lists.

QoL as a Sensitizing Concept: Changing Paradigms

In the mid 1990s a paradigm shift took place in the disabilities field in Western Europe (including The Netherlands) and the majority of the Anglo Saxon countries. In the Netherlands, the perspective changed from viewing people with intellectual disabilities as patients, towards viewing them as citizens, and the support systems changed from institutional care towards community support (Van Gennep, 1994, 2000). Van Gennep (2000) pointed out a difference between a so-called scientific and a civil paradigm shift. He stated that in the Netherlands the scientific and civil paradigm are not as congruent as in other parts of western society. In the Netherlands supporting people with intellectual disabilities is less influenced by scientific knowledge and is more influenced by social views. The physical–structural design dominates, not the content of the paradigm shift; e.g. 'community care' instead of 'inclusion'. Recently, there have been some promising initiatives such as the Coalition for Inclusion (2008), an association of individuals dedicated to striving for the inclusion of people with disabilities, who are trying to influence policy and decision-makers.

In contrary to The Netherlands, at an EU-level science does influence policy. The EASPD, an NGO (non-government organization) of European Service providers for Persons with Disabilities, produced a memorandum on a European Quality Principles Framework based on scientific insights (EASPD, European Association of Service providers for Persons with Disabilities, 2006). This memorandum is aimed at improving the quality of services to improve the quality of life for people with (intellectual) disabilities. It is the result of 'a fundamental shift' that has taken place from the medical model that stresses disability to a social and human rights model that aims at full citizenship; a paradigm shift from patient to citizen, from segregation to inclusion (EASPD, European Association of Service providers for Persons with Disabilities, 2006). The EASPD is proposing to adopt QoL principles as the defining values. 'What such principles hold dear are elements such as equality, full participation, inclusion, empowerment, creating opportunities, offering choices and supporting people with disabilities in shaping their own lives' (EASPD, European Association of Service providers for Persons with Disabilities, 2006).

QoL as an Organizing Concept: Changing Roles

In the same period that the paradigm shift took place (the 1990s), quality assurance became an important issue in the disabilities field. Quality assurance owed its rise to the same developments in the general health-care field ('cure') and the service industry. Professional service providers took the lead in developing quality systems, driven by the idea that quality assurance was a means to be more (cost) effective. Influenced by the paradigm shift at least two developments took place in this so-called 'quality decade'; both implied changing roles of stakeholders in the disabilities field.

First, in the early 1990s quality assurance and improvement of support was process-driven. From the mid-1990s quality systems became more output and outcome-driven, based on QoL. This change can be clearly illustrated by the increased emphasis on professional support plans as an important part of a quality system. This instrument, initially meant to monitor the professional process, also became an instrument for 'clients' to evaluate the support provided, reflecting the empowerment and citizenship of people with intellectual disabilities.

Second, the service providers developed quality systems that were not only cost effective, but also improved their professionalism. Quality improvement was mainly internally focused. During the aforementioned structural changes to the Dutch health-care system (in the first section), quality systems became more of an instrument to justify the provided support to several stakeholders, including clients, insurance companies and the government. Quality improvement became more externally focused, implying changes in quality assurance from processes to output and outcome. The concept of QoL proved to be useful in defining those outcomes.

QoL as a Reflecting Concept: Reference Framework

During the change towards a more outcomes-focused system, the concept of QoL was not only used as an organizing concept, but also as a reflecting concept. The QoL paradigm is broadly used in The Netherlands. For instance, the Dutch Association of Care providers in Disabilities defined professional support in terms of the contribution of support to the QoL of people with disabilities(VGN, 2007).

A major effort is achieved by the development of a so-called 'quality framework' (Kwaliteitskader Gehandicaptenzorg, 2007). All stakeholders of the disabilities field were involved in the development, including client organizations, care providers, professional organizations, Health Care Inspectorate, the Ministry of Health, Welfare & Sports and the Health Care Insurance organizations. The aim of this quality framework is to be transparent, evaluate, justify, optimize and enhance the level of quality of the support provided in the disabilities field. The two major principles of this framework are QoL and self-direction. The principles are operationalized in the eight domains described by Schalock and Verdugo (2002) and four quality themes that are basic conditions for providing support. The quality domains and themes are the following: physical well-being, psychological well-being, interpersonal relationships, social integration, personal development, material well-being, self-direction, rights, support arrangements & support plan, physical, social and emotional safety, quality of staff and organization and consistency in support. The domains and themes will be further operationalized through indicators and implemented in the field. Some pilot studies have been conducted recently highlighting numerous applications and best practices in the field (Wijngaarden, Kok, & Sixma, 2008). We will focus on some of these pilot studies in the next section.

Practice

In applying the concept of QoL, we find a parallel with the well-known phases of change management: unfreezing, moving and freezing (Lewin, 1947). The first implication of using the concept of QoL is awareness and a sense of urgency to change, similarly with the unfreezing phase. In other words, QoL is a sensitizing concept. In the moving phase the awareness becomes action; things need to be changed. Similarly, the sense of urgency to strive for QoL outcomes leads to action; QoL as an organizing concept. Finally, the concept of QoL is used in the freezing phase of internalization and evaluation; QoL as a reflecting concept. In this section we will clarify the three phases of the concept of QoL by describing some best practices, mostly from The Netherlands and some from the EU.

Applications in Sensitizing

The concept of QoL leads to awareness. The 'state of happiness' is important on a personal level, but also on a meso level for organizations and on macro level for countries. Governments not only refer to QoL in, for instance, the fight against poverty and the war on terrorism, but also in recent disabilities policy, as highlighted in the previously mentioned example of the EU (macro level). A totally different example of sensitizing can be found in the recreation industry. A Dutch chain of holiday resorts brands itself with the slogan: 'a State of Happiness'.

Many service providers in health care, including the disabilities field, mention QoL in their mission statements. Several good practices can be found at this meso level in the disabilities field. For example, one service provider which supports over 4,000 people with psychiatric or intellectual disabilities states in their mission statement that people with disabilities deserve support enabling them to live an inclusive life in which they experience optimal QoL (Pameyer, 2009). The service provider's starting point is to support the client in directing his or her own life. At personal (or micro) level, one can find striving for a better QoL in personal support plans of people with disabilities (Schippers, 2003).

Another good practice is from the umbrella organization of clients associations, which mention in their website that they strive for participation in society and self-direction (LFB, 2009). The umbrella organization of parents associations promotes that people with intellectual disabilities are part of our society and that they have to live their own lives and participate in their own way. Freedom of choice for all life domains is also promoted (Platform VG, 2009).

At an EU level, the Disability High Level Group, representing all the EU members states under the European Commission presidency, has drawn up a position paper on the 'Quality of the Social Services of General Interest'. The purpose of this chapter is to 'provide guidance and inspiration on how to promote quality social services addressing the particular needs of people with disabilities'. Guidance and inspiration is found in the QoL concept including the following key features: rights, person-centred services, comprehensiveness and continuity, participation, partnerships, results orientation and good governance (Disability HLG, 2007).

The examples of good practices in using the concept and domains of QoL in general information is numerous throughout the disabilities field. The overall conclusion is that the concept of QoL played and is still playing an important role in 'unfreezing' the opinions on people with intellectual disabilities.

Applications in Organizing

The new paradigm seems to have had an impact in the Dutch and EU disabilities field, but the proof of the pudding is always in the eating. Does the concept of QoL change services, programmes and interventions for people with intellectual disabilities? Implementations of the concept in practice show that this is the case.

A good example of using QoL as an organizing concept is given by a service provider in the south western part of the Netherlands, supporting approximately 600 people with intellectual disabilities. This service provider drew up a vision on living and working, formulated the objectives of the programmes, and made them concrete. Essential in this process was that people with intellectual disabilities should be enabled to direct their lives themselves. This insight made it necessary to organize their services in a different way: the individual person became the smallest organizational unit, including the splitting up of supported home living and providing care. Specifically, the emancipation and self-determination of people with intellectual disabilities was the most important starting point for improving QoL (Van Loon & Van Hove, 2001). A focus on QoL was continued during the programme changes. The concept of QoL was operationalized and implemented through eight domains of QoL (Schalock & Verdugo, 2002). From a large action research study, the service provider concluded that three out of those eight domains were important in the changes made; these being, inclusion, self-determination and personal development (Van Loon & Van Hove, 2001).

Another service provider in the north western part of The Netherlands focuses strongly on communication of core values in their programme changes towards optimal QoL of their clients (approximately 2,500). QoL is operationalized in five elements: relations, respect, skills, participation and choices. Staffing and recruitment policy does not specifically target experience or level of education but the person's attitude and personal values. Both staff and clients are continuously and consistently coached. Personal initiatives, a flat organizational structure and a human face for organizational areas are critical in orientating the organization towards quality support. Staff members have the freedom to find their own ways, and are coached and stimulated to do so. Support planning is used to have a dialogue with clients and reflection is systematically organized on all levels (Van Dalen, 2007).

Applications in Reflecting

Since the 'quality decade' in health care, described in section 2, assessment of products and services is not only process-based, but more and more outcome-based. This has led the way for using QoL as a reflecting concept.

A terrific example of using the concept of QoL in evaluating services is an EU study aimed at measuring QoL in programmes on employment (QoL measures project, qol.euproject.org, 2009). This study needs to be mentioned for more than one reason. First, the emphasis in this study is on employment, one of the major issues in achieving QoL. There is not much research done on employment as a critical part of QoL (Schalock & Verdugo, 2002). Second, the fact that both western and eastern European countries took part in the study, including Austria, Belgium, Croatia, Finland, Hungary, Ireland, The Netherlands, Portugal and Sweden. Important indicators that contribute to QoL in the workplace included working conditions, job characteristics and environment, job match, support, social interaction and integration at the worksite, positive effects of the job (e.g. wages), perceived role and performance at work. One of the conclusions of this chapter is that specific employment indicators should be embedded in other QoL domains because the domains are interdependent. QoL at work should not be discussed in isolation from other life spheres. As this study was focused on instrument development, the country samples from the pilot studies were too limited to draw conclusions at (inter)national level (Astegger, 2008).

In a Dutch study on family-related QoL, the concept was used to interpret results from an action research model, aimed at developing partnerships to support nine families with a family member with an intellectual disability. The objective was to contribute to the experience of QoL, namely: ensuring personal needs were met, employment/satisfaction, personal meaning, positive self-image, social inclusion and improved well-being (Brown & Brown, 2003). The development of various partnerships, for instance with employers, schools, relatives, support organizations and volunteers, led to a change in experienced QoL and improved well-being (Schippers & Van Boheemen, 2009).

These good practices show that the changes influenced by the concept of QoL are becoming internalized in the minds of policy-makers and practitioners in the field of intellectual disabilities: they are becoming 'freezed'.

Discussion: Chicken, Egg or Polder?

In conducting the above review of Dutch and EU examples of policy and practice in applying the concept of QoL, one can ask the question: 'Which came first, the chicken or the egg?' It appears that we may have a clue to the answer in that this chapter started with a description of Dutch health-care system and legislation, followed by a description of changing paradigms in the field of intellectual disabilities. But this is not the case. It seemed so simple and straightforward, first giving an overview of the Dutch health-care system and afterwards zooming in on the disabilities field, in the meantime illustrating some changing views. In describing those developments, it became ambiguous and the chicken and egg question arose. It appears that the developments were mutually influenced; as the changing paradigms in the field do not occur in isolation, but are influenced by changes in society in general. Moreover, in general Dutch legislation is following societal developments, rather than initiating them. In the EU, however, legislation is more often initiating or sometimes even forcing developments.

The time frame that is used to describe the Dutch and EU developments and practices covers the past few decades. In this time frame we described changes referring to Lewin's phases of change, unfreeze, move and freeze. However, by analogy with legislation that follows societal changes, developments in the practice of applying a QoL approach will change over time. Having said this, it would be a 'contradiction in terms' to state that a QoL approach involves 'freezing' good practices, meaning that the status quo will remain forever. Good practices will change over time, because a QoL framework changes over time. However, we are living in this decade and therefore it is important to have an actual focus on QoL outcomes for people with intellectual disabilities.

In the described examples and practices we could drain from a reservoir of practices on sensitizing practices, somewhat less-organizing practices were available and little reflecting practices. What matters in real-life for people with intellectual disabilities is not issues such as the chicken or egg question, but real QoL outcomes. The concept of QoL is definitely of use in progressing towards a reflecting model; namely, to justify policy and practice in contributing to and improving of the quality of life of people with intellectual disabilities.

The Dutch polder model is aimed at consensus, not necessarily at consistency. In the past the richest farmers mostly stipulated how and where the dikes were built. The ultimate objective for the future in the disabilities field is to strive not only for consensus, but consistency as well. Consensus is reached in sensitizing, organizing and reflecting applications of the QoL concept; at least at macro level in the Netherlands and the EU. The described practices in this chapter look like separate flowers, not making a well-arranged bunch of flowers – another famous Dutch export. If stakeholders at all levels become partners, a world could be won.

References

Astegger, K. (2008). *Quality of life measures. Measuring quality of life in the workplace for people with intellectual disabilities. Research report.* EU Leonardo da Vinci program.

Brown, I., & Brown, R. I. (2003). *Quality of life and disability. An approach for community practitioners*. London: Jessica Kingsley Publishers.

Brown, R. I., & Schalock, R. L. (2006). *The concept of QoL and its application to persons with intellectual disabilities. Volume 1: Introduction and overview*. Dickson: IASSID Special Interest Research Group on QoL.

Coalition for Inclusion. (2008). *Speerpunten coalitie*. (*Spearheads coalition*). Retrieved December 12, 2008, from http://www.coalitievoorinclusie.nl/speerpunten.html

Disability High Level Group. (2007). *Quality of social services of general interest*. Brussels: Disability HLG.

EASPD, European Association of Service providers for Persons with Disabilities. (2006). *Memorandum on a European quality principles framework*. Brussels: EASPD.

Kwaliteitskader Gehandicaptenzorg. (*Quality framework disabilities*). (2007). Utrecht: VGN.

Landelijke Federatie Belangenverenigingen Onderling Sterk. (2009). *Wat willen wij? (What do we want?)*. Retrieved February 16, 2009, from: http://www.onderling-sterk.nl/index.php?id=1076

Lewin, K. (1947). Group decision and social change. In T. M. Newcomb & E. L. Hartley (Eds.), *Readings in social psychology* (pp. 340–344). New York: Henry Holt and Co.

Ministry of Health, Welfare & Sport. (2006). *The new care system in the Netherlands*. Den Haag: Ministerie van VWS.

Pameyer (2009). *Vision & mission statement*. Retrieved February 16, 2009, from http://www.pameijer.nl/

Platform VG (2009). *Algemene informatie*. Retrieved February 16, 2009, from http://www.platformvg.nl/Platform_VG/Algemeen

Quality of Life Measures. (2009). *Quality of life measures in employment*. Retrieved March 9, 2009 from http://qol.euproject.org

Schalock, R. L., & Verdugo, M. A. (2002). *Handbook on QoL for human science practicioners*. Washington, DC: AAMR.

Schippers, A. P. (2003). *Het spel en de knikkers. Kwaliteit van ondersteuningsplannen voor mensen met een verstandelijke beperking*. (*It's all in the game. Quality of support plans for people with an intellectual disability*). Nunspeet: Stichting Philadelphia Zorg. Dissertation.

Schippers, A., & Van Boheemen, M. (2009). Family QoL empowered by family-oriented support. *Journal of Policy and Practice in Intellectual Disabilities*, *6*(1), 19–24.

SCP, Social and Cultural Planning Office of the Netherlands. (2005). *Zorg voor verstandelijk gehandicapten. Ontwikkelingen in de vraag. (Care for intellectual disabled. Developments in the demand)*. Den Haag: SCP.

Van Dalen, A. (2007). *Het kan anders en het werkt*! *Esdégé-Reigersdaal: kiezen voor anders besturen*. (*A different way proved to be possible*! *Esdégé-Reigersdaal: Choosing for different steering*.). Amsterdam: Annemarie van Dalen.

Van Gennep, A. (1994). *De zorg om het bestaan. Over verstandelijke handicap, kwaliteit en ondersteuning* (*Caring about life. About intellectual disability, quality and support*). Amsterdam/Meppel: Boom.

Van Gennep, A. (2000). *Emancipatie van de zwaksten in de samenleving. Over paradigma's van verstandelijke handicap* (*Emancipation of the weakest in the society. About paradigms of intellectual disability*). Amsterdam: Boom.

Van Loon, J. H. M., & Van Hove, G. (2001). Emancipation and self-determination of people with learning disabilities and down-sizing institutional care. *Disability & Society*, *16* (2), 233–254.

VGN Dutch Association of Careproviders in Disabilities. (2007). *De professionele gehandicaptenzorg. In dialoog werken aan de kwaliteit van bestaan* (*The professional disabilities field. Contributing in dialogue to quality of life*). Utrecht: Author.

Wijngaarden, Bv. an, Kok, I., & Sixma, H. (2008). De bruikbaarheid van een CQ-index voor de ggz, verslavingszorg en gehandicaptenzorg: eerste bevindingen (The feasibility of a Customer Quality index for the psychiatric field, the addiction field and the disabilities field: first findings). *TSG: Tijdschrift voor Gezondheidswetenschappen*, *86*(8), 463–470.

Wikipedia. *The polder model*. Retrieved December 8, 2008, from http://en.wikipedia.org/wiki/Polder_model

WHO (World Health Organization). (1993). *WHO QoL Study Protocol*. Geneva: Author.

Chapter 9
Differences in Variables Influencing the Ratings of Importance and Use of Quality of Life Domains and Indicators by Polish Services Users and Their Parents

Wojciech Otrębski

Introduction

After 20 years of the socio-economic transformation, community-based services for people with ID in Poland are still in need for further development and improvement. The psychological category of quality of life seems to be one of the best suited for application in the process of building the new service delivery systems for various target groups, including people with ID (Bańka, 2005; Keith & Bonham, 2005; Kowalik, 2001; Oleś, 2002; Wołowicka, 2001). In the context of using the concept of QOL as the basis for developing and providing services for persons with ID, it seems crucial to analyse how service users and their parents evaluate the importance and use of QOL indicators. On one hand, these two groups are the first to benefit from improvements, and on the other hand, they exert an extensive influence on the way the services are provided (Jenaro et al., 2005; Otrebski, 2000, 2005).

Method

Participants

The results of this chapter are a part of a larger community-based research project carried out in a range of both rural and urban settings in Poland (villages, major and minor towns) where contacts were made with 67 intellectually disabled service users (53.70% women and 46.30% men) and 73 parents (60.30% women and 39.70% men). The number of parents was bigger than that of intellectually disabled individuals since in six cases both parents filled up the survey questionnaires (Table 9.1).

W. Otrębski (✉)
Department of Rehabilitative Psychology, Institute of Psychology, John Paul II Catholic University of Lublin, Lublin, Poland
e-mail: Otrebski@kul.pl

R. Kober (ed.), *Enhancing the Quality of Life of People with Intellectual Disabilities*, Social Indicators Research Series 41, DOI 10.1007/978-90-481-9650-0_9,

Table 9.1 Demographic characteristics of the service users group

Variables	Frequency (f)	Percentage (P)
Gender		
Female	36	53.70
Male	31	46.30
Age		
16–20	18	26.90
21–25	14	20.90
26–30	16	23.90
31 or more	19	28.30
Level of ID		
Mild	35	52.20
Moderate or lower	32	47.80
Multiple disorders		
Not present	22	32.80
Present	45	67.20
Place of living		
Villages	17	25.40
Small towns	20	29.80
Big cities	30	44.70
Family situation		
Both parents	43	64.20
One parent missing	23	34.3
Married couple	1	1.80
Number of siblings		
No sibling	5	7.50
One	14	20.90
Two	19	28.40
Three or more	18	26.80
Missing data	11	16.40
Economic well-being		
Bad	1	1.50
Average	46	68.70
Good	20	29.90

The individuals with ID were in the age range from 16 to over 31 years. The level of intellectual disability was described as mild in 52.20% and as moderate or higher in 47.80%. The majority of the investigated service users (67.20%), suffered from other co-occurring disorders in addition to their intellectual disability. More than half of them (64.20%) lived with both parents. Approximately, 70% of the subjects described their family economic status as average and the remaining as good (Table 9.1).

Parents of the individuals with intellectually disabilities were aged 38 years and above. Approximately, the half of the parents sample were parents of children

Table 9.2 Demographic characteristics of the parents group

Variables	Frequency (f)	Percentage (P)
Gender		
Female	44	60.30
Male	29	39.70
Age		
38–50	27	37.00
51–60	29	39.70
61 or more	17	23.30
Level of child's ID		
Mild	39	53.40
Moderate or lower	34	46.60
Level of education		
Primary school	11	15.10
Vocational school	25	34.20
High school	32	43.80
Diploma, undergraduate, or postgraduate	5	6.80
Place of living		
Villages	20	27.40
Small towns	21	27.80
Big cities	32	43.80
Employment status		
Employed	18	24.70
Retired/disability pension	45	61.60
Unemployed	10	13.70
Economic well-being		
Bad	9	12.30
Average	45	61.60
Good	19	26.10

with mild and moderate ID. The parents' education was at high school diploma (43.80%), vocational school (34.20%), primary school (15.10%) and undergraduate and graduate (6.80%) levels (Table 9.2).

Survey Instrument

The Cross-Cultural Survey on Quality of Life Indicators (Verdugo & Schalock 2001) was translated into Polish by the author. Two types of equivalence were established: conceptual and linguistic. The survey instrument is based on the 24 core indicators and eight QOL domains identified in the international QOL literature (Schalock & Verdugo 2002). For each of the 24 indicators, two sets of questions are asked which address both the importance and the use of a given indicator: (I) "How important is it (the indicator) for people with ID in your country?" And (II) "How much is it used in services/supports received or delivered". A 4-point Likert scale is used to scale the response dimensions for both sets of questions:

- Importance: not important (1), not very important (2), somewhat important (3), and very important and
- Use: never (1), sometimes (2), frequently (3), always (4).

Two types of reliability were established: Cronbach's alpha coefficients ranged from 0.92 to 0.95 with the average of 0.94 (SD = 0.01); split-half coefficients ranged from 0.84 to 0.92 with the average of 0.89 (SD = 0.03). These values indicate high reliability, and are consistent with comparable studies (Jenaro et al., 2005).

Survey Procedure

First, the contacts were made with the respective service users and then their parents were asked to participate in the survey. Both groups were familiarized with the chapter's purpose and procedure. Generally, the groups demonstrated favourable attitudes towards the survey.

Data Analysis

The following statistical analyses were applied to the data. For the description of the depended variable, mean scores and standard deviations were calculated for each of the eight QOL domains based on the Likert ratings across the indicators for a given domain. These data were analysed through the use of *t*-tests or Mann–Whitney tests, parametric one-way ANOVA, and Kruskall–Wallis ANOVA, as suitable for the variables properties.

Results

Importance

As shown in Tables 9.3 and 9.5, the evaluations of the importance of eight QOL domains were associated with different sets of variables in the group of the service users and in the group of their parents. The evaluations were significantly higher in the group of individuals with ID than in the parent group.

In the group of service users, the perception of the importance of interpersonal relationships, as indicative of their QOL, were associated with the level of intellectual disability and the place of residence. Subjects with mild ID and those living in big cities perceived this domain as significantly more important than those with moderate or lower levels of ID ($p \leq 0.01$), and those living in villages and small towns ($p \leq 0.05$). The evaluation of the importance of material well-being by the service users was related only to the place of residence, where, again, those living in

Table 9.3 Mean scores and standard deviations obtained by the service users in Cross Cultural Perspective Survey – part I

	Em. Well. – 2		Int. Rel. – 1		Mat. Well. – 1		Per. Dev. – 1		Phy. Well. – 1		Phy. Well. – 2		Self. Det. – 1		Self. Det. – 2		Soc. Inc. – 1		Right – 1		Right – 2	
Variables	M	SD	M	SD	M	SD	M	SD	M	SD	M	SD	M	SD	M	SD	M	SD	M	SD	M	SD
Level of ID																						
Mild			3.70*	0.72			3.61*	0.55	3.65**	0.40	3.16**	0.65	3.54*	0.44	2.77**	0.67	3.47*	0.61	3.63*	0.63		
Moderate or lower			3.30	0.59			3.10	0.72	3.40	0.58	2.84	0.61	2.95	0.81	2.46	0.62	2.95	0.68	3.19	0.83		
Age																						
16–20	24.78**	0.68					38.92**	0.47					43.92**	0.38								
21–25	36.29**	0.72					33.36**	0.53					26.11**	0.72								
26–30	44.56**	0.46					41.09**	0.56					37.34**	0.62								
31 or more	32.16**	0.59					23.84**	0.85					27.61**	0.85								
Level of disability																						
Mild							40.18**	0.62					42.25*	0.53								
Moderate							27.76**	0.74					30.28*	0.73								
Severe							33.63**	0.79					23.13*	0.79								
Place of living																						
Villages	20.76*	0.57	23.03**	0.81	32.50**	0.68			20.74**	0.63												
Small towns	37.35*	0.73	36.70**	0.57	25.00**	0.46			39.25**	0.44												
Big cities	39.27*	0.54	38.42**	0.45	40.85**	0.52			38.02**	0.35												
Family situation																						
Both parents									3.60	0.43												
One parent missing									3.82**	0.23												
Number of siblings																						
One	33.14*	0.39							34.11**	0.29											34.89*	0.68
Two	29.26*	0.48							26.11**	0.34											26.11*	0.59
Three or more	17.00*	0.63							19.58**	0.47											18.97*	0.58

$^{*}p \leq 0.01$; $^{**}p \leq 0.05$.

Table 9.4 Mean scores and standard deviations obtained by the service users in Cross Cultural Perspective Survey – part II

	I		II		III		IV		V		VI		VII		VIII	
	M	SD	M	SD	M	SD	M	SD	M	SD	M	SD	M	SD	M	SD
Gender																
Female	29.63	2.09							38.58*	2.03						
Male	39.08*	2.47							28.68	1.83						
Level of ID																
Mild			29.21	2.22					40.07**	2.02						
Moderate or lower			39.23*	1.97					27.36	1.74						
Age																
16–20																
21–25																
26–30																
31 or more																
Multiple disorders																
Not present					25.91*	2.43										
Present					37.96*	2.30										
Place of living																
Villages			44.00*	2.35												
Small towns			32.75*	1.74												
Big cities			29.17*	2.27												
Level of disability																
Mild									41.21*	2.06						
Moderate									27.09*	1.65						
Severe									32.71*	2.02						
Family situation																
Both parents																
One parent missing																
Number of siblings																
One					35.25**	1.65			17.43*	1.44	22.96*	1.70				
Two					26.37**	1.92			28.84*	2.08	33.61*	2.65				
Tree or more					18.42**	2.22			29.67*	2.04	20.33*	2.71				

*$p \leq 0.05$; **$p \leq 0.01$.

Table 9.5 Mean scoresand standard deviations obtained by the parents in Cross Cultural Perspective Survey – part I

	Em. Well. – 2		Int. Rel. – 2		Mat. Well. – 2		Self. Det. – 1		Right – 1	
Variables	M	SD	M	SD	M	SD	M	SD	M	SD
Gender										
Female					2.45	0.77				
Male					2.84*	0.61				
Level of the child's ID										
Mild	3.26**	0.58	3.19*	0.63	2.76*	0.71	3.37*	0.59	3.49**	0.65
Moderate or lower	2.77	0.63	2.80	0.66	2.37	0.75	3.04	0.73	2.79	0.98

$^{*}p\leq 0.05$; $^{**}p\leq 0.01$.

big cities assessed this domain as significantly more important than did those living in villages and small towns ($p\leq 0.05$).

The possibility of personal development was evaluated as significantly more important for the description of QOL by the service users with mild levels of ID than by those with moderate or lower levels of ID ($p\leq 0.001$). Similarly, this QOL domain assessed as significantly more important by the service users in the age range between 26 and 30 years as compared with the subjects from other ranges ($p\leq 0.05$), and for those with mild levels of disability as compared with individuals with greater levels of disability[1] (moderate or severe) ($p\leq 0.05$). The evaluation of the importance of physical well-being by the service users was again associated with the level of intellectual disability and place of residence but additionally with the familial situation and the number of siblings. For those who had mild levels of ID, lived in small towns, stayed with only one parent and had only one sibling this domain was significantly more important than for the others ($p\leq 0.05$).

The differences in self-determination were found related only to three demographic variables characterizing service users: the level of ID, age and level of disability. For the service users with the mild levels of ID as well as for those with mild levels of disability this domain was significantly more important than for those with lower levels of ID and disability ($p\leq 0.01$). A similar difference was observed between the service users in the age range of 16–20 and those from other age ranges ($p\leq 0.05$). The evaluation of the importance of social inclusion and rights in the group of subjects with ID differed significantly with regard to only one demographic characteristic: the level of ID. Those individuals with mild ID assess them as more important then did the others ($p\leq 0.01$).

[1] In Poland there are different classifications for levels of ID and for level of disability. In regards to levels of ID, Poland follows DSM-IV. Level of disability is assessed based on an individual's ability to live an independent life. Thus, although the names of the levels are the same (mild, moderate, severe), the constructs are measuring different criteria.

With regards to the evaluation of the importance of QOL domains for the parents group, only two of the domains were found to be associated with one demographic characteristic: the level of child's ID. For the parents of the children with mild levels of ID, self-determination and rights were significantly more important QOL domains than for the parents of children with greater levels of ID ($p \leq 0.05$ and $p \leq 0.01$, respectively).

Use

As presented in Tables 9.3 and 9.5, the service users and their parents' evaluations of the use were less differentiated than for the importance regarding their demographic characteristics. Differences were found in six domains for the individuals with ID and in three domains in the parents groups.

In the group of service users, the differences in the emotional well-being as an indicator of their QOL were associated with age ($p \leq 0.05$), place of residence ($p \leq 0.01$) and number of siblings ($p \leq 0.05$). For those who were between 26 and 30 years of age, for those living in big cities, and for those who had one sibling, this domain was significantly more useful than for other groups of responders.

The differences in physical well-being and self-determination were found to be related to only one demographic variable characterizing the service users: level of ID ($p \leq 0.05$ and $p \leq 0.05$). Those with mild levels of ID perceived this domain as of significantly more use in service delivery than did those with moderate or lower levels of ID. For two other domains, social inclusion and rights, the associations were observed only with the number of siblings. These domains were seen as significantly more useful by those service users who had one sibling than by those with more siblings.

With regard to the evaluation of the use of QOL domains among the parents, three of the domains were found to be associated with the level of the child's ID, and one of these three domains was additionally associated with the parent's gender. Emotional well-being ($p \leq 0.01$), interpersonal relationship ($p \leq 0.05$) and material well-being ($p \leq 0.05$) were rated as being of significantly more use by the parents of children with mild ID than for by the parents of children with moderate or lower levels of ID. Additionally, the last mentioned domain was rated by males as being used significantly more often as compared with females ($p \leq 0.05$).

Ranks

As a part of the Survey, each participant was asked to rank the eight domains with respect to their importance for the description of QOL for persons with ID (Tables 9.4 and 9.6). The findings from the service users indicated that:

- emotional well-being was ranked as significantly more important by male than female responders ($p \leq 0.05$),

Table 9.6 Mean scores and standard deviation obtained by the parents in Cross Cultural Perspective Survey – part II

	Emotional well-being		Interpersonal relationship		Material well-being		Personal development		Social inclusion	
	M	SD	M	SD	M	SD	M	SD	M	SD
Gender										
Female							30.44	2.06		
Male							46.95*	2.05		
Level of child's ID										
Mild					40.55*	2.26			40.88*	2.23
Moderate or lower					27.78	2.22			27.35	2.09
Employment status										
Employed			40.14**	4.22						
Retired/ disability pension	16.89**	3.11	28.74	2.98			17.31*	4.51		
Unemployed	10.20	1.80					9.45	3.00		
Economical well-being										
Average									35.56**	2.18
Good/very good									25.26	2.25

*$p \leq 0.01$; **$p \leq 0.05$.

- interpersonal relationships were ranked as significantly more important by those with moderate or lower levels of ID ($p \leq 0.05$) and by those living in villages ($p \leq 0.05$) as compared with those with mild levels of ID and living in non-rural areas,
- the service users with multiple disorders gave higher ranks to the material well-being domain than those without ($p \leq 0.05$), additionally, the highest ranks were ascribed to this domain by those having one sibling and the lowest ranks by those having three or more siblings ($p \leq 0.05$),
- physical well-being was the domain associated with the biggest number of variables: the female service users, those with the mild levels of ID and disability, and those with two or three siblings evaluated this domain as more important than, respectively, the males ($p \leq 0.01$), those with lower levels of ID ($p \leq 0.01$) and disability ($p \leq 0.05$), and those having one sibling ($p \leq 0.05$),
- the service users having two siblings assessed the self-determination domain as more important than did the others (with one or three siblings) ($p \leq 0.05$).

There were less statistically significant associations between the demographic characteristics and the domains ranks among the parents. The findings from the parents indicated that:

- emotional well-being was perceived as the domain most important for the evaluation of QOL in person with ID significantly more frequently by those parents who were retried or lived on disability pension than those who were unemployed ($p \leq 0.05$),
- interpersonal relationships were viewed as important for QOL evaluation significantly more frequent by the employed parents than by those retried or living on disability pension ($p \leq 0.05$),
- material well-being and social inclusion were two domains which were perceived as important for the evaluation of QOL in person with ID significantly more frequently by the parents of children with lower levels of ID ($p \leq 0.01$); additionally, the importance of the second of these domains was associated also with the parents' economic status, were those who reported average financial conditions viewing this domain as more important than those who reported good or very good financial condition ($p \leq 0.01$),
- personal development was the last domain whose rankings showed significant differences as a function of such variables as the parents' gender and employment status. The fathers and the parents who were retried or lived on disability pension perceived this domain as important for the evaluation of QOL in persons with ID more frequently than the mothers ($p \leq 0.01$) and unemployed parents ($p \leq 0.01$).

Cross-Group Analyses: Importance, Use and Ranks

Comparisons between the assessments of the eight QOL domains made by the service users and their parents revealed several significant differences (Tables 9.7 and 9.8). When evaluating the *importance* of the domains, the group of service users perceived two of them – material well-being and physical well-being – as significantly more important than the group of parents ($p \leq 0.01$ and $p \leq 0.05$, respectively). With regard to the evaluations of the *use* of the domains by the service providers, social inclusion and rights were the two which service users perceived as significantly more important than their parents ($p \leq 0.05$ and $p \leq 0.01$, respectively).

The analysis of the QOL domains *ranking* showed that there was only one significant difference between evaluations of the service users and their parents (Table 9.9).

Table 9.7 Mean scores and standard deviations obtained by the service users and their parent in Cross Cultural Perspective Survey – part I (importance) and differences between the groups

	Em. Well.	Int. Rel.	Mat. Well.		Per. Dev.		Phy. Well.	Self. Det.		Soc. Inc.		Right
	M	M	M	SD	M	SD	M	M	SD	M	SD	M
Parents	66.14	66.82	2.60	0.76	3.26	0.65	64.23	3.21	0.66	3.21	0.63	65.30
Service users	75.25	74.51	3.35*	0.57	3.37	0.68	77.34**	3.26	0.71	3.22	0.70	76.16

*$p \leq 0.01$; **$p \leq 0.05$.

Table 9.8 Mean scores and standard deviations obtained by the service users and their parents in Cross Cultural Perspective Survey – part I (use) and differences between the groups

	Em. Well.		Int. Rel.		Mat. Well.		Per. Dev.		Phy. Well.		Self. Det.		Soc. Inc.		Right	
	M	SD	M	SD	M	SD	M	SD	M	SD	M	SD	M	SD	M	SD
Parents	3.04	0.64	3.02	0.66	2.60	0.74	2.90	0.75	2.95	0.71	2.68	0.61	2.78	0.63	2.76	0.80
Service users	3.13	0.60	3.12	0.70	2.65	0.76	3.06	0.58	3.01	0.65	2.62	0.66	3.05*	0.71	3.11**	0.70

*$p \leq 0.05$; **$p \leq 0.01$.

Table 9.9 Mean scores and standard deviations obtained by the service users and their parents in Cross Cultural Perspective Survey – part II and differences between the groups

	Em. Well. M	Int. Rel. M	Mat. Well. M	Per. Dev. M	Phy. Well. M	Self. Det. M	Soc. Inc. M	Right M
Parents	68.73	71.92	65.97	67.84	69.67	69.56	63.64	73.98
Service users	72.43	68.96	75.43	73.40	71.40	71.52	77.98*	67.49

*$p \leq 0.05$.

The group of service users ranked the domain of social inclusion significantly higher in evaluating QOL in persons with ID than their parents did ($p \leq 0.05$).

Discussion

According to Schalock (2004), what we know and will continue to learn bout QOL, specifically about its application to people with ID, can make a difference in both peoples' lives and in policies and practices that impact those lives. The results of the current chapter presented above may extend our knowledge about QOL. The results indicate that demographic variables play a significant role in differentiating the perception of the importance and use of some QOL domains among service users and their parents. This chapter also yielded a finding that there are certain differences between these two groups in this aspect.

All those who deliver the services/support to the individuals with ID and their families should be aware that perception of the importance and use of QOL domains may vary depending on such personal characteristics as: the level of ID, age, level of disability; and on such social characteristics as: place of residence, family situation, number of siblings. Among the parents of the individuals with ID, this variation appears to be associated with such variables as gender and the level of the child's ID.

Second, it would be useful for service providers to remember that ratings of the QOL domains among service users and their parents also fluctuate depending on demographic characteristics. For the persons with ID it may be gender, level of ID, multiple disorders, level of disability – as personal characteristics – and place of living and number of siblings – as social characteristics. In contrast, for the parents, it is only gender out of personal characteristics, and the level of the child's ID, employment status and economical well-being out of social variables that are associated with QOL domains ratings.

With regard to the well-known common wisdom that differences between generations always exist, we partially obtained empirical confirmation for this in the field of QOL. The differences between the service users and their parents were revealed with respect to two QOL domains in the case of the perception of importance and use of QOL domains, and with respect to one QOL domain in the case of ranking.

It may safely be concluded that the presented results of this chapter, similarly to the previously published work by Keith and Bonham (2005) enrich our knowledge about the possibilities of the application of QOL concepts into organizations that provide services for people with ID and their families.

References

Bańka, A. (Ed.). (2005). *Psychology of the quality of life*. Poznań: Association Psychology & Architecture.

Jenaro, C., Verdugo, M. A., Caballo, C., Balboni, G., Lachapelle, Y., Otrebski, W., et al. (2005). Cross-cultural study of person-centered quality of life domains and indicators: A replication. *Journal on Intellectual Disability Research, 49*(10), 799–805.

Keith, K. D., & Bonham, G. S. (2005). The use of quality of life data at the organization and systems level. *Journal on Intellectual Disability Research, 49*(10), 734–739.

Kowalik, S. (2001). Usefulness of the quality of life concept in the rehabilitation practice of disabled. In L. Wołowicka (Ed.), *Quality of life in the medical sciences* (pp. 54–77). Poznań: Medical Accademy Press.

Oleś, P. (2002). The quality of life in health and sickness. In P. Oleś, S. Steuden, & J. Toczołowski (Eds.), *How I can see less world. Vision impairments and quality of life* (pp. 37–42). Lublin: TN KUL.

Otrebski, W. (2000). Quality of life of people with mental retardation living in two different environments in Poland. In K. D. Keith & R. L. Schalock (Eds.), *Cross-cultural perspective on quality of life* (pp. 83–92). Washington, DC: American Association on Mental Retardation.

Otrębski, W. (2005). Variables influencing the ratings of importance and use of quality of life domains and indicators by Polish professionals. *Journal of Intellectual Disability Research, 49*(10), 750–755.

Schalock, R., & Verdugo, M. A. (2002). *Handbook on quality of life for human service practitioners*, Washington, DC: AAMR.

Schalock, R. L. (2004). The concept of quality of life: What we know and do not know. *Journal of Intellectual Disability Research, 48*(3), 203–216.

Verdugo, M. A., & Schalock, R. L. (2001). *Cross-cultural survey of quality of life indicators*. Salamanca, Spain: Institute on Community Integration, Faculty of Psychology.

Wołowicka L. (Ed.). (2001). *Quality of life in medical sciences*. Poznań: Medical Academy Press.

Chapter 10
Quality of Life of Individuals with Intellectual Disabilities and Their Families in China: Research and Applications

Mian Wang

Introduction

The notion of disability and special education has been first studied in China since antiquity. About some 2,000 years ago, the ancient Chinese texts recorded the call of philosophers and educators for treating individuals with disabilities with tolerance and for understanding the causes of disabling conditions (Pang & Richey, 2006). However, not until the late nineteenth century did the modern history of China's special education really begin when the first special schools were founded by US and European missionaries. Special education in China has undergone a slow and gradual development process in transition from a "charitable protection and training" stage to a "segregated special education" stage, and further to inclusive education era ever since. Especially since 1990s, the Chinese society has witnessed a greater paradigm shift on special education system in accompany with China's dramatic social change and economic growth.

However, many new challenges emerged as a result of the transition from a solely segregated special education system to an integrated system where special education schools, special classes in regular schools, and suiban jiudu ("Learning in Regular Classrooms", deemed as the Chinese version of inclusion) coexist. Chief among these challenges are: scarcity of educational opportunities for students with disabilities, scarcity of qualified special educators, lack of instructional quality (e.g., lack of adaptive curricula and instructional strategies) and accountability (lack of specific evaluation for students with disabilities), and lack of family and professional collaboration. The concept of quality of life (QOL) was introduced to China at the time and soon became an emerging area of study that is believed to offer solutions to some of the special education challenges (Xu, Wang, Xiang, & Hu, 2005). In this chapter, I will provide an overview of individual and family quality of life (FQoL) research in China and a summary of important applications of QOL and FQoL framework to order to address the challenges that China's special education faces.

M. Wang (✉)
Education Department, Gevirtz Graduate School of Education, University of California, Santa Barbara, CA 93106, USA
e-mail: mwang@education.ucsb.edu

R. Kober (ed.), *Enhancing the Quality of Life of People with Intellectual Disabilities*, Social Indicators Research Series 41, DOI 10.1007/978-90-481-9650-0_10,

Overview of QOL Research in China

Quality of Life (QOL) studies began in China since 1980s and focused primarily on the objective well-beings of the elderly people and persons with chronic illness (Luo & Sun, 1995). The exploration of the QOL of people from disadvantaged families was undertaken by sociologists in order to develop social welfare policies and guide practices (Xia, 1999). At the time, the QOL research had its priorities on studying objective well-being that pertains to family income, living conditions and family relationships given the improvement of quality of life of the population in relation to China's rapid economic growth in the past decades. As the QOL research continued to expand in the twenty-first century, Chinese scholars have shifted the focus of study to the subjective well-being and have incorporated happiness about life in the QOL study (Zhou, 2008). In particular, numerous attempts were made to study the QOL concept and how to apply it in the field of special education and disability to improve social services for people with intellectual disabilities (ID) (see Xu, 2002, 2003, 2004; Xu, Wang, Xiang, & Hu, 2005).

Xu and colleagues have written a few conceptual papers in which they introduced the QOL framework developed in the international literature and discussed about how the QOL framework would affect the special education reform in China in order to embrace inclusion and improve service delivery system for individuals with disabilities (Xu, 2002, 2004). However, Shek and colleagues (2005) pointed out that culture plays an important role in the process of defining QOL in the Chinese context. While happiness and satisfaction are viewed substantial components of quality of life for people in the American culture, forbearance, endurance and contending mentality are emphasized more in the Chinese culture in terms of its importance and value to QOL (Shek et al., 2005). As a common belief in the Chinese traditional culture, happiness of life consists of four core elements: FU, LU, SHOU, and XI. As delineated by Xu et al. (2005), FU refers to well-being and good fortune; LU refers to benefits of officials in feudal China, but it denotes physical and financial well-being in a broader sense; SHOU means long life (denoting good health and longevity); and XI pertains to happiness. Chinese people believe four words altogether represent their dreams or expectations for a happy life. Interestingly, such a belief accords with some of the key elements of the QOL concept. In addition, as the modern Chinese society recognizes an emerging trend in the disability field where advocacy focuses on enhancing the independence and productivity of people with ID there is an urgent need to study all the important aspects of QOL concept in the Chinese context. In particular, it is important to understand how the QOL core domains and indicators identified in the international literature can be examined in the Chinese context to inquire about the etic (universal) and emic (cultural-bound) properties of QOL. Xu and colleagues conducted a survey study to specifically explore how the QOL core domains and indicators are understood in the Chinese context through the lens of individuals with ID, their families, and professionals (Xu et al., 2005).

A total of 355 participants were recruited from four cities in the different regions of China: Beijing, Harbin, Ningbo, and Chengdu. Of those participants, there were

87 individuals with moderate ID (46 males and 41 females), 58 parents (52% of whom were mothers) of individuals with ID, and 210 professionals (teachers or rehabilitation personnel who provide service to the individuals with ID). Xu et al. (2005) used the Chinese version of the *Cross-Cultural Survey of Quality of Life Indicators* (Verdugo & Schalock, 2003) which is a 4-point Likert scale including both Importance and Use ratings of the 24 core QOL indicators. The survey was made in three forms for individuals with ID, parents, and professionals, respectively. Data from the three respondent groups were analyzed by running exploratory factor analysis (principal component analysis).

The results of factor analysis showed that seven factors emerged in the respondent group of individuals with ID accounting for 67.3% of total variance. Two of the eight QOL domains (personal development and physical well-being) were highly correlated ($r = 0.74$, $p<0.01$) and loaded onto one component in the analysis. The fact that seven principal components of QOL of Chinese respondents with ID are consistent with the eight core domains of QOL identified in the international QOL literature suggests the etic properties of QOL concept (Schalock et al., 2002). In addition, all three respondent groups reported similar ranking of the importance of 8 QOL domains. In particular, individuals with ID ranked importance of the 8 QOL domains in a descending order as: Physical well-being, Rights, Material well-being, Emotional well-being, Personal development, Social inclusion, Interpersonal relations, and Self-determination.

A subsequent study that included a total of 541 participants recruited from six cities (Beijing, Shanghai, Chongqing, Chengdu, Harbin, and Ningbo) was conducted to reexamine the factor structure of QOL (Xiang, Xu, & Wang, 2007). As an extension of their prior inquiry endeavors in determining the major domains of QOL in the Chinese context, they found in this study that individuals with ID do have some different opinions as compared to their parents and professionals in rating the importance and use of the QOL domains. However, individuals with ID, their parents, and teachers concurred that health (physical well-being) is the most important QOL domain in their rankings. The results of factor analysis show that there is a 7-factor structure of QOL for individuals with ID, a 5-factor structure of QOL for their parents, and a 3-factor structure of QOL from the professionals' point of view.

Overview of FQoL Research in China

In response to the increasing emphasis in family-centered service model and the development and advancement of QOL research since 1980s, Family Quality of Life (FQoL) research has emerged as a new field of study in the field of developmental and intellectual disabilities (Poston et al., 2003, Schalock, 2004, Brown & Brown, 2004). In the United States, leaders have advocated for the family-centered approach that focuses on quality of life of families of children with disabilities as a desired outcome measure of disability policy and service system (Bailey et al., 1998; Dunst & Bruder, 2002; Turnbull, 2003). A series of studies were carried out by the researchers at the Beach Center to conceptualize the FQoL and develop the measure of FQoL. The findings of their studies suggest a 5-factor FQoL construct that contains domains of Family Interaction, Parenting, Physical/material well-being, emotional well-being, and disability-related supports (Park et al., 2003; Poston et al., 2003; Summer et al., 2005).

As the FQoL research continues to evolve, there is a remarkable increase of international interest in studying FQoL cross-culturally (Aznar & Castanon, 2005; Brown, Anand, Fung, Isaacs, & Baum, 2003; Tang et al., 2005; Turnbull, Brown, & Turnbull, 2004). A group of international researchers from Australia, Canada, Israel, the UK, and the United States involved in a collaborative project to study FQoL and developed a survey tool (Isaac et al., 2007). Bayat (2005) studied the perception of FQoL of Indian parents who have a child with autism and effect of autism on their FQoL. Verdugo, Cordoba, and Gomez (2005) examined the reliability and validity of the Spanish version of the Family Quality of Life Scale (FQOL) and found the FQOL scale was a valid instrument for the research of families with children with disabilities in Spanish-spoken countries.

Some family studies done in the Chinese context were somewhat related to some of FQoL domains. Researchers have investigated the Chinese parents' concerns about education opportunities and independence of their children with ID (Lei & Wu, 2000), and parenting styles and its influences on their mental health (Jiang, 2004). Yet other family studies focused on family needs of children with ID and found the most urgent family needs are professional support and emotional support (Wang, 1993; Mu, 1995; Zhang, Chen, He, & Liu, 2004), Xu (2001, 2003) studied the QOL of Chinese families of children with ID and found that there are significant positive correlations among stress, self-blaming, and imaginative coping styles of fathers, as well as positive correlations among stress, self-blaming, and withdrawing coping styles of mothers. He also found that there is a significant negative correlation between parental stress and their quality of life (Xu, 2003). Researchers from Taiwan developed the Family Quality of Life Questionnaire for Young Children with Special Needs (FQOLQ-YCSN) which was partly based upon the domain structure of the FQOL scale developed by the Beach Center on Disability (Tang et al., 2005). However, little is known about the FQoL of families of children with ID in China.

Hu and Wang (2008) conducted a survey study to examine the factor structure of FQoL of Chinese families with child with ID and influencing factors of FQoL in China. In this study, we randomly selected 560 participants (mothers or fathers) from the families whose children with ID attend 12 special schools (six schools from the urban area and six from the suburban area) in Beijing. Of 560 families who received the survey, 442 parents actually returned the completed survey and the return rate is 78.9%. The Chinese version of the *Family Quality of Life Scale* (Beach Center, 2004) was used in the study. The Family Quality of Life Scale (FQOLS, Beach Center, 2004) measured family perceptions of both the importance and satisfaction of different domains of FQOL in a 5-point Likert-type scale. The FQOLS contains 25 items grouped into five subscales: Family Interaction, Parenting, Emotional Well-being, Physical/Material Well-being, and Disability-related Support, and the scale has excellent psychometric properties (see Hoffman et al., 2006; Wang et al., 2006). The Chinese version of the FQOLS was pilot studied and field tested, and as a result two scale items were modified for cultural appropriateness.

We used the Structural Equation Modeling (SEM) techniques to run a confirmatory factor analysis (CFA) to test the factor structure of FQoL in the Chinese sample. We also employed MANOVA to examine group difference of families with different demographic features: living conditions (e.g., housing situations and transportation means), family income, and severity of disability of child with respect to their perception of FQOL. The CFA results showed that there is a good model fit for the 5-factor FQoL model in the Chinese sample ($\chi^2(265, n = 442) = 784.17$, $p = 0.0$, RMSEA = 0.072 (0.067|0.078), CFI = 0.97, NNFI = 0.97). Such results suggest that there is a similar 5-factor structure of FQoL construct of Chinese families of children with ID as compared to that of American families. In addition to the proof of good construct validity of the scale, the FQoL survey (Chinese version) was also found to have good reliability (e.g., the Cronbach's alphas of all five subscales and the overall scale varying from .77 to .91). Our study offers evidence to the assumption about the etic property of FQoL construct across cultures.

The results of MANOVA show that there is a significantly statistical difference between families with different housing situations and between families with different transportation means on their satisfaction ratings of FQoL domains. Significant differences were also found between families with different family income levels and between families of children who have different levels of severity of disability. These findings are consistent with studies done to families in other cultures (Wang, Mannan, Poston, Turnbull, & Summers, 2004; Schalock & Verdugo, 2002; Felce & Perry, 1995). The previous studies suggested that severity of intellectual disability has impact on family quality of life (Wang et al., 2004). We confirm such findings in the Chinese context. Feng and Yi (2002) suggested that family's socio-economic status is one of the key indicators of family well-being. The findings in our study confirm such suggestion.

The fact that Chinese families of children with ID living with different housing options differ significantly from each other about their perception of FQoL confirms the earlier study findings about the effect of housing conditions on quality of life of adults with ID (Felce & Perry, 1995). In addition, The findings that Chinese families of children with ID who have different transportation means to access to service differ significantly from each other in perceiving the importance of and satisfaction with FQoL are consistent with the early study conclusion that transportation is an important influencing factor of family quality of life of individuals with ID (Schalock et al., 2002).

Applications of QOL and FQoL in China

The concept of QOL has significantly impacted the social integration, education opportunities, employment, and personal development of individuals with ID in China. The impacts are well reflected in the reforms and changes regarding curriculum development, intervention and rehabilitation models, and employment.

As special education rapidly grew in 1980s in China, lack of adaptive and functional curricula became a huge problem for making an education plan for students with ID. Special education schools simply adopted the general curriculum used in the regular schools and hoped the teachers could modify as needed when they teach students with ID. The key foci of the general curriculum are academic subject knowledge and skills that prepare students to perform well in the tests in order to advance to secondary education and higher education. No surprising, the use of general curriculum could not accommodate the individual learning needs of many students with ID. Chinese educators started to study and try to develop a functional curriculum for students with ID. The QOL framework was used to guide the development of new QOL-oriented curriculum (Xu, 2001). On the basis of QOL research, the QOL-oriented curriculum emphasized the importance of recognizing the expectations and needs of students with disabilities. The QOL-oriented curriculum focused on helping students with ID to realize their own dreams and expectation, develop a positive self-concept and interpersonal relationships, increase opportunities of community integration, and enhance their achievement and happiness. For the fulfillment of these goals, the new curriculum emphasized maintaining the consistency and harmony between the individual with ID and the environment. The core QOL domains identified in the research literature were used as the basis to guide the process of QOL-oriented curriculum development and application of such a curriculum.

The QOL concept has also made important influence on the reform of special education and rehabilitation service models in China. Special education for students with ID began to expand in the 1980s. However, at the time, segregated special education schools were still the "mainstream" of the China's special education system. With the strong call for more inclusive education, more schools seemed to have embraced the "Learning in Regular Classroom" model. However, implementation of inclusion in a multi-mode special education system faces many challenges and barriers. Along with the new AAMR definition system which emphasizes support system, the QOL concept was introduced to Chinese special education. Chinese educator began to understand and learn from the QOL research about how to establish the support system to help improve QOL for people with ID. As a result, a supported education framework for people with ID in China was proposed (Xu, 2005). Supported education model includes the following elements and characteristics: a dynamic and pluralistic education placement system for students with ID that has replaced the former single placement model (special education school), a functional curriculum that should replace or complement the solely academic subject-oriented curriculum, a community-based teaching model that should substitute the classroom-teaching model, the emphasis of children-centered learning strategies that should substitute the teacher-centered teaching strategies, the emphasis of active parents involvement that has been lacking in China's education system, and the multi-component and multi-method evaluation that should be established to substitute the grade passing and knowledge test model. The supported education model is still in the early stage of development and implementation. However, the QOL framework has provided a solid foundation to promote the development of such a model as well as a multi-subjects rehabilitation model.

The QOL framework has also impacted the thinking of employment and career development for people with ID. A QOL-oriented rehabilitation model emphasizes the areas of independence, productivity, and community integration for people with ID to be able to improve. This gives rise to the emphasis of supported employment and supported living model for adults with ID to be able to implement. In the former planned economy in China, sheltered employment was the predominant option for people with disabilities. The manufacturing factories sponsored through the social welfare system of the Chinese government offered limited opportunities for people with disabilities, particularly for those with hearing impairments and physical disabilities, and sometimes for a few people with ID to work and self-sustain. However, with the advent of a market economy system in China, the former welfare-based employment model encountered fundamental challenges. The supported employment model for people with ID has become a well-recognized model to resolve those challenges and lead to the fulfillment of goal for helping adults with ID to live a quality of life.

Overall, the paradigm shift of service delivery model from process-focused to outcome-oriented reveals the need of embracing a more comprehensive framework to guide the reform of education and social service system at both policy-making and practice levels (Xu, 2002). So the QOL concept has become a sensitizing concept in today's Chinese society and an important theoretical framework for the reform of education and rehabilitation for people with ID.

Families have been the major source of support to their child with a disability in China due to the lack of service delivery system. So supporting families to support their children with disabilities should become an important priority in both policy and practice in China. Community-based education and support is a vehicle of support for improving quality of life of families living in most rural areas of China. The results of Hu and Wang's study (2007) show that Chinese families are not satisfied with the outside support and safety in community. In recent years, professionals in China have given more attention to the important role of community education and related services as to improve family support (Huang & Liu, 2006; Lei, 2001). Education agencies should promote community education in practice to increase the public's knowledge about intellectual disabilities, organize activities for families of children with ID, their siblings and relatives, to make families more involved in and integrated into the community.

Professionals and practitioners should take the family-level support into consideration in order to enhance the overall FQoL. Family support service should be emphasized in policy and implemented fully given that Chinese families have ranked Disability-Related Support as the most domain of FQoL which is often lacking in their life. In China, there is still no recommended individualized family service plan or family-centered service system directed to families that are defined in the government policy.

In addition, a better health care system with more health insurance options available should be established to provide more and better opportunities of service to families of children with ID because families have indicated in our survey study that they are least satisfied with the medical services. At present, Chinese families have to use only one major insurance plan that is available to their children with ID and is often limited to families living in urban areas. Vocational training to increase working opportunities for individuals with ID is another important issue related to FQoL because the results of our survey study show that families were very concerned about the difficulty of employment for children when they are in transition to the adult service system.

Research provides important guidance to effective applications of FQoL. The FQoL studies of Chinese families have limited generalizability given the limitation of study samples. Future study is particularly needed to include Chinese families from other geographic regions in China especially those families from rural areas to reexamine the domains/indicators of FQoL. In addition, besides some family demographic variables that have been already studied (e.g., income, housing, disability condition, etc), many other factors related to services need to be studied in the future. For example, the future study should focus on investigating the service impact as a moderator on the relationship between risk factors (e.g., poverty, severity of disability, etc.) and FQoL. Understanding such relationships has very important implications for practices toward improving FQoL. In addition, FQoL has been used as an outcome measure of service delivery with the aim to promote family-centered service delivery system and enhance families' participation in services. More studies need to be carried out to evaluate the ongoing supports and services for families of children with ID and lead to data-driven decision making for developing better service delivery system. After all, there is still so much remaining unknown in the field and needing to be explored to inform our practices to enhance the quality of life of individual with ID and their families.

References

Aznar, A. S., & Castanon, D. G. (2005). Quality of life from the point of view of Latin American families: A participative research study. *Journal of Intellectual Disability Research, 49*(10), 784–788.

Bailey, D. B., McWilliam, R. A., Darkes, L. A., Hebbeler, K., Simeonsson, R. J., Spiker, D., et al. (1998). Family outcomes in early intervention: A framework for program evaluation and efficacy research. *Exceptional Children, 64*(3), 313–328.

Bayat, M. (2005). *How family members' perceptions of influences and causes of autism may predict assessment of their family quality of life*. ProQuest Information & Learning. Dissertation Abstracts International: Section B: The Sciences and Engineering, 66 (6–B).

Brown, I., Anand, S., Fung, W. L. A., Isaacs, B., & Baum, N. (2003). Family quality of life: Canadian results from an international study. *Journal of Developmental and Physical Disabilities, 15*(3), 207–229.

Brown, I., & Brown, R. (2004). Concept for beginning study in family quality of life. In A.Turnbull, I. Brown, & R. Turnbull (Eds.), *Families and people with mental retardation and quality of life: International perspectives* (pp. 27–47). Washington, DC: American Association on Mental Retardation.

Center, B. (2004). *Family quality of life scale*. Lawrence, KS: Beach Center on Disability, University of Kansas.

Dunst, C. J., & Bruder, M. B. (2002). Valued outcomes of service coordination, early intervention, and natural environments. *Exceptional Children, 68*(3), 361–375.

Felce, D., & Perry, J. (1995). The extent of support for ordinary living provided in staffed housing: the relationship between staffing levels, resident dependency, staff: resident interactions and resident activity patterns. *Social Science and Medicine, 40*, 799–810.

Feng, X. T., & Yi, S. G. (2002). Family quality of life for citizens: Indicators and structure. *Research on Sociology, 2000*(4), 107–118.

Hoffman, L., Marquis, J. G., Poston, D. J., Summers, J. A., & Turnbull, A. P. (2006). Assessing family outcomes: Psychometric evaluation of the Family Quality of Life Scale. *Journal of Marriage and Family, 68*, 1069–1083.

Hu, X., & Wang, M. (2007). *Cross-cultural family quality of life study on Chinese families with a child with an intellectual disability*. Paper presented at the IASSID Quality of Life Roundtable meeting, San Diego, CA.

Huang, J. J., & Liu, Y. H. (2006). Report on family support from society for exceptional children. *Journal of Chinese Special Education, 70*(4), 3–7.

Isaacs, B. J., Brown, I., Brown, R. I., Baum, N., Myerscough, T., Neikrug, S., et al. (2007). The international family quality of life project: Goals and description of a survey tool. *Journal of Policy and Practice in Intellectual Disabilities, 4*(3), 177–185.

Jiang, Q. D. (2004). The relationship of parenting style and mental health of students with mild MR. *Journal of Chinese Special Education, 2004*(7), 38–41.

Lei, J. H. (2001). Review and analysis of quality standard of special education. *Journal of Chinese Special Education, 36*(4), 7–11.

Lei, J. H., & Wu, C. Q. (2002). What issues parents with child with MR are concerned about? *Journal of Chinese Special Education, 2000*(4), 16–17.

Luo, J., & Sun, Y. (1995). Quality of life for people with cancer. *Journal of Cancer Studies in China, 22*(2), 19–23.

Mu, K. L. (1995). Study on parents' needs of students with MR. *Research on Exceptional Children and Teachers in China, 1995*(3), 18–22.

Pang, Y., & Richey, D. (2006). The development of special education in China. *International Journal of Special Education, 21*(1), 77–86.

Park, J., Hoffman, L., Marquis, J., Turnbull, A. P., Poston, D., Mannan, H., et al. (2003). Toward assessing family outcomes of service delivery: Validation of a family quality of life survey. *Journal of Intellectual Disability Research, 47*(5), 367–384.

Poston, D., Turnbull, A., Park, J., Mannan, H., Marquis, J., & Wang, M. (2003). Family quality of life: A qualitative inquiry. *Mental Retardation, 41*(5), 313–328.

Schalock, R. L. (2004). Quality of life from a motivational perspective. *International Review of Research in Mental Retardation, 28*, 303–319.

Schalock, R. L., & Verdugo, M. A. (2002). *Handbook on quality of life for human services practitioners*. Washington, DC: American Association on Mental Retardation.

Schalock, R. L., Brown, I., Brown, R., Cummins, R. A., Felce, D., Matikka, L., et al. (2002). Conceptualization, measurement, and application of quality of life for persons with intellectual disabilities: Report of an international panel of experts. *Mental Retardation, 40*(6), 457–470.

Shek, D. T. L., Chan, Y. K., & Lee, P. S. N. (2005). *Quality of life research in Chinese, Western, and Global Contexts*. Dordrecht: Springer.

Summers, J. A., Poston, D. J., Turnbull, A. P., Marquis, J. G., Hoffman, L., Mannan, H., et al. (2005). Conceptualizing and measuring family quality of life. *Journal of Intellectual Disability Research, 49*(10), 777–783.

Tang, C., Lin, K., Lin, J., Chen, Y., Lou, S., & Jean, Y. (2005). Family quality of life for young children with special needs: The measurement tool development in Taiwan. *Research on Disability in Taiwan, 13*(1), 33–52.

Turnbull, A. P. (2003). Family quality of life as an outcome of early intervention services: Research and practice directions. In B. F. Williams (Ed.), *Directions in early intervention and assessment* (pp. 477–498). Spokane, WA: Spokane Guilds' School and Neuromuscular Center.

Turnbull, A., Brown, I., & Turnbull, H. R. (Eds.) (2004). *Families and people with mental retardation and quality of life: International perspectives*. American Association on Mental Retardation, Washington, DC.
Verdugo, M. A., Cordoba, L., & Gomez, J. (2005). Spanish adaptation and validation of the family quality of life survey. *Journal of Intellectual Disability Research, 49*(10), 794–798.
Verdugo, M. A., & Schalock, R. L. (2003). *Cross-cultural survey of quality of life indicators*. Salamanca, Spain: Institute on Community Integration, Faculty of Psychology-University of Salamanca.
Wang, T. M. (1993). Study on family needs of children with MR. *Journal of Special Education Research in Taiwan, 1993*(9), 73–90.
Wang, M., Mannan, H., Poston, D., Turnbull, A. P., & Summers, J. A. (2004). Parents' perceptions of advocacy activities and their impact on family quality of life. *Research & Practice for Persons with Severe Disabilities, 29*, 144–155.
Wang, M., Turnbull, A., Little, T., Summers, J. A., Poston, D., & Mannan, H. (2006). Perspectives of fathers and mothers of children in early intervention programs in assessing family quality of life. *Journal of Intellectual Disabilities Research, 50*, 977–988.
Xia, G. M. (1999). Family quality of life for citizens of China. *Academic World, 74*(1), 40–46.
Xiang, Y., Xu, J., & Wang, M. (2007). Reexamination of core indicators of Quality of Life for Chinese individuals with mental retardation. *Chinese Journal of Special Education, 89*, 41–48.
Xu, J. (2002). The evolvement of the new definition of mental retardation: New tendency oriented to function, support and quality of life. *Chinese Journal of Special Education, 40*(4), 19–23.
Xu, J. (2004). Quality of life of Chinese people with mental retardation. *Chinese Journal of Special Education, 50*(8), 41–45.
Xu, J., Wang, M., Xiang, Y., & Hu, X. (2005). Quality of life for people with intellectual disabilities in China: A cross-culture perspectives study. *Journal of Intellectual Disability Research, 49*(10), 745–750.
Xu, M. Z. (2001). Study on cognitive and behavior problems of MR children with quality of life of their parents. *Journal of Chinese Special Education, 4*, 49–57.
Xu, M. Z. (2003). Study on stress coping style with quality of life for parents with MR child. *Journal of Chinese Special Education, 2*, 23–30.
Zhang, Y., Chen, Y. Q., He, W. H., & Liu, Y. H. (2004). Report on preschool family education for exceptional children in Beijing. *Journal of Chinese Special Education, 11*, 73–78.
Zhou, C. C. (Eds.). (2008). *Subjective quality of life: Indicators and evaluation*. Beijing: Social Science Publishing House.

Chapter 11
Begging to Live: The Strategy of Survival for People with Intellectual Disabilities in Nigeria

Patrick A. Edewor, Oluremi H. Abimbola, and Olujide A. Adekeye

Introduction

The link between intellectual disability and begging has received little attention in scholarly works in Nigeria. What is usually found in literature on the subject is the lumping together of all manners of disabilities (physical, mental, and intellectual). This situation has not helped in bringing to the fore, the imperatives of the seriousness the subject deserves both in academic and public policy parlance.

This chapter examines the various descriptions of intellectual disability in the Nigerian context; classification of street begging and the interface between the phenomenon of street begging and intellectual disability. The chapter concludes by suggesting how the quality of life of the intellectually disabled persons can be enhanced.

Intellectual Disability Described

Intellectual disability has been a subject of interest to scholars over the ages. The many dimensions of the subject (causes, detection, prevalence, and treatment/management) have been subjected to different strands of academic and practitioner-based analyses. For example, medicine has largely been concerned with the causes, epidemiology with the prevalence while psychology, sociology, and other related disciplines, with treatment and therapy/management.

Perception of causes of intellectual disabilities and treatment adopted are intertwined. In societies where most families conceive of the problem as a result of effect of demons, efforts are usually channeled toward either appeasing the demons or warding them off. A different approach of treatment is adopted in societies where the problem is viewed as a medical situation that can be managed.

It is interesting to note that cause-attribution of intellectual disability has followed a trend. In pre-progressive era, demonology had largely explained the cause.

P.A. Edewor (✉)
Department of Sociology, Covenant University, Ota, Ogun State, Nigeria
e-mail: edeworpat@yahoo.com

R. Kober (ed.), *Enhancing the Quality of Life of People with Intellectual Disabilities*, Social Indicators Research Series 41, DOI 10.1007/978-90-481-9650-0_11,

In most Nigerian societies, until recently, the cause of intellectual disabilities was attributed to gods who were out to avenge a parent's misdemeanor or sent to afflict the parent for no particular offence. This pattern of attribution goes a long way in mitigating parents of the persons with intellectual disabilities from making open to the public, the incidence of intellectual disability for fear of stigmatization by members of society.

Advances in medicine and education have, however, changed this perception to a large extent. The change in perception occasioned by advancement in medicine and education has not, however, translated to improvement in the quality of life of the intellectually disabled. This situation is not farfetched from lack of coordinated efforts by government, low level of education of parents, undisclosing nature of Nigerian families, lack of family-based care and pervasive poverty, among others.

The World Health Report (2001) contends that the prevalence level of intellectual disabilities in the world is between 1 and 3%. This implies that about 190 million people battle with intellectual disabilities as at the time of the report. One feature of intellectual disability is that its prevalence is not specific to a particular race, color, gender, educational group, or socio-economic background. However, World Health Organization (WHO) (2007) reports that location, socio-economic background, and ethnicity determine, to a large extent, access to treatment and management of intellectual disabilities. Aside from the above, education of parents also bear heavily on attitude to care and management.

One peculiarity with the Nigerian case in the area of intellectual disability is near absence of focus on intellectual disability, as evidenced in the WHO report (2007:67):

> There is very little information available about intellectual disabilities. For now, the focus is more on physical disability. There is no co-coordinated or concentrated effort to look into the area of intellectual disabilities at present.

This situation is in agreement with the lack of focus noticed by Adewuyi (2007) in the 1984 National survey of the disabled. The survey lumped together all categories of disabilities. The lack of specificity is manifest in the description of disability by the survey as reported by Adewuyi (2007):

> A disabled person is one who on account of injury (accidental or otherwise), disease or congenital malformation, is substantially handicapped in obtaining and/or keeping employment or in undertaking normal chores of daily life on his own or of a kind which, apart from the impairment, would be expected of a person of his socio-economic status.

According to American Association on Intellectual and Developmental Disabilities as cited in Schalock, Luckasson, and Shogren (2007), an individual is considered to have an intellectual disability when: (1) the person's intellectual functioning level (IQ) is below 70–75; (2) the person has significant limitations in adaptive skill areas as expressed in conceptual, social, and practical adaptive skills; and (3) the disability originated before the age of 18. "Adaptive skill areas" refer to basic skills needed for everyday life. They include communication, self-care, home living, social skills, leisure, health and safety, self-direction, functional academics (reading, writing, basic math), and work. Intellectual disabilities will vary in degree

Table 11.1 Terminology used to refer to intellectual disabilities across countries

	Africa (%)	Americas (%)	South-East Asia (%)	Europe (%)	Eastern Mediterranean (%)	Western Pacific (%)	*N*
Developmental disabilities	14.7	16.0	20.0	29.8	23.1	27.3	146
Intellectual disabilities	47.1	60.0	80.0	59.6	46.2	63.6	146
Learning disabilities	35.3	32.0	60.0	27.7	23.1	36.4	146
Mental deficiency	26.5	12.5	60.0	19.1	0	4.5	145
Mental disability	55.9	44.0	0	34.0	46.2	22.7	146
Mental handicap	61.8	16.0	80.0	34.0	46.2	31.8	146
Mental retardation	82.4	80.0	80.0	70.2	92.3	63.6	146
Mental subnormality	11.8	12.0	60.0	6.4	23.1	4.5	146

Adapted from Atlas global resources for persons with intellectual disabilities 2007.

and effect from person to person, just as individual capabilities vary considerably among people who do not have an intellectual disability.

It is noteworthy that intellectual disability is described using different terminologies, which is context-related. In Nigeria, the phenomenon is known as mental retardation. The World Health Organization (2007) reports the various terminologies by which the term is referred (see Table 11.1).

Types of Begging

The phenomenon of begging in Nigeria has been subjected to various classificatory schemes. Instructive in this regard are the works by Aliyu (1972), Okediji (1972), and Arnold (2007). The different classifications are either premised on the motives for begging or the mode of carrying out the act. The various descriptions clearly show that begging cannot be linked only to economic situation but has the character of a multidimensional sociological situation (Adewuyi, 2007).

Aliyu (1972) delineates begging into three classes: compulsive beggars, pupil beggars, and inevitable beggars. He describes compulsive beggars as those begging on a temporary basis. This category of beggars may be victims of rightsizing or outright unemployment. Adewuyi (2007, p. 16), while elaborating on Aliyu's (1972) description of compulsive beggars posits that they "are clean, healthy, able-minded, able-bodied individuals that beg as a temporary solution to loss of employment or disguised unemployment." Pupil beggars are those children, who, due to begging-enabling environment or institutionally disabling conditions, consider begging as a credible alternative.

The last classification by Aliyu is the inevitable beggars. This class of beggars comprises individuals who suffer one form of disadvantage or the other and, whose social safety valves have been blocked by social dislocations (poverty, unemployment, family problems, etc.). Beggars in this category may be those suffering from social, mental, or physical disability and with no social support to alleviate their disabilities. Though not stated by Aliyu in his work, there is a link between pupil beggars and inevitable beggars. The former can serve as a veritable feeder for the latter. In other words, the presence of pupil beggars represents a supply pool for graduation into inevitable begging. This is, however, without prejudice to other causes of inevitable begging.

The classificatory approach adopted by Okediji (1972) is, however, different from the one presented above. He broadly classifies beggars into two categories; those who are not threats to society's existence (ritual-beggars) and those who constitute a social problem. The first category derives legitimacy from cultural practices that encourage or tacitly support begging. For example, begging by masquerades and mothers of twins among others are culturally derived and individual agents in such practices are not considered threats to social fabrics. The other category comprises beggars who constitute a social problem to the society. These are individuals who have no means of surviving. In the words of Adewuyi (2007, p. 16), "persons that have lost touch with their relations and have resigned to alms-collection." In the second category may be people with intellectual disabilities. This is because begging by this category of people is not culturally derived but a situation given by hardships.

Another classification of begging is that reported by Arnold (2007). This he classifies as passive begging and aggressive begging. According to him "passive begging involves solicitation that is non-threatening and often non-verbal, with the beggar for example simply holding out a hand (or a cup) or sitting in front of a cap for receipt of coins and notes," while he describes aggressive begging as "'coercive solicitation' that features some degree of intimidatory action (such as following a potential donor down the street) and implied or actual threats."

The Interface Between Intellectual Disability and Begging

Street begging is one of the most apparent symbols of social exclusion in any society. It has been established that begging is a survival strategy overwhelmingly driven by need and not greed (Briefing Paper, 2003; Ebigbo, 2003). The intellectually disabled are found in almost every country of the world, however, perception of the phenomenon, treatment, and management is context-related. In most cases, economic situation and level of development of a society may be determining factors in how intellectual disabilities are viewed and treated.

The attention the intellectually disabled receive either help them lead life positively or find themselves at the other end, which may mean begging on the street. Most people with intellectual disabilities in Africa suffer dire consequences arising from lack of care, lack of educational opportunity, lack of any form of empowerment, and a life devoid of growth and development. Some of these people with disabilities in Nigeria leave home due to lack of parental support manifesting in inadequate means of livelihood. Consequently, they end up on the street to survive by begging and scavenging the street for food. It must be noted, however, that the plight of the intellectually disabled resulting from lag in parental care may be due to the helpless situations of the parents themselves.

The helpless situations of some parents notwithstanding, most parents, due to ignorance, shame, and fear of stigmatization often do not make public a disabled child (Ajobiewe, 2000; Olawale, 2000; Akinpelu, 2004). This may not be unconnected with what Esen, as cited in Obayan (1995) refers to as "undisclosing nature" of the Nigerian family. Because of fear of stigmatization, families in the Nigerian context prefer to shield from outsiders information that may attract negative feeling to them. Hence, people with intellectual disabilities end up on the street due to this fear and in most cases combined with poverty, ignorance, insensitivity, and illiteracy on the part of the parents. Ordinarily, it looks absurd to have a large number of the disabled population on the street begging, considering the abundance of natural resources in Nigeria. Reality, however, shows that some parents of people with intellectual disabilities, as a result of poverty, often send these children to beg on the streets and in neighborhoods. However, studies (Briefing Paper, 2003; Ebigbo, 1989a) have suggested that this only adds to the already present disabling condition with consequences such as brutal diseases, further exacerbating low-thinking ability, promoting the poverty mentality and exposing the children to street hazards including bullying, accidents, sexual assaults, and sexually transmitted infections including HIV.

The indifference of government and other policy-makers to the plight of people with disabilities leave many of these persons unserved. Hence, majority of people with a disability resort to street begging for alms to survive. Studies such as Briefing Paper (2003), Ebigbo (2003), Fitzpatrick and Kennedy (2000) and Kennedy and Fitzpatrick (2001), have confirmed that begging, whether by the able or person with a disability, is a survival strategy and is overwhelmingly driven by "need" not "greed." People with disabilities in Nigeria beg because of the expensive nature of surviving on the street.

Kisekka (1981) notes that most states in northern Nigeria have outlawed street begging, but the number of despondents begging on the streets makes a mockery of the ban on street begging. Recently, the government of Jigawa State promised appropriate legislation to prohibit anyone from begging on the streets of Jigawa State, while Kwara State has signed the bill on street begging into law.

People with disabilities have the highest rates of unemployment in most countries of the world (Kosciulek, 2004; Randall & Brown, 1999). They also make up a large percentage of people living in poverty (Ebigbo, 2003). People with disabilities beg on the streets of Nigeria often in the form of asking for money without an exchange of services in a public place. The disabled not only beg for money, but also they beg for anything they need – food, clothes, and shoes, among others. Discrimination, stigmatization, and ignorance have been adjudged as reasons why employers of labor are reluctant to employ persons with intellectual disability. Anyagafu and Iwenjora (2006) note that in Nigeria, there is a class of children who neither feel good nor are happy. Their outlook paints a vivid picture of their state of helplessness. They appear unkempt and totally hopeless in regards to what the future holds. These people find homes and shelter in the filthy and awkward places like abandoned buildings, under overhead bridges and school premises. They often retire to these "abodes" at dusk and leave early in the morning before the prying eyes of security agents or the rightful owners of the structures turn out for business. This piece encapsulates the life and plight of people with intellectual disabilities in Nigeria, who, due to lack of education, care and love found respite on the street.

People who beg are among the most damaged and vulnerable people in our society (Briefing Paper, 2003). Just like the context in Nigeria, the Briefing Paper reports that the vast majority of people on the streets are homeless, suffer from poor skills, low income, poor housing, ill health, and family breakdown. One big task of the intellectually disabled child is getting him to come to terms with the evident disability. The level of success for people with disabilities is premised on their mindset concerning the disability, attitude toward the disabling condition, and psychosocial support from friends and families.

In Nigeria, as in other parts of the world, the sight of children selling chewing gum, sachets of pure water, or shining shoes in street corners are commonplace, but the dynamic mechanism that prompts some of these disabled children to find solace on the street is yet to be analyzed deeply or comprehensively (Lauter, 1998). Many studies (Oloko, 1989; Ebigbo, 1989b; UNICEF, 2006) have posited that dire poverty and parents' divorce are common to all street children in all developing countries, Nigeria inclusive.

Special schools are available for persons with special needs in Nigeria including the people with intellectual disabilities. These types of schools are, however, in very limited number. Ajobiewe (2000) notes that special education policies have remained too dependent on general education policy. The National Policy on Education, though a broad statement of government intent capable of being implemented by other agencies or commission assigned or designated, dishearteningly has not been reviewed for many years. Ajobiewe (2000) avers that while Britain and the United States of America have kept on reviewing their general and special education laws on a general basis, Nigeria has had an unstable legislative base since 1981, making it difficult to consider new trends in the field.

Consequently, it can be argued that begging, disability, and poverty are profoundly intertwined. Like crime, juvenile delinquency and prostitution; begging represents a lack of adjustment to the normal operation of the individual and the group.

Conclusion

Education is central to overcoming the various problems posed by the phenomenon of intellectual disability. In most developed economies, where education policy and implementation focus not only on general education but also on special education, people with intellectual disabilities are found to be living a good quality life. Plausible policy on special education is in place, but commitment to its implementation is missing in Nigeria's education landscape. Government and other stakeholders should, therefore, pursue vigorously implementation of policies and programs aimed at enhancing the quality of life of people with intellectual disabilities. This will go a long way in reducing the incidence of street begging by this category of people.

Education and enlightenment programs should also be instituted as to the manageability of intellectual disability. If these are in place, perception of stigmatization will reduce and the tendency to abandon people with intellectual disabilities on the streets will drastically reduce.

Street begging is a menacing plague that must not survive. Hence, all hands must be on deck to ensure that children with intellectual disabilities are educated to their full mental capacity and taught other life skills and self-management skills to lead a life devoid of begging. Begging is dehumanizing especially to the "differently-abled" population. Begging under any condition does not dignify a person or nation; rather, it erodes ones self-esteem.

References

Adewuyi, T. (2007). *Street begging in Nigeria*. Ibadan: Spectrum Books Limited.

Ajobiewe, T. (2000). *Management of disability in the family and community*. Ibadan: Teton Educational Services.

Akinpelu, O. F. (2004). Handling handicapped and disadvantaged students in schools. In A. I. Idowu (Ed.), *Guidance and counselling in education*. Ilorin: Indemac (Nigeria Publishers) Ltd.

Aliyu, A. (1972). Political and administrative implications of rehabilitation of beggars. In F. O. Okediji (Ed.), *Rehabilitation of beggars in Nigeria*. Ibadan: University Press.

Anyagafu, C., & Iwenjora, F. (2006). Sorry story of Nigeria's street kids: Wasted by poverty in the land. *Vanguard Newspaper, Saturday,* February 4.

Arnold, B. (2007). http://www.caslon.com.au/beggingnote.htm

Ebigbo, P. O. (1989a). Psychosocial aspects of child abuse and neglect in Africa. In K. Peltzer and P. O. Ebigbo (Eds.), *Clinical psychology in Africa (South of the Sahara), the Caribbean and Afro-Latin America: A textbook for universities and paramedical schools*, Nigeria, 401–424.

Ebigbo, P. O. (1989b). Situation analysis of child abuse and neglect in Nigeria: Making use of Nigerian daily newspapers. *Journal of African Psychology*, *1*, 95–101.

Ebigbo, P. O. (2003). Street children: The care of child abuse and neglect in Nigeria. *Children, Youth and Environment*, *13*(1), Retrieved on July 13, 2007 from http://cye.colorado.edu

Fitzpatrick, S., & Kennedy, C. (2000). *Getting By: Begging, rough sleeping and the big issue in Glasgow and Edinburgh*. Bristol: The Policy Press.

Kennedy, K., & Fitzpatrick, S. (2001). Begging, rough sleeping and social exclusion: Implications for social policy. *Urban Studies*, *38*(11), 2001–2016.

Kisekka, M. N., ed. (1981). *Children in Kaduna State, Nigeria: Problems and needs*. Zaria: Department of Sociology, Ahmadu Bello University, Kaduna Child Welfare Committee.

Kosciulek, J. F. (2004). Empowering people with disabilities through vocational rehabilitation counseling. *American Rehabilitation*. Retrieved August 4, 2007, from http://findarticles.com/p/articles/mi_m0842/is_1_28/ai_n8681410

Lauter, L. (1998). 'Street children' in Children in need of special protection: GOC – UNICEF Mid-term Review Final Report, UNICEF Beijing.

Nigeria. (1984). *Survey of disabled persons in Nigeria*. Nigeria: Federal Ministry of Information, Social Development, Youths and Sports.

Obayan, A. O. I. (1995). Changing perspectives in the extended family system in Nigeria: Implications for family dynamics and counselling. *Counselling Psychology Quarterly*, *8*, 3.

Okediji, O. (1972). Sociological aspects of rehabilitation of beggars. In F. O. Okediji (Ed.), *Rehabilitation of beggars in Nigeria*. Ibadan: University Press.

Olawale, S. G. (2000). *Counselling exceptional children: A handbook for professionals and parents working with exceptional children*. Ibadan: HMS Publications Inc.

Oloko, B. (1989). Children's work in urban Nigeria: A case study of young Lagos Street traders. *UNICEF Staff Working Paper*, *4*, 19–30.

Paper, B. (2003). *Compassion not coercion: Addressing the question of begging*. London: Crisis.

Randall, G., & Brown, S. (1999). *Homes for street homeless people: An evaluation of the rough sleepers initiative: An evaluation*. London: DETR.

Schalock, R. L., Luckasson, R. A., & Shogren, K. A. (2007). The renaming of mental retardation: Understanding the change to the term intellectual disability. *Intellectual And Developmental Disabilities*, *45*(2), 116–124.

UNICEF (2006). *A new approach to Egypt's street children*. Retrieved from http://www.unicef.org/sowc/egypt30616.html

WHO. (2007). *Atlas: Global resources for persons with intellectual disabilities*. Geneva: WHO Press.

World Health Report (2001). *Mental health: New understanding, new hope*. Geneva: World Health Organization.

Part IV
Children with Intellectual Disabilities

Chapter 12
Life Satisfaction for Children with Profound Intellectual and Multiple Disabilities

Gordon Lyons and Michele Cassebohm

> *Tell me honestly, I challenge you – answer me: Imagine that you are charged with building the edifice of human destiny, the ultimate aim of which is to bring human happiness, to give them peace and contentment at last, but that in order to achieve this it is essential and unavoidable to torture just one little speck of creation, that same little child beating her chest with her little fists, and imagine that this edifice has been erected on her expiated tears. Would you agree to be the architect under those conditions? Tell me honestly! (from Fyodor Dostoevsky's The Brothers Karamazov).*

Introduction

> (Quality of life)... the slipperiest creature in the conceptual zoo! (Compton, 1997, p. 120)

The concepts of quality of life (QOL) and life satisfaction have been enmeshed in the fabric of human existence since mankind stepped out of the primeval miasma and beyond the daily struggle for mere survival. In the more peaceful moments of living, humans undoubtedly pondered whether their slice of the giant pie was sufficient to meet more than just their basic needs... Was this as good as it gets? Historically, a considerable number of humankind would have considered that their quality of life was rich, but for others – inevitably the poverty stricken and disenfranchised – this would remain a question not worth to ask.

Since antiquity people have sought a "life of quality". Aristotle and Plato reflected extensively on eudaemonia – happiness and living well. Traditional Eastern philosophies put that a personally balanced "Yin" and "Yang" brings the best QOL. This pursuit of goodness of life, wellbeing, life satisfaction or QOL remains enduringly – notwithstanding diverse cultural interpretations and emphases.

G. Lyons (✉)
The University of Newcastle
e-mail: gordon.lyons@newcastle.edu.au

R. Kober (ed.), *Enhancing the Quality of Life of People with Intellectual Disabilities*, Social Indicators Research Series 41, DOI 10.1007/978-90-481-9650-0_12,

Superficially, QOL presents as a simple concept. The ubiquitous question "How are you?" generally transcends nationality, culture, socio-economic status and gender and has remained a most common first question people ask as an expression of interest in another's health, welfare and goodness of life. The question conveys a fundamental concern of humans for each other. However, life satisfaction and quality of life are not phenomena or terms subject to consensus. Some authors have used terms such as QOL, life satisfaction, psychological wellbeing and subjective wellbeing interchangeably. Others refer to QOL as a multidimensional concept that encompasses these other concepts, whilst others have used the term globally to subsume these.

QOL became a field of social scientific research in the early 1960s and a research discipline in the later 1960s. During the late 1950s and 1960s, the human rights movement gained popular support in Western countries and research into intellectual and developmental disability (services) gained professional impetus. During this period the wider community became better informed about the frequently impoverished lives of many persons with (intellectual) disabilities who lived in institutions. More recently, the evaluation of the processes, standards and outcomes in disability support programmes within a QOL rubric has gained popularity.

Life satisfaction is an individual phenomenon that cannot be readily compared, whereas QOL is more closely related to standard of living, is measured using culturally appropriate social indicators and is more about understanding and improving the standard of living of population groups. Life satisfaction is more about how individuals feel about their lives, so life satisfaction research is more about understanding the nature of personal feelings, cognitive appraisal and personality.

To find out about another person's life satisfaction, researchers can generally just ask how satisfied that person is with their life. This is usually done in person or by means of a questionnaire, using a validated instrument or technique. Learning about another person's life satisfaction is obviously problematic though when that person cannot readily communicate his/her (level of) satisfaction, for example, when that person has profound intellectual and multiple disabilities (PIMD). Many would consider the quality of life for these people to be of the lowest. However, it is our position, based on the evidence of our continuing research agenda, that life satisfaction of children (and adults) with PIMD can be discerned, recognised and understood, and that the philosophy and ethics of life satisfaction and QOL for children with PIMD are no different from that of others.

This chapter is built around an explanation of the first author's doctoral and continuing research studies and reflects a core belief that educators and service providers should, like most parents do, recognise and respond to the centrality of life satisfaction and happiness when making decisions with and for children with PIMD, rather than "just" responding to the "best interest principle" as widely reflected in the literature on normalisation, integration and inclusion. This chapter also represents a distillation of the authors' philosophical and ethical energies that contend that children (and indeed adults) with PIMD can experience a reasonable life satisfaction and quality of life.

This chapter commences with a brief explanation of the design of the first author's doctoral study, summarises some of the diverse literature around the topic, then presents a grounded theory on the nature of life satisfaction for children with PIMD. The chapter concludes by presenting some challenging issues and questions to the reader.

The Study

> To be labeled retarded (sic) is to have a wide range of imperfections imputed to you. One imperfection is the inability to analyse your life and your current situation. Another is the inability to express yourself – to know and say who you are and what you wish to become (Bogdan & Taylor, 1989, p. 136).

The first author's doctoral study investigated two research questions: What is life satisfaction for children with PIMD, and how do we learn about this? A basic starting point for designing the study was to select a facilitative inquiry paradigm. Grounded theory, one variant under the socio-logical tradition of ethnography, proved so. Given also that the purpose of the study was to build knowledge, understanding and theory about life satisfaction for children with PIMD, and that the central concepts of symbolic interaction are the self, the world and social action, symbolic interaction presented as a most appropriate theoretical perspective. Furthermore, ethnographic research, with its holistic emphasis, was adopted because it was synchronous with symbolic interaction. Finally, Straussian grounded theory emerged as the most appropriate research methodology.

The study focused on 22 children, all with high support needs (13 having PIMD) and 77 of their communication partners including parents, other family members, paid and volunteer carers, teachers, teacher aides, support professionals. Participant observation and semi-structured interviews were the primary research methods for gathering field data. Most of the fieldwork was carried out over 8 months with field data collected via repeated participant observations, primarily in school settings and by interview. Both the children and their communication partners were observed and their communicative interactions were discussed during and after observation sessions, and during interview sessions. Inquiry into the first research question involved 126 (mostly single) interview sessions with all communication partners. Inquiry into the first research question involved up to three consecutive interviews with 15 communication partners, most of whom were relatively unfamiliar with the children.

The key finding from the study was a grounded theory about the nature of life satisfaction for children with PIMD.

The Literature

> We know all too little about the quality of [the lives of persons with intellectual disabilities], and next to nothing about their satisfaction with those lives (Edgerton, 1990, p. 153).

Society generally has little knowledge about, or understanding of, people with PIMD (Atkins, 1999). It often devalues those with impairments, disabilities and handicaps, and associates these with a lower quality of life (Barber, 1990; Wolf, 1990). Finkelstein's (1993, p. 13) definition of disability, "the loss or limitation of opportunities that prevents people who have impairments from taking part in normal life in the community on an equal basis with others due to physical and social barriers", aligns with the socio-political model, has broad international support and reflects the usage of the term in Australia (Bigby & Ozanne, 2001; Butow, 1993).

Generally, the term "children with PIMD" refers to children aged up to 18 years who have diagnoses that describe and include severe developmental disability, severe cognitive, functional and behavioural deficits, and no language-based communication (Goode, 1997). They are generally attributed an "untestable" IQ of less than 20 (Arthur, 1998), but considerable uncertainty remains about the validity of these assessments. Remarkable children who have discredited such assessments include Helen Keller, Annie McDonald (Crossley & McDonald, 1980) and Christy Brown (1989). Many of these descriptions, however, reflect the "deficit perspective" of disability that does not acknowledge or appropriately emphasise the social place, humanity and abilities of children with PIMD.

An understanding of the communication challenges faced by children with PIMD is central to understanding PIMD, and communicative competence is crucial to the QOL of children with PIMD (Butterfield, Arthur, & Linfoot, 1992), so establishing meaningful communication and intersubjectivity represents a major challenge for families, carers and service providers (Feil, 1993). Many children with PIMD lack formal symbolic, vocal or gestural language, and often rely on pre-symbolic, action-based, idiosyncratic communication gestures and utterances (Goode, 1990a, 1994). Carter and Hook (1998), however, concluded that research about communication training recognised the potential communicative intent of subtle, idiosyncratic and non-symbolic behaviours, and that some learners communicated effectively without the need for conventional symbols.

Landesman (1986) suggested that life satisfaction and QOL were distinct concepts, whereas Romney, Brown, and Fry (1994) and Cummins (personal communication, 21 June, 1999) argued that QOL was more than the subjective experience of life satisfaction. Life satisfaction is a personal phenomenon closely linked to the broader phenomenon of QOL and the first author's prior research has shown that an examination of the QOL literature provides the best scaffold for investigating and understanding life satisfaction.

In the 1990s, qualitative research about persons with intellectual disabilities focusing on individuals and specific populations became prevalent. During this period the broad purpose of QOL research was to improve population QOL and in general terms, and the QOL research agenda for those with intellectual disabilities paralleled this agenda for the wider population.

Scores of theories and models of QOL have been proposed, however, three prevalent and widely documented perspectives – the social indicators perspective, the psychological perspective and the goodness of fit/social policy perspective – were clearly identifiable in the literature (Halpern, 1993b; Schalock, 1990). Two principal schools of thought emerged amongst theorists about QOL/life satisfaction measurement and assessment. The most widely supported upheld a holistic approach, inclusive of both qualitative and quantitative approaches. The second argued that QOL could be described but not measured. Felce and Perry (1996) argued that subjective evaluations of emotional wellbeing had been neglected in the intellectual disability literature because of the difficulties these persons had in communicating the nuances and complexities of abstract feelings and emotions. Hence QOL/life satisfaction assessment and measurement for individuals with PIMD brings about specific and complex challenges for researchers, decision-makers and practitioners and the nature of life satisfaction and QOL remains subject to continuing debate.

It is our view that QOL is a multidimensional phenomenon that encompasses life satisfaction. Life satisfaction may be viewed as subjective QOL, wherein it is "the degree to which the individual's life is perceived to match some implicit or explicit internal standard or referent" (Evans, 1994, p. 53). Life satisfaction is more about how individuals feel about their lives, and life satisfaction research about understanding the nature of personal feelings, cognitive appraisal and personality. QOL is more about understanding and improving the standard of living of population groups. Life satisfaction, like personality, cognitive process and affect, cannot be measured objectively. Life satisfaction may, however, be compared to subjective QOL wherein the individual weights a variety of life domains in accordance with their personal relevance and importance.

A Grounded Theory

> Whether or not people with severe disabilities who cannot speak experience the world like other people is probably improvable. However, it is just as reasonable to presume that they have subjective experiences as to assume that they do not (Taylor & Bogdan, 1996, p. 20).

The first author's grounded theory about the life satisfaction of children with PIMD is summarily explained in three layers. The first is the Conceptual Scaffold (Fig. 12.1) which lists the theory's key conceptual categories. The second is the Storyline, which describes all 19 categories. The Central and each Main Category are described through their respective part of the Storyline, and through samples of the Field and Literature Data. The Subcategories are described only through samples of the Field Data, i.e. in vivo quotes from the study interviewees. The Literature Data consists of quotes from the literature review conducted throughout the study and are presented in themes. (The first author's doctoral study (Lyons, 2003) describes and explains this theory in detail, and is available online from the first author.) The third layer, the Relational Scaffold (Fig. 12.2), posits explanations for the interrelationships between these categories.

Central Category – Doing enjoyable things... Life satisfaction for children with PIMD is primarily about doing enjoyable things. It is about being engaged in activities that, and with people who, are needed, wanted, liked and/or preferred.

Central Category - Doing enjoyable things
Life satisfaction for children with PIMD is primarily about doing enjoyable things. It's about being engaged with people who, and in activities that, are needed, wanted, liked and/or preferred.

Main Category - Just like other children but personal
Life satisfaction is the same for all children,
but for children with PIMD it is often expressed in very personal ways.

Subcategory - Life satisfaction discourses
Life satisfaction doesn't make sense for children with PIMD,
but quality of life and happiness do.

Subcategory - Disability discourses
Disability is understood in different ways.
Unfamiliar others often only see disability in children with PIMD,
and not how they are feeling, learning and growing.

Subcategory - Childhood and adulthood
Children with PIMD are developing.
They have a future, but they live in the here and now.

Subcategory - Individuality
Children with PIMD are individuals,
and have their own characters and expressions.

Main Category - Happiness and contentment
Life satisfaction is about feeling both happiness and contentment.

Subcategory - Day-by-day
Happiness and contentment should be experienced daily,
and life lived one day at a time.

Subcategory - Just taking it all in
Contentment can be just taking it all in.

Subcategory - Balance
Happiness and contentment is about personal balance.

Main Category - Comfort and wellbeing
Life satisfaction is about feeling both comfort and wellbeing.

Subcategory - Physical health
Relief from acute/chronic pain is prerequisite.

Subcategory - Daily wellbeing
Just having a good day is valued.

Sub-category - Belonging
Relationships are central.

Main Category - Favourite things
Life satisfaction is doing and having favourite things.

Subcategory - Being with others
Is caring and sharing.

Subcategory - Special things
Is doing special things with special people.

Subcategory - Water play
Playing with water is freedom, fun and belonging.

Subcategory - Fun
Is having a 'wicked' sense of humour!

Fig. 12.1 The conceptual scaffold

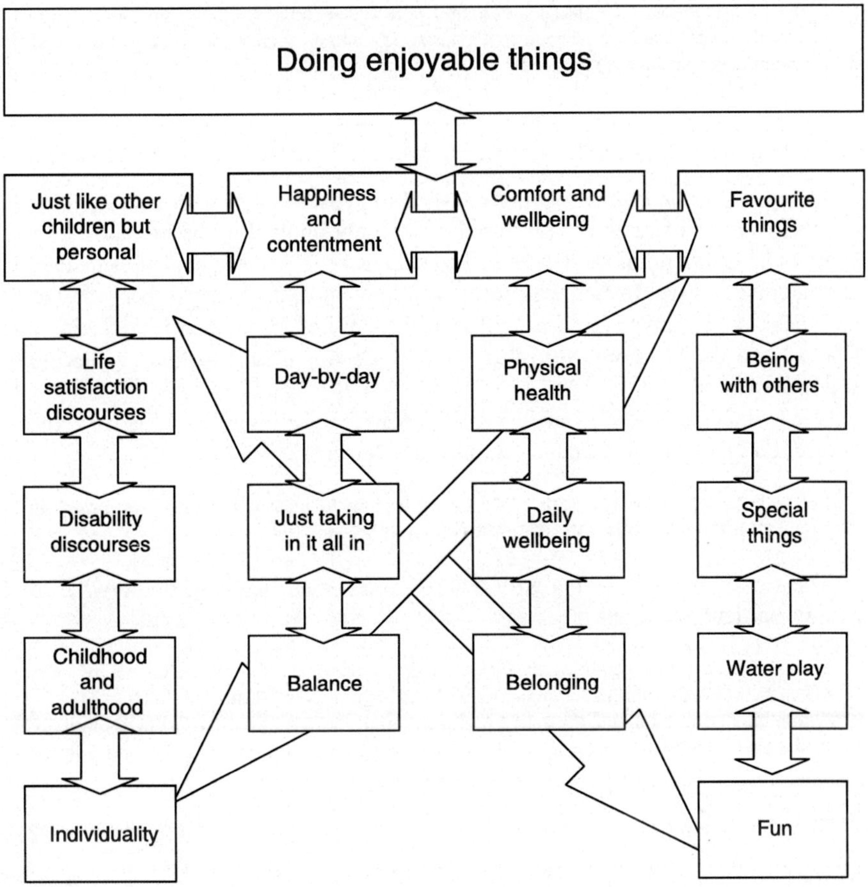

Fig. 12.2 The relational scaffold

This central category has four main categories: Just like other children but personal; Happiness and contentment; Comfort and wellbeing and Favourite things – and 14 subcategories. Doing enjoyable things usually requires engagement with people, as children with PIMD have a limited capacity to self-engage in activities, other than isolative self-stimulatory behaviours. Communication, through intersubjectivity and understanding, "opens doorways" to doing enjoyable things. Parents and other primary carers emphasised doing enjoyable things that were wanted and liked, whereas school staff emphasised doing things that were needed.

> She likes to move around in different environments. She likes to be around her family and friends. She loves to be around the kids and people. (Mother)
>
> She wants to be able to do things and feel things... so I think being busy, doing different things, not being quietly in a corner anywhere (Teacher)

If she's lying there doing her positioning... I go and set up a switch toy and she will just start bashing at it madly... as soon as it's there she's into it... she wants to be part of it and she wants to be doing it. (Therapist)

He enjoys being at school.... he likes being around people and he likes active things... he likes lots of people buzzing around. (Teachers' Aide)

What makes his day? Doing exactly what [he] wants to do, all the time! (Respite Carer)

Doing enjoyable things – being engaged in activities and with people, that are needed, wanted, liked and/or preferred – is widely implied in the literature to be a central characteristic of (and even prerequisite to) a life of quality, life satisfaction and happiness. Five themes with three positions on each emerged from the literature data. These themes are: Doing; Doing with others; Enjoyment; Interaction and Choice, and the positions were that each theme was either: A right; A necessity and/or Beneficial.

The first theme – Doing – included references to meaningful and creative activity, purposeful involvement, stimulation, play and leisure, i.e.

Like other people, [people with PIMD] have a right to pleasurable activities aimed at stimulation and relaxation. (Vlaskamp & Nakken, 1999, p. 101)

The second theme – Doing with others – refers specifically to doing with other people, particularly adults, i.e.

Persons with PIMD "need to experience a quality of life that is built on relationships with others, full of opportunities for engaging with the environment" (Carnaby, 2001, p. 4).

It is important to include the active participation of these students [with PIMD] in integrated environments because this offers them the greatest opportunity of achieving a better quality of life. (Guess, Roberts, & Behrens, 1998)

The third theme – Enjoyment – centred on enjoyment that might arise from thinking (reminiscing and imagining), doing and/or doing with others, i.e.

Only recently... have publications on enjoyment of leisure begun to appear, acknowledging the right and desirability of people with profound and multiple learning disabilities to what is now a central activity for many people in developed countries. (Lambe & Hogg, 2001, p. 3)

Education is only part of their [children with PMLD] lives. For them, and their parents, enjoyment of free time, leisure activities, is also of major concern. (Lambe & Hogg, 2001, p. 1)

The fourth theme – Interaction – centred on interrelationships between children with PIMD and others, i.e.

To achieve satisfaction, children with severe intellectual disability need social interaction with their communication partners on an everyday, routine basis (Butterfield & Arthur, 1995).

For some individuals [with PIMD] happiness can be increased dramatically by very simple social interactions. (Favell, Realon, & Sutton, 1996, p. 47)

The fifth theme – Choice – included reference to choice, decision-making, autonomy and empowerment:

Today one of the most commonly heard shibboleths in services for people with cognitive disability is that they have the right to make choices and determine things for themselves. (Goode, 1995, p. 1)

Self-determination has a critical place as a right and quality of social wellbeing. (Bach, 1994, p. 139)

[G]ood days are those in which [people] feel more competent and autonomous in their daily activities. (Sheldon, Ryan, & Reis, 1996, p. 1270)

Main Category – Just like other children but personal... Life satisfaction is the same for all children, but for children with PIMD it is often expressed in very personal ways.

This main category has four subcategories: Life satisfaction discourses; Disability discourses; Childhood and adulthood and Individuality. Children with PIMD were the focus of this study, but children with severe intellectual disabilities also participated. Life satisfaction was expressed in both similar and obvious, and idiosyncratic and subtle ways. Children with PIMD tended to use more subtle and personal expressions.

I think it's the same with these kids as it is with the other kids. I don't think it's got anything to do with disability. The disability comes in the way they can express that, but I don't think the feelings are any different. (Teacher)

Well it's a lot of body language, a lot of facial expressions... if she's excited about something she sort of tends to... her whole body seems to move and her arms flap around a bit... if she wants to be in something then its that... "Yeh I'm wanting to be in that!"... Yes, yes [it's obvious]. (Teacher)

When she's happy she stiffens, and when she's unhappy she stiffens, but there just seems to be a subtle difference. (Teacher's Aide)

We didn't expect it of [our daughter] because being handicapped, we always think that she's not going to be like normal kids, but she's very much like a normal child. (Father)

Seven themes emerged from the literature data. The first six refer to the similarities of life satisfaction for children with PIMD, whereas the seventh refers to the differences. These are:

Growth and development

It seems reasonable to take the position that children with PIMD develop psychologically and emotionally in the same way as other children. The developmental path of children with PIMD is "remarkably similar" to other children, although this development is "extremely prolonged". (Hogg & Lambe, 1997, pp. 220–221)

Relationships are the same

The qualities of good relationships for children [with PIMD] seemed quite comparable to those for all children. (Goldstein, Kacmarek, & English, 2002, p. 143)

Experiencing feelings is the same

Children with PIMD seem to experience feelings and emotions like other children. People with developmental disabilities have personal preferences, likes and dislikes "just like others". (Rawlings, Dowse, & Shaddock, 1995, p. 137)

Expressing feelings is the same

Children with PIMD frequently express their feelings and emotions in the same ways as other children. For people with PIMD, individual affect ratings can be predicted by just seven readily identified behavioural cues. (Reeves, Hogg, Roberts, & Mudford, 2000)

Unhappiness and dissatisfaction are the same

Much of the literature on affect amongst people with PIMD explains that comparisons about expressions of unhappiness and dissatisfaction are the same as comparisons about expressions of happiness and satisfaction. (Hogg, Reeves, Roberts, & Mudford, 2001)

Ethics and rights are the same

The prevailing principles and practices of normalisation, social role valorisation and inclusion support equitable rights for children with and without disabilities. (Perrin & Nirje, 1985; Wolfensberger, 1995; Foreman & Arthur, 2002 respectively)

Expressing feelings is also unique

There is now broad professional recognition of the diversity and validity of the idiosyncratic communicative behaviours used by persons with PIMD. (Arthur, 1994, p. 183; Felce, 1997)

Subcategory – Life satisfaction discourses... Life satisfaction does not make sense for children with PIMD, but quality of life and happiness do.

But life satisfaction ... that's hard isn't it. For me (as his mother) I want it to be for him. I want life satisfaction to be happy in what he does and to enjoy life, as he knows it, if I can make it happy for him and get him to do as many things as he possibly can with me and enjoy it. (Mother)

I think [my student's] quality of life... if you really look into her eyes... they're telling you something... she thinks her quality of life is beautiful... Well I think it is. (Teachers' Aide)

It's really important because it's all about the family and the child. It's not really about what you think ultimately, it's about what's important to them. (Therapist)

Subcategory – Disability discourses... Disability is understood in different ways. Unfamiliar others often only see disability in children with PIMD, and not how they are feeling, learning and growing.

It's strange how (our son), the way he is, how unfortunate... it's strange how I cope with him being disabled, that he will never have the pains that a lot of people do, and he will never know the disappointments in life. In a way he's protected from life's little hiccups and major happenings as well. So in a way it's almost good, perversely blessed... well that's how we've rationalised it. (Parents)

I've never looked at kids not being able to do things. I always look at the things they can do... and I think when you say to people you work with children with disabilities they always say "Oh I don't know how you could do that. It's never entered my mind because they're just children and we just do the things that they can do and enjoy." (Teachers' aide)

Subcategory – Childhood and adulthood... Children with PIMD are developing. They have a future, but they live in the here and now.

But you know his kick in the face comes over and over again, because he's trying to fit into the teenage social aspect, but he can't fit into it. (Teachers' Aide)

[My student] at that age might have had a smile on his face, a happy boy, but as he got older and his body's got twisted and his spine's got worse... (Teachers' Aide)

Subcategory – Individuality... Children with PIMD are individuals, and have their own characters and expressions.

> But what I'm saying is (my granddaughter) exudes something, something nice. Given all the bad things that she's got wrong with her, she must be exuding something in her own personality for people to react this way. (Grandfather)
>
> I think every child is different because with (my student) you have to get to know [her] first before you start doing things with her. You have to get in her circle. There's no other way you're ever going to know her. (Teachers' aide)

Main Category – Happiness and contentment... Life satisfaction is about feeling both happiness and contentment.

This main category has three subcategories: Day-by-day; Just taking it all in and Balance. For children with PIMD, being happy and contented is what life satisfaction is really all about, and their communication partners not only wanted them to be so but viewed their happiness to be a right of childhood. Discerning happiness in children with PIMD is generally not problematic but with children with PIMD living with acute and chronic pain, discerning contentment is generally problematic. Communication partners found it hard to discern between contentment and boredom, and it took them more time to get to know children with more disablement. Being contented is more a state of being rather than doing, and can be "just taking it all in".

> I think that generally speaking they are [happy], and if they're doing the things that make them happy... I mean if they're allowed to express themselves the way they can, or are allowed to enjoy the activities that make them feel good, then they are happy. (Teacher)
>
> I think [my student would] think [life] was pretty good, pretty normal. You know, there are lots of things that she doesn't want to do and she's got to do. But that's pretty normal for most kids, and I think that most of the time she's fairly content or happy and enjoying herself. (Teacher)
>
> There's a contentment about it. It's not frantic movements or whatever. It's just that quiet... contentment. (Mother)

Six themes emerged from the literature data. These are – The nature of happiness and contentment

> There is a fair degree of consensus amongst researchers that "happiness is probably composed of three related components, positive affect, absence of negative affect, and satisfaction with life as a whole... happiness is better conceptualized as a trait rather than a transient emotional state". (Lu & Shih, 1997, p. 249)

Assessing happiness and contentment

> It has become increasingly accepted that an important, perhaps most important, factor (or measure, indicator) of a person's happiness is that individual's own, subjective feeling of contentment, well-being, and satisfaction with life. (Szymanski, 2000, pp. 352–353).

The importance of happiness and contentment

> Engagement in an activity for the sheer joy of the experience is an essential part of defining self and one's personal worth. Developing an activity repertoire with no strings attached except for the fun and enjoyment in the doing is one important dimension of

> getting to know self, developing an awareness of one's skills, capabilities, ability to commit, caring about self, and discerning one's capacity for joy and pleasure. (Fidler, 1996, p. 144).

Sources of happiness and contentment

> There are as many sources of happiness as there are human activities and interests... Three major areas are creative activity, affectionate relationships and sense usage. In practice the sources of happiness rarely, if ever, fall neatly within such categories. (Davison, 1977, pp. 13–14)

The pursuit of happiness and contentment

> People with mental retardation or developmental disabilities are driven by largely the same basic desires as the general population... In terms of happiness they have the same needs as all people have. (Reiss, 2001, p. 378)

Research on happiness and contentment for people with intellectual disabilities

> Happiness/unhappiness [for people with PIMD] can be reliably judged through careful observation of facial expression and bodily movement... (but these observations) do not ultimately tell us anything about the subjective experience of happiness. (Hogg, 1998, pp. 6–7)

Subcategory – Day-by-day... Happiness and contentment should be daily and life one day at a time.

> (Her mood) could change then after lunch, it depends. Like if there's something good on, like a movie she loves, and she loves her books... so that might totally change her around. (Teachers' Aide)
>
> I've certainly noticed that, he seems to know which day of the week it is. On Wednesday he knows Dad's coming. How he knows that I'm not sure but he certainly seems to know the day Dad's coming. (Respite Carer)

Subcategory – Just taking it all in... Contentment can be just taking it all in.

> Yeah and then if (my daughter's) happy, she might have just a little smile on her face, and her eyes will be bright, and you'll see she'll just be content. She'll be still, and her eyes will be wider open, and she'll just have a little cheeky-like kind of grin on her face. You can see she's just taking it all in. (Mother)

Subcategory – Balance... Happiness and contentment is about personal balance. Life satisfaction for children with PIMD is about feeling both happiness and contentment.

> He is in his own world quite a bit, but I think he's usually pretty happy. I mean, as I said, disruptions to his routine and things like that would get him quite upset and agitated. But usually, no, he's a good kid actually, yeh. (Teacher)

Main Category – Comfort and wellbeing... Life satisfaction is about feeling both comfort and wellbeing.

This third main category has three subcategories: Physical Health; Daily Wellbeing and Belonging. For children with PIMD, comfort is primarily about physical comfort, but also about emotional comfort. Wellbeing is primarily about emotional wellbeing. Physical health, daily wellbeing and belonging seem to inform an understanding of the feelings of comfort and wellbeing for children with PIMD and are comparatively easy to discern through mood, disposition, and degrees of relaxation, engagement and attentiveness.

> With therapy... (my student) was very sensory defensive. It was very extreme. If you tried to touch her arms other than just picking her up, like if you did brushing or dressing and undressing, she'd go very stiff in the arms. It wasn't just her having a startle. It would be 'Just get this stuff off me!' She gave very definite reactions to that. Her face would sort of screw up and she'd get some bubbly saliva around her mouth. (Therapist)
>
> I don't have a specific (routine). (My niece) is so rarely out of sorts, honestly, so it's difficult for us to give you an answer to that because she's just such a contented little kid. But I check her clothing to see nothing is caught or her jumper is not up her back. Things like (her) nappy. It's just a comfort thing for her because she can't move herself. (Aunty)
>
> (My student's) body was a bit of a mess, so finding something that was comfortable for him; just to able to be comfortable would be good. (Teachers' Aide)

The two themes emerged from the literature data: Comfort and wellbeing are important, and Comfort and wellbeing are interrelated. Physical and emotional comfort and wellbeing are principal components of theories and models about QOL relating to children, and people with (intellectual) disabilities. Comfort and wellbeing are also interrelated. That is in general, comfort and wellbeing enhance each other, and specifically, physical comfort and wellbeing and emotional comfort and wellbeing enhance each other.

Comfort and wellbeing are important

> For persons with intellectual disabilities, "wellness and well-being are a result of participation in personally and socially relevant activities". (Velde, 1996, p. 15)
>
> Comfort is viewed as a buffer against the physical impairments and chronic health problems of people with severe multiple impairments. (Atkins, 1999, p. 156)

Comfort and wellbeing are interrelated

> Relationships are postulated between happiness (positive mood, optimism) and physiological health... Positive beliefs have been found to be beneficial for health... even protective effects on wellbeing. (Crocker, 2000, p. 320)
>
> The conceptual structure of physical touch in caring centred around five aspects of physical touch: promoting physical comfort; promoting emotional comfort; promoting mind–body comfort, performing social role; and sharing spirituality. (Chang, 2001, p. 820)
>
> The body and emotions are interactional... The emotions, therefore, are expressions of the body's experience of life... Emotional well being's got a lot to do with these people's quality of life. (Atkins, 1999, p. 158)

Subcategory – Physical health... Relief from acute/chronic pain is prerequisite

> I think that [my student's] first feeling was that life was pretty good was when he woke up and wasn't in pain, and that would've been the biggest starting block. Because it's so hard to offer him experiences that he might find joyful if he's in pain... and there's probably lots more things, now that he's not in pain, that he can do that will make his life satisfaction higher. (Therapist)
>
> I think [my granddaughter's] been more comfortable because they put her on a tablet that stopped the pain. And we weren't aware that she must have been in constant pain for five years. And suddenly off her own bat she started laughing much more. Like much more. (Grandmother)

Subcategory – Daily wellbeing... Just having a good day is valued

[When my son] comes home from school [and] he's happy, we know he's had a happy day. He's had a great day and you can pick it up when he comes home. (Mother)

This probably goes back to what we were saying before, whether that day they're "cued in" or whether this is going to be a bad day when they just want the world to go away. (Mother)

Subcategory – Belonging... Relationships are central

[My student] knows that there are people around, but it needs to be people that he's familiar with before he'll express his emotions, like his happiness or... He'll express his dislikes to whoever's there, but I think too if you're going to get to see him being happy, you need to be someone who's going to stick around for a while. I've noticed that. Because he doesn't care who he shows that he's "peed" off with or annoyed with, but if you're going to see him joke around and be happy, you're going to have to be there for the long haul. (Teacher aide)

[T]here's a whole slate of new people and [my student's] not reacting so well. I came in [and] she was crying all day one day. I came in, just walked up to her, and she stopped crying because it was someone familiar. (Teacher)

Main Category – Favourite things... Life satisfaction is doing and having favourite things.

This fourth main category has four subcategories: Being with others; Special things; Water play and Fun. These subcategories bring uniqueness to this theory, by putting forward aspects that are clearly particular to the children who participated in this study.

When [my daughter] was younger, she'd get a toy that she'd almost become, not obsessed with, but you know, there would be something about that particular thing that would really get her attention I mean you never knew what it was, and you could never predict which toy it would be that would do it for her. (Mother)

[My student will] giggle and gurgle at toys and things that are going on, and she's got her favourites, and she goes straight to the favourites. (Teacher)

[My daughter's] favourite pastime would be listening to music or watching her videos, and conversing with us. She loves being with people. She loves spending time with us and playing with us. (Mother)

Three themes emerged from the literature data: Preference assessment for learning; Preference assessment for enjoyment and Just leisure. The first theme draws attention to the short history of preference assessment for people with PIMD. The second theme refers to a more recent trend in research on preference assessments for these people. This trend in research is associated with an equally recent interest in the third theme – recreation and leisure activities for people with PIMD.

Preference assessment for learning

The most critical feature in establishing functionality [in people with profound disabilities] is identifying the potential reinforcing objects, activities, or people. (Campbell, 1989, p. 168)

Preference assessment for enjoyment

Comprehensive assessments of individuals with PIMD should identify behaviours that include indications of favourite and special things, especially sensory experiences. (Barber, 2001, p. 5)

Just leisure

For people with, "leisure time use is increasingly recognised as an important determinant of quality of life. Leisure includes free time, a variety of interests and activities, freedom, choice and relaxation. It is intrinsically rewarding". (Cavet & Lacey, 1998, pp. 204–205)

Subcategory – Being with others... Is caring and sharing.

[Child] seeks out your face and your hands. He touches and holds your hand or arm, looks closely at your face with a huge smile, especially if your response is animated and positive. If you respond with a hug, a stroke of his hair or a kiss, he makes no attempt to move away. Sometimes though he grabs you and seems to want to take you with him. (Respite Carer)

Subcategory – Special things... Is doing special things with special people.

[O]ver at [my wife's] dad's place he has these particular placemats with lots of little dots on it and [our daughter] will actually, if you walk her through the kitchen, she will stop at that table and play with those table placemats... And that's the first thing she wants to do every time she goes to Poppy's, Play with those placemats. (Parents)

Subcategory – Water Play... Playing with water is freedom, fun and belonging.

I think if [my granddaughter] could spend the day any way she wanted, she would spend a whole day in the hydrotherapy pool. I think she loves that pool and the bath and the water. I think that's (her) greatest love. (Grandmother)

Subcategory – Fun... Is having a "wicked" sense of humour!

[My student] gets silly, goes through silly stages, where he might try and keep putting his foot out to trip you over. Yeh, he goes through silly little things like that. And it's on purpose. He knows it's silly. He thinks that's funny. (Teacher Aide)

Key Interrelationships Between and Within Categories

The interrelationships between these 18 categories are complex. The Relational Scaffold (Fig. 12.2 below) summarises these. This scaffold draws upon the metaphor of a "mobile" wherein life satisfaction may be said to be best when the mobile is in balance, that is, when the categories and interrelationships between them result in a personal balance for the individual child.

Key Interrelationships Between the Central and Main Categories

Key interrelationships give "structure" to this theory when they link at the first and broadest level between the central category and the four main categories. The central category, Doing enjoyable things, embraces and permeates all of its four main categories. A "best" life satisfaction comes when children with PIMD experience a personal balance of all elements of Life Satisfaction. This balance is "centred" when the central and 14 main categories coincide. The "position" of this balance is primarily influenced by the "weight" contributed by the main categories of Happiness and contentment, and Comfort and wellbeing.

The position of this balance is very personal, and often difficult for others to ascertain. The greatest challenge is for communication partners to find and respond to this personal balance. To experience a best life satisfaction, children with PIMD need communication partners who know them well.

Key Interrelationships Within – Just Like Other Children but Personal

Life satisfaction discourses explains what other people understand life satisfaction might be for children with PIMD, and indeed for all children, however, children with PIMD are like most other children in terms of the (lack of) meaning and utility of this term. Similarly, Disability discourses are about how others view, interpret and/or understand disability, especially PIMD. Individuality, like Disability discourses, juxtaposes against Just like other children but personal in contrasting ways. First and foremost, children with PIMD are just like other children and similarly are demonstratively individual. Implicit in Childhood is growth, development and change, and future Adulthood. Similarly, implicit in Childhood is an orientation towards the here and now.

Key Interrelationships Within – Happiness and Contentment

Happiness and contentment is what life satisfaction is really all about. It is what the children want and what their close others want (and expect) for them. Children with PIMD appear, and are reported, to be happy children (unless they are in pain). Contentment is often just taking it all in. Clearly, finding a personal Balance for children with PIMD is important if they are to experience life satisfaction. Children with PIMD, just like other children, cannot be happy or contented all day, every day, they cannot be just taking it all in, all day every day, but children with PIMD, just like all children, should experience happiness and contentment at least every day.

Key Interrelationships Within – Comfort and Wellbeing

Comfort and wellbeing are essential prerequisites for happiness and contentment, and are what children with PIMD need. Physical health, especially relief from acute and/or chronic pain, is prerequisite to feeling comfort and having wellbeing. In fact, for many of children with PIMD, Daily wellbeing, just having a good day, occurs simply when their pain is relieved. Comfort and wellbeing come from Belonging. Without belonging and valued relationships, daily wellbeing and even continuing physical health are unlikely.

Key Interrelationships Within – Favourite Things

Being with others, caring and sharing, is the most favoured thing. For most of the children being with others is the consistent theme that "adds value" to their other favourite things, that is, Doing special things is best when it involves being with others, Water play is freedom and fun and Being with others, and just having Fun is sharing a wicked sense of humour through Being with others. Caring and sharing are the links that are common to all these subcategories

Being with others is a frequent experience for children with PIMD. This can explain in part why the children seem quite happy, because they experience their most favoured things frequently. Conversely, Special things and Water play are experienced less frequently, and are maybe valued in part because of this. Being with others and Water play are usually initiated by others, whereas Special things and Fun are frequently initiated by the children.

The Grounded Theory: Its Significance and Potential Implications

This theory has potential implications for a diversity of policies, practices and research that relate to the lives of children with PIMD, and which might ultimately improve their life satisfaction and quality of life. First, the "take home message" is that the life satisfaction of children with PIMD can be discerned. Second, the theory gives weight to widespread parental and carer claims that they generally know their children well enough to discern their life satisfaction – including their happiness, wants and preferences – despite a body of professional opinion claiming that this knowing is overstated. Third, it suggests that unfamiliar others, who often shy away from engaging with children with PIMD, can come to know them and can come to understand their inner states.

This theory could encourage further basic research into the nature of life satisfaction (subjective wellbeing and subjective quality of life) for children with PIMD, and/or for other persons for whom communication and understanding about feelings and emotions is challenging. These could include younger children, adults with PIMD, older persons with severe dementia and/or people with severe acquired brain damage.

That the life satisfaction of children with PIMD can be described and explained has substantial implications for their welfare. Learning about (the life satisfaction of) persons with PIMD takes time, and staff changes and turnover in support services are quite high. As a result, knowledge and understanding about these individuals is often lost, so a better knowledge of the processes by which others come to know about the life satisfaction of these individuals would obviously be valuable.

This theory could inform the development of a more thorough process to transfer information and understanding from existing (or departing) to new communication partners. Second, it could contribute to improving the initial training for and/or familiarisation of education personnel, residential care and support workers, and health professionals. Third, this could assist parents, family and other primary carers to learn more quickly and/or thoroughly about the wants, likes and preferences of their children.

A number of other issues and challenges emerge from this research. . .

- Children with PIMD, like all children, want to do enjoyable things. Given their pervasive dependence on those close to them, just how actively engaged are they? Given that a "full life" seems a good life, how can we make routine activities of daily living, which occupy so much of the day (more) enjoyable for both the children and their carers?
- Children with PIMD can be content to "just take it all in". Obviously, it is essential that communication partners can discern between contentment and boredom. It is about a personal balance. . . Is it OK for children with PIMD to just enjoy their own time and space?
- Children with PIMD seem quite reasonably happy, at least in comparison to other children, but their (objective) quality of life is totally in other's hands. In general, infanticide and euthanasia, particularly as they relate to infants with PIMD, are argued for primarily on the basis that children with PIMD will experience an unbearably poor quality of life. How justified is this view?
- Children with PIMD, like all children, enjoy fun. They often have a wicked sense of humour and display some considerable emotional intelligence. Can prevailing discourses of disability be revised to embrace emotional intelligence as an indicator of social validity or value?
- Children with PIMD, like all children, go to school to learn. Special education curriculum generally embraces a "common" curriculum with a functional skills orientation. If a core goal of education is to empower individuals to pursue a better quality of life as a contributing citizen, is education for fun, not (just) education with fun, worth reconsidering?
- Children with PIMD regard water play as a favourite thing, and as meaning freedom, fun and belonging. Water play seems to have an almost universal appeal. How prominent is water play in the lives of most children with PIMD?
- Children with PIMD have "special things" – special ways of engaging with particular people. So often these special and valuable things remain undisclosed. This demonstrates a unique quality of intersubjectivity – a communicative strength to work with to empower them as social beings. Could communication training embrace these special things, and adopt rather than adapt them to empower other communication partnerships?
- Generally, children with PIMD are happy children – when they are not in pain and when they experience a balance in doing enjoyable things. If the quality of life paradigm prevailed, could this be seen as some reassurance to parents and other primary carers that they are "doing a good job"?
- Children with PIMD need communication partners who can respond to their wants, interests and preferences. Turnover amongst staff in respite care services, support services and schools can be high – sometimes as a result of policy. Should services encourage and support greater staff stability, possibly at the expense of other apparent priorities?

- Relationships are central to life satisfaction. How can we make sure that children with PIMD "belong"?
- For children with PIMD, life satisfaction is very much about happiness, and happiness is relatively easy to discern. Is the assessment of the happiness of children with PIMD a priority?
- The life satisfaction of children with PIMD can be discerned. Individual Plans should focus on an individual's wants, interests and preferences, rather than (just) their "best interests". Is Person Centred Planning the right way to go?
- For many of children with PIMD pain is pervasive. Until this pain is addressed, a focus on life satisfaction seems to lose importance for carers. Are frequent regular (preventative) medical checkups a priority for children with PIMD?
- Children with PIMD, who usually live at home, are generally happy. Adults with PIMD, who more usually live in supported congregate care, seem less so. (A personal observation and judgment.) Is something going wrong?

The "final say" about life satisfaction for children with profound multiple intellectual disabilities comes from the children themselves. If they were asked just what life satisfaction was, they might reply...

> You can come to know us, and about our life satisfaction. (The term doesn't make much sense, but quality of life and happiness do!) It's mostly about doing fun things with the people that we like. It's the same for us as it is for other children, but we show how we think and feel in very personal ways.
>
> Different people see us in different ways. It depends on how they understand our disabilities. People who don't know us usually only see our disabilities, and not how we are feeling, learning and growing. We are individuals in what we do and how we feel. We are children and we have a future, but we live mostly in the here and now.
>
> A good life is having happiness and contentment each day, although contentment can be as simple as just taking it all in. It's about being in balance. A good life is also about comfort and wellbeing. Many of us have lots of pain, so our health is very important. Just having a good day is great.
>
> Being friends is most important. It's about belonging. A good life is also about our favourite things. This can be just caring and sharing, or doing special things with special people, or playing in water, or just joking around!
>
> It can be hard to come to know us, and this is hard to explain. It's the same as with other children, but takes longer. Eventually, the penny will drop for you! To come to know us, you need to do three things at the same time.
>
> First, you need to watch and listen for how we show our feelings, for "patterns" in what we do every day, and for changes in these patterns. You need to be able to look back to learn to understand the little things we do.
>
> Second, you need to spend time being with us and playing with us. You need to do the usual, simple things with us, and then put yourself in our shoes. What you do will probably be just trial and error, but you can experiment on purpose.
>
> Third, you need to talk to the people who know us, and ask the right questions, and work together with others. This takes some planning.
>
> How well you come to know us depends upon how well you know yourself. Your time with other children can help, and how you feel about us and what you presume about us is important. For some people this is hard, and for others it's easy. Some people have just got it!

References

Arthur, M. (1994). Communicative instruction in the 1990's: An overview of future directions. In K. Linfoot (Ed.), *Communication strategies for people with developmental disabilities: Issues from theory and practice* (pp. 177–197). Artarmon: MacLennan & Petty.

Arthur, M. (1998). *Socio-communicative variables and behaviour states in students with the most severe and multiple disabilities: An observational study*. Unpublished PhD thesis, Macquarie University, Sydney.

Atkins, C. (1999). *Just little things: Nurses' perceptions of quality of life for people with severe multiple impairments*. Unpublished PhD thesis, University of Sydney, Sydney.

Bach, M. (1994). Quality of life: Questioning the vantage points for research. In M. H. Rioux & M. Bach (Eds.), *Disability is not measles: New research paradigms in disability* (pp. 127–152). North York, ON: Roeher Institute.

Barber, P. (1990). *Literature review: Medical decision-making for newborns with disabilities. Quality of life as a criterion*. Lawrence, KS: Beach Center on Family and Disability, The University of Kansas.

Barber, M. (2001). *Affective Communication Assessment: An Owners Manual*. P.M.L.D. Link, 13(1).

Bigby, C., & Ozanne, E. (2001). Shifts in the model of service delivery in intellectual disability in Australia. *Journal of Intellectual and Developmental Disability, 26*(2), 177–190.

Bogdan, R. C., & Taylor, S. J. (1989). Relationships with severely disabled people: The social construction of humanness. *Social Problems, 36*(2), 135–148.

Brown, C. (1989). *My left foot*. London: Mandarin.

Butow, H. (1993). Australian disability strategy. *Australian Disability Review, 93*(4), 5–11.

Butterfield, N., & Arthur, M. (1995). Shifting the focus: Emerging priorities in communication programming for students with a severe intellectual disability. *Education and Training in Mental Retardation and Developmental Disabilities, 30*, 41–50.

Butterfield, N., Arthur, M., & Linfoot, K. (1992). Meeting communication needs in communication programming for students with severe intellectual disability: The creating communicative contexts manual. *Special Education Perspectives, 1*(1), 35–43.

Campbell, P. H. (1989). Dysfunction in posture and movement in individuals with profound disabilities: Issues and practices. In F. Brown & D. H. Lehr (Eds.), *Persons with profound disabilities: Issues and practices* (pp. 163–189). Baltimore, MD: Paul H. Brookes.

Carnaby, S. (2001). Editorial. *Tizard Learning Disability Review, 6*(2), 2.

Carter, M., & Hook, J. (1998). Communication programming for students with high support needs: A model for deciding what to teach. *Special Education Perspectives, 7*(1), 42–55.

Cavet, J., & Lacey, P. (1998). Leisure and the arts. In P. Lacey & C. Ouvry (Eds.), *People with profound and multiple learning disabilities: A collaborative approach to meeting complex needs* (pp. 204–214). London: David Fulton.

Chang, S. O. (2001). The conceptual structure of physical touch in caring. *Journal of Advanced Nursing, 33*(6), 820–827.

Compton, D. A. (1997). (Ed.). *Issues in therapeutic recreation: a profession in transition.* Champaign: Sagamore Press.

Crocker, A. C. (2000). Introduction: The happiness in all our lives. *American Journal on Mental Retardation, 105*(5), 319–325.

Crossley, R., & McDonald, A. (1980). *Annie's coming out*. Ringwood: Penguin.

Davison, I. (1977). *Values, ends and society*. St. Lucia: University of Queensland Press.

Dostoyevsky, F. (1950). *The brothers Karamazov*. Translated from the Russian by C. Garnett. New York: Random House.

Edgerton, R. B. (1990). Quality of life from a longitudinal research perspective. In R. L. Schalock & M. J. Begab (Eds.), *Quality of life: Perspectives and issues* (pp. 149–160). Washington, DC: American Association on Mental Retardation.

Evans, D. R. (1994). Enhancing quality of life in the population at large. *Social Indicators Research, 33*, 47–88.

Favell, J. E., Realon, R. E., & Sutton, K. A. (1996). Measuring and increasing the happiness of people with profound mental retardation and physical handicaps. *Behavioral Intervention, 11*(1), 47–58.

Feil, N. (1993). *The validation breakthrough*. Sydney: McLennan & Petty.

Felce, D. (1997). Defining and applying the concept of quality of life. *Journal of Intellectual Disability Research, 41*(2), 126–135.

Felce, D., & Perry, J. (1996). Assessment of quality of life. In R. L. Schalock (Ed.), *Quality of life: Volume 1: Conceptualization and measurement* (pp. 63–72). Washington, DC: American Association on Mental Retardation.

Fidler, G. S. (1996). Life-style performance: From profile to conceptual model. *The American Journal of Occupational Therapy, 50*(2), 139–147.

Finkelstein, V. (1993). The commonality of disability. In J. Swain, V. Finkelstein, S. French, & M. Oliver (Eds.), *Disabling barriers – Enabling environments* (pp. 13–16). London: Sage.

Foreman, P., & Arthur, M. (2002, November). *Perspectives on educational programming for students with high support needs*. Paper presented at the Australian Society for the Study of Intellectual Disability 35th Annual Conference, Melbourne, Australia.

Goldstein, H., Kacmarek, L. A., & English, K. M. (2002). *Promoting social communication: Children with developmental disabilities from birth to adolescence*. Sydney: Paul H. Brookes.

Goode, D. A. (1990). On understanding without words: Communication between a deaf-blind child and her parents. *Human Studies, 13*, 1–37.

Goode, D. A. (1994). *A world without words: The social construction of children born deaf and blind*. Philadelphia, PA: Temple University Press.

Goode, D. A. (1995). *Self-determination and choice by people with severe intellectual disability*. New York: College of Staten Island.

Goode, D. A. (1997). Assessing the quality of life of adults with profound disabilities. In R. I. Brown (Ed.), *Quality of life for people with disabilities: Models, research and practice* (2nd ed., pp. 72–90). Cheltenam: Stanley Thornes.

Guess, D., Roberts, S., & Behrens, G. A. (1998). Response to Mudford, Hogg, and Roberts on continuous recording of behavior state. *American Journal on Mental Retardation, 103*(1), 75–79.

Halpern, A. S. (1993, July). *Evaluation of the transition process from a qualitative process*. Paper presented at the Second International Transition Conference, Sydney, Australia.

Hogg, J. (1998). Competence and quality in the lives of people with profound and multiple learning disabilities: Some recent research. *Tizard Learning Disabilities Review, 3*(1), 6–14.

Hogg, J., & Lambe, L. (1997). An ecological perspective on the quality of life of people with intellectual disabilities as they age. In R. I. Brown (Ed.), *Quality of life for people with disabilities: Models, research and practice* (2nd ed., pp. 201–227). Cheltenham: Stanley Thornes.

Hogg, J., Reeves, D., Roberts, J., & Mudford, O. C. (2001). Consistency, context and confidence in judgments of affective communication in adults with profound intellectual and multiple disabilities. *Journal of Intellectual Disability Research, 45*(1), 18–29.

Lambe, L., & Hogg, J. (2001). *Creative arts and people with profound and multiple learning disabilities: Education, therapy and leisure*. Brighton: Pavilion.

Landesman, S. (1986). Quality of life and personal satisfaction: Definition and measurement issues. *Mental Retardation, 24*(3), 141–143.

Lu, L., & Shih, J. B. (1997). Personality and happiness: Is mental health a mediator? *Personality and Individual Differences, 22*(2), 249–256.

Lyons, G. S. (2003). *Life satisfaction for children with profound multiple disabilities*. Unpublished PhD thesis, University of Newcastle, Callaghan, Australia.

Perrin, B., & Nirje, B. (1985). Setting the record straight: A critique of some frequent misconceptions of the normalization principle. *Australia and New Zealand Journal of Developmental Disabilities, 11*(2), 69–74.

Rawlings, M., Dowse, L., & Shaddock, A. (1995). Increasing the involvement of people with an intellectual disability in choice making situations: A practical approach. *International Journal of Disability, Development and Education*, *42*(2), 137–153.

Reeves, D., Hogg, J., Roberts, J., & Mudford, O. C. (2000). *On what do staff base judgments of affective communication with adults with profound intellectual and multiple disabilities?* Unpublished manuscript, University of Manchester, Manchester, UK.

Reiss, S. (2001). A sensitivity theory of end motivation: Implications for mental retardation. In H. N. Switzky (Ed.), *Personality and motivational differences in persons with mental retardation* (pp. 373–392). Mahwah, NJ: Lawrence Earlbaum Associates.

Romney, D. M., Brown, R. I., & Fry, P. S. (1994). *Improving the quality of life: Recommendations for people with and without disabilities*. Dordrecht: Kluwer Academic.

Schalock, R. L. (1990). Attempts to conceptualize and measure quality of life. In R. L. Schalock & M. J. Begab (Eds.), *Quality of life: Perspectives and issues* (pp. 141–148). Washington, DC: American Association on Mental Retardation.

Sheldon, K. M., Ryan, R., & Reis, H. T. (1996). What makes for a good day? Competence and autonomy in the day and in the person. *Personality and Social Psychology Bulletin*, *22*(12), 1270–1279.

Szymanski, L. S. (2000). Happiness as a treatment goal. *American Journal on Mental Retardation*, *105*(5), 352–362.

Taylor, S. J., & Bogdan, R. (1996). Quality of life and the individual's perspective. In R. L. Schalock (Ed.), *Quality of life: Volume 1: Conceptualization and measurement* (pp. 11–22). Washington, DC: American Association on Mental Retardation.

Velde, B. P. (1996). Quality of life through personally meaningful activity. In R. L. Schalock (Ed.). *Quality of life: Perspectives and issues* (pp. 12–26). Washington, DC: American Association on Mental retardation.

Vlaskamp, C., & Nakken, H. (1999). Missing in execution: Therapies and activities for individuals with profound multiple disabilities. *British Journal of Development Disabilities*, *45*(2), 99–109.

Wolf, N. (1990). *The beauty myth*. London: Vintage.

Wolfensberger, W. (1995). Social role valorization is too conservative. No, it's too radical. *Disability & Society*, *10*(3), 365–367.

Chapter 13
Aspects of Quality of Life for Children with a Disability in Inclusive Schools

Joanne Shearer

Introduction

Quality of life has been conceptualized and presented by researchers in the field of disability studies as a useful model for lifestyle assessment, planning, and intervention (Brown et al., 2000; Schalock et al., 2002). It has been described as a sensitizing concept and a holistic phenomenon, which is lifespan-oriented and subject to the complexity of interacting forces (Brown, 1997; Parmenter, 1994; Renwick, Brown, & Nagler, 1996; Schalock, 1996; Taylor, 1994). Certain aspects of quality of life for individuals have been found to be culturally specific, pertaining to the country in which they live, their religious foundations, and the dominant philosophies and ideologies of their time in history (Goode, 1994a). The international consensus document, reported in *Mental Retardation* by Schalock et al. (2002), discussed the growing interest in quality of life as an influential concept in the field of disability, and set out guidelines for conceptualizing, measuring, and applying quality of life to all groups. As quality of life research developed, it became clear that a consensus document, such as this, was needed to bring together the variation in literature which had accumulated internationally. The purpose for the consensus document was to demonstrate unity and provide a clear framework for further quality of life applications (see Schalock et al., 2002).

In the early years (i.e., the 1980s) quality of life studies in the field of intellectual disabilities focused mostly on the lives of adults. These studies found the quality of life approach to be culturally relevant – taking into account environmental variables, individual perceptions, and personal values. The quality of life perspective shed new light on the progress being made toward community living for people with intellectual disabilities and their access to mainstream vocations. The differences between proxy responses and the perceptions of the individuals themselves also became evident through quality of life research. Concepts such as choice and empowerment, personal preferences, self-determination, and the relationship between risk-taking

J. Shearer (✉)
Flinders University, Adelaide, South Australia, Australia
e-mail: joanneshearer@aapt.net.au

R. Kober (ed.), *Enhancing the Quality of Life of People with Intellectual Disabilities*, Social Indicators Research Series 41, DOI 10.1007/978-90-481-9650-0_13,

and human development were debated. In addition, researchers leading these early studies grappled with how best to measure an individual's quality of life (see Brown, Bayer, & MacFarlane, 1989; Cummins, 1991; Goode, 1994b; Renwick, Brown, & Raphael, 1994; Schalock, Keith, Hoffman, & Karan, 1989), and contributed a great deal to the discussion and development of Quality of Life (QOL) as a tool for practical application in service developments.

Developments in the area of quality of life measurement have been clearly documented in the literature and have progressed even further to describe how quality of life can be used for evaluation and service development, professional training, intervention, and in the assessment of Family Quality of Life (Turnbull, Brown, & Turnbull, 2004; Brown & Brown, 2003; Schalock, Gardner, & Bradley, 2007; Schalock & Verdugo, 2002). In 2005, an issue of the *Journal of Intellectual and Disability Rehabilitation* focused exclusively on the theme of quality of life applications, and more recently Schalock and his colleagues have shared their insights on applying quality of life based on decades of combined research and experience (Shalock et al., 2007).

As confidence in using the quality of life model has grown, and increased understandings shared, inquiry and discussion has broadened to family life and other disability groups, including children. (Exceptionality Education Canada, 2000; Isaacs et al., 2007; Turnbull, Brown, & Turnbull, 2004). The Beach Center at the University of Kansas has taken a lead in understanding and discussing various aspects of quality of life for families who have a member with a disability (see www.beachcenter.org), as have a group of international research colleagues, in their development of the International Family Quality of Life study (Isaacs et al., 2007).

In 1993, Timmons, in her study on the quality of life of adolescents living in Calgary, noted that, at the time, of almost 1,000 studies concerned with quality of life for people with a disability, less than 30 were concerned with children. While there has been considerably more discussion on quality of life for children with a disability (Exceptionality Education Canada, 2000; McKenzie, 2000) since then the topic remains one of the less-explored aspects of quality of life research and a specific focus on the unique aspects of quality of life for children with a disability remains minimal in the literature.

The study on which this chapter is based sought information about quality of life for children with a disability, the relevance of Quality of Life as a means of measuring children's experiences, and its relevance to their future lives. The chapter shares insights from the children and their parents and describes aspects of their life experiences which have enhanced their quality of life. The chapter is divided into discrete sections to share this information within the study's context. First, the participants and methods for inquiry and analysis are described, and then comments on the findings of using the Quality of Life model and its concepts are expressed. The study used a mix of quality of life concepts and the Felce and Perry (1993) Quality of Life framework. The remainder of the chapter is devoted to discussing the quality of life experiences of these children.

The Participants

The study was based in Adelaide, South Australia, and draws on the experiences of five young children with a disability who attended inclusive school settings. Four children had Down syndrome and one child cerebral palsy. All five children were included in a mainstream school, were girls, and were aged from 9 to 12 years.

The families were invited to contribute through their disability service provider. The criteria for participation were clearly stipulated, and the families' participation was voluntary. The child with a disability had to be in their primary years of schooling (i.e., 8–12 years old); attending a mainstream school; able to respond verbally to oral questions in a face-to-face situation; and both their mother and father needed to be living in the same home as their children.

The aim of the study was to explore the application of the quality of life model as an approach to research the lives of children with a disability and inform decisions about intervention and service development.

Method of Investigation and Analysis

The Felce and Perry (1997) quality of life framework was the structure employed in this study. Felce and Perry (1993) contributed to the conceptualization and measurement of quality of life by reviewing the voluminous amount of literature on the topic of wellbeing, then synthesizing the concept into a functional framework, with the aim of developing a common approach to quality of life applicable across societal groups. Their framework has three major elements, subjective and objective measurement, life domains, and the influence of personal values.

The methodology involved interviews with children and adults (face-to-face) to seek their perceptions of the children's lives. This approach represents a subjective method of measuring quality of life. In addition to the data collected by interview questions, information was also gathered incidentally and informally in pre-interview and post-interview visits to the families' homes. Observations of housing quality, material possessions, and the number of members in each family contributed to the overall picture of the children's lifestyle and their family structure.

The children themselves and their parents were interviewed separately and each person answered questions designed to seek information about the child's past and current life experiences, as well as their vision for the future. The children all had an intellectual disability. They were keen to participate in the interview process, so their motivation was high and they responded well to questioning. In some instances the children would assert themselves to correct the interviewer's interpretation of their responses – when it was wrong. This behavior is likely to have increased the reliability of the data, the accuracy of the data recorded (which was on audiotape and in written note form) and therefore, the validity of the findings. Collecting information from the children, while important, did prove limited with regard to the amount of information they provided. It was important to collect information from the parents also to enhance and enrich the understanding of these children's lives.

The parents' responses were not intended as substitutes or to provide proxy responses to that of their children, but rather to provide additional, and possibly different, perceptions that supplemented their child's view of the world. Parents' responses tended to be similar – complementing and enhancing their child's. In no instances did an individual's response greatly contradict the information provided by another member of the same family; however, there were a few occasions when the children's views were slightly different from that of the parents'. In the majority of cases, each interviewee confirmed the reliability and validity of each other's comments, even though they were not privy to the responses of another beforehand. Interviewing the families in their own home added to their level of comfort when interviewed.

Interviewing fathers about their child with a disability was another distinct aspect of this study because mostly mothers had been the primary source of information when investigating the life experiences of children with a disability. Often the mothers of this study knew more about practical aspects of the child's life, like the child's schooling and leisure activities, whereas the fathers provided their perspectives on their relationship with their child, the role they played in their child's life and their lifestyle, and reflected on their own values about their child's disability.

The children provided wonderful insight into their private view of the world. However, each of them also found some of the questions difficult to comprehend and answer. In these cases the children would often respond with brief answers or not respond to questions at all. It was important to elicit as much information from the children as possible because they were considered to be the key participants in the research (because the study was essentially about the children's own lives), and their perceptions were highly valued for this reason. Often when more information was required, spontaneous and idiosyncratic additional questions were prompted. Discretionary judgments were made also not to include some of the questions, because they became repetitive, too complex, or the children tired.

Particular themes emerged from the adults' and children's responses, such as the influence of health and physical status, participation in leisure activities, community involvement, skills development, family relationships, school as a meeting point for developing friendships, teachers' professional knowledge and competence, the importance of open communication, and concern for the safety and security of the children. The variation in abilities and competencies of each of the children was also considered, as well as their childhood inexperience, the prevalence of choice in childhood, and a vision for their futures. The impact of the school experience and the perceived benefits and limitations of inclusive schooling, while acknowledged as important influential factors, were secondary considerations to the aim of the study, which focused on understanding how the quality of life model applied to children with a disability.

Reflections on the Quality of Life Model and Concepts for Children with a Disability

The five life domains, of the Felce and Perry quality of life framework (productive, material, social, emotional, and physical wellbeing), together with the agreed conceptual principles of Quality of Life (choice and empowerment, self-image, a lifespan orientation, holism, human variability, and the interaction of environments), guided the development of questions and the analysis of the data.

In relation to life domains, there were differences between children's and adults' responses, in some areas of wellbeing. For example, *teachers* were not listed under the social wellbeing domain, yet the social relationships between teachers, children, and families were integral to the study. It seems important that *teachers* are included as a specific group when assessing the personal relationships of school age children and their families because the frequency of contact between teachers, children, and their families is so high. Similarly, emotional security was often discussed in the context of the parent–child relationship but this dimension was not listed as a subcategory of the emotional wellbeing domain. According to the framework, *security* is an indication of material wellbeing. This nuance in interpretation of the word *security* would need to be explained, and *emotional security* or alternatively *attachment* be added to the list of subcategories under the domain of emotional wellbeing when used to assess the lives of children with a disability.

In addition, some difficulties arose when trying to separate the data into life domains because the activities and experiences of children with a disability apply to more than one domain. For example, leisure activities such as swimming and walking could have been classified into the domains of productive wellbeing as well as physical wellbeing. Similarly, activities with family and friends could have been classified into both the emotional and social wellbeing domains. This finding reflects the holistic nature of the quality of life model and the interactive effects of life experiences. It also exposes a degree of artificiality when interpreting and classifying life into areas of wellbeing.

The impact of disability across the lifespan in relation to the rapidly changing dynamic of childhood was openly discussed by the parents when questioned. Their responses illustrated their awareness of the kaleidoscope of disability in the context of their family and community life. Knowledge of children's social structure in relation to their emotional wellbeing, their health in relation to their productive wellbeing, and their competencies in relation to their safety, and so forth, are important considerations because these interactions are likely to influence how others respond to them, which, in turn, can positively or negatively influence their quality of life. To understand the development of children as they grow and change enables recognition of their positive contributions and their future potential. This information is necessary when making decisions about how best to provide support to the child, so that they can achieve in their areas of strength, resolve difficulties, and establish a firm foundation for continued successes into adolescence and adulthood.

Brown, Bayer and Brown (1992) and Timmons and Brown (1997) discussed the link between choice, risk-taking and levels of achievement. They also discussed the impact of the provision or restriction of such opportunities on empowerment, self-image and motivation across all areas of an individual's life. The children of this study were provided with some choices to make for themselves and others were restricted by their parents. The parents made major decisions, such as which school to attend but in their decision-making would consider the needs of the child and the family and their decisions reflected their philosophy of inclusion. Over time, opportunities for the children to make choices would become broader and more frequent, as their knowledge and experiences increased and they came to understand the consequences of their choices.

Felce and Perry (1997) also emphasized the holistic nature of Quality of Life in relation to objective circumstances, subjective appraisal of circumstances and personal values, which are potentially interdependent at all times and the relationships between them are neither static nor uniform. They suggest that the interaction of these aspects contributes to an individual's quality of life and a change in one aspect may affect another.

This was true of the experiences of the children of this study. Their school lives affected their home life. The friends they made at school were most often the friends that they played with out of school; the need to complete homework affected the time they had available to pursue other activities at home or in the community. Conversely, home and community life also affected school life.

The positive or negative affect of school life on home life and vice versa was largely determined by the degree to which teachers, parents and the children communicated, planned and worked collaboratively. Behavior management was one area common to both settings and a consistent approach to communication was essential. One child's parents discussed their suspicion that their child's relationship with her teacher at school was not healthy because her behavior at home had changed. They described how at home, if she did something wrong, "She would actually go and sit and face the corner," which was not an expectation of her parents. This situation was resolved with the involvement of the principal and, ultimately, the child was moved to a different class with a different teacher.

When variation in rules and regulations between environments is necessary, these should be clearly communicated with the child, so they are able to distinguish between expectations in different settings. Collaborative partnerships and opportunities to share information between teachers, parents and others involved in the child's life are necessary to enhance the quality of life of the child. Teachers and parents need to work collaboratively and teachers are likely to benefit by learning about the importance of positive parent–teacher partnerships in their training.

Variability among families of children with a disability was prevalent – both intra-family variability and inter-family variability. Some of the inter-family variations noted from this study included housing type, socio-economic status, work roles, religion, activities, family dynamics and values. Intra-family variability included variables such as age, gender, personality, health, capability, knowledge, responsibility and position in the family.

It is important that the variation in families and the influences on quality of life be acknowledged. It is equally important to understand individuals' personal contexts, their perceptions and to recognize the unique characteristics of families of children with a disability when considering their quality of life assessments. Knowledge and acceptance of variability is a contributing factor for maintaining and developing quality of life. The challenge is how such variability can be accommodated in structured environments, such as schools. This challenge appeared to be taken up by the schools associated with the families of this study because on more that one occasion parents expressed with gratitude the support they received from their children's school teachers, teaching assistants and the principal, to include their child and family as valued members of the school community.

The Quality of Life Experiences of Children with a Disability

The children's life experiences are discussed in terms of their leisure and educational activities, health, family interaction and friendships – and these aspects have been classified according to the five life domains of the quality of life framework (i.e., physical, material, social, emotional and productive wellbeing). For families with more than one child, the parents' desire to treat each of their children similarly was evident and their children with a disability were fully included. They were involved in a range of activities to enhance their development, some individually and others with family and friends.

Of particular interest, was the way in which the children spoke about *here and now* when they reflected on the events that shaped their lives. They talked about their most recent activities, those that were freshest in their minds, the things that happened that day or in the very recent past and they provided concrete examples in response to the questions asked of them. In addition to talking about specific activities, all of the children spoke fondly about their friends, family and other relationships.

Comments on Inclusion

Parents had a desire for their children with a disability to be included in mainstream education but this was not without its dilemmas. Positive elements of inclusive schooling considered by the parents were that their children were challenged to do their best; and mostly their children learnt appropriate social behaviors through the modeling of their non-disabled peers. Parents also saw their children developing skills to participate in mainstream society that were considered useful for later years and their adult life.

The concerns of inclusive schooling were to achieve a balance between the pressure of keeping up with the other children academically and maintaining the children's self-worth and happiness, particularly as their delay in intellectual competence became more evident with age. The parents expressed some concern over long-lasting friendships because they feared that the number of their children's friends and the frequency of their contact would diminish. In addition, parents mentioned the shortfall of one-on-one instruction time at school to supplement the additional educational needs of their children, and they expressed concern over the limited skills of some teachers in their knowledge on how to include their children in the class, even though many of the teachers were very committed. The "battle" to educate the school community, teachers, teaching assistants, and other parents about the value and suitability of children with disabilities in mainstream education was a wearing demand on these families. Parents were not as concerned about the attitudes of their children's peers, which were mostly positive and inclusive.

The parents offered some very practical suggestions on how to enhance the quality of the inclusive process and how to provide effective support for their children with a disability. For example, hands on assistance at school, daily communication between home and school through diaries, consultation regarding the modification of curriculum and extra-curricula activities, and the need to recognize behavior as an indication of contentment or distress, to name just a few. These practical suggestions of what works to enhance the quality of life experiences of children with a disability are likely to vary according to each situation, and collaborative problem solving is often required. More importantly, is the emphasis on overarching principles and broader concepts. These include, knowing the child, their family and community life; maintaining collaborative partnerships; and emphasizing the positive attributes and capabilities of the child. These principles are transferable across situations and are readily integrated within the education system.

Life Domains

Productive Wellbeing

The differences between academic, social, and physical competencies for these children with a disability were evident and openly discussed by their parents. Two of the children were particularly well coordinated and good at physical activities like skipping, gymnastics, swimming, and other sports. These children highlight the need to be mindful of the variation in abilities across children with a disability and the importance of looking at children's positive assets, so their potential abilities and self-image can be nurtured.

Each of the children had a modified curriculum at school that was negotiated in consultations between teachers, principals, and the family. Sometimes, physical activities were modified, for example, some children were given a head start in the running race on sports day so they could finish with their peers. However, in contrast, another family discussed how they were not consulted about whether or not their child was to participate in the school's swimming carnival. Without consultation such modifications could be inappropriate. From this family's perspective, their child with a disability had an opportunity to show her competency at swimming, however, because she was unable to independently put on her bathers (and regularly received help from a school assistant to undertake this task), the school made the assumption that the child would not be physically capable to compete in the swimming events. They did not realize that she was a very capable swimmer and according to her parents was able to hold her own in competition. The child had trained during her private swimming lessons for the upcoming carnival but when the time arose, she was not provided with the opportunity to participate in the competitive races, instead she was included in the non-competitive activities. The family was disappointed that the school staff had not asked if she wanted to be included or not.

This example emphasizes the need for communication between everyone, the school, the parents and the child themselves, regarding children with a disability's productive and physical wellbeing. Consultations should seek out knowledge of children's capabilities in order to enhance their competencies and provide advice on which are the most appropriate opportunities for their development. They also offer an opportunity to incorporate the child and their parent's choices.

Independence was listed as a subcategory of the productive wellbeing domain and once again, the study showed variability across the group of children. From one perspective, all children in this age group are dependent – their family structure and parents provide for their fundamental needs, such as food, housing, clothing, transportation, health, and so on. Over the course of childhood and into adulthood it is usual for individuals to acquire life skills and become increasingly independent. However, the degree of independence that is possible for the children with a disability, relative to that of their non-disabled peers was of interest to this study.

All of the children from this study were independently mobile and capable of communicating verbally with others, although some had a speech impediment. These competencies (in communication and mobility) appeared to have enhanced the children being accepted and aided their assimilation into inclusive schools. The children were able to make friends and attend their friends' birthday parties without the support of their parents (other than for transportation). One of the children participated in mainstream acting and dance classes and had recently returned from an all inclusive school camp.

However, analysis across the families' showed the trend that the children's capacity for independence affected their opportunity to access certain groups, activities, and settings. At times, extra supports were needed for the children to be included and achieve the highest level of independence possible. Without this extra help some of the children would not have been able to participate in a mainstream curriculum.

The children's health status also influenced their independence. One of the children had epilepsy and consequently, extra staff were required for excursions because of the responsibility of the school to ensure she was safe in unfamiliar surroundings. Another child had a sleep disorder, which required her to use a specialized machine at night while she slept. Fortunately, her condition was not life-threatening and she did not need to do this every day so she was still able to go on school camps. Had she needed to use the machine every day and take it on camp, her participation may have been restricted. Parents also expressed some concern about their children not always having well-developed sense of physical boundaries, and they would wander. Potentially, this restricted their ability to participate in some school activities because extra supervision was needed, e.g., for school excursions, so they did not become lost.

Choice and control are also subcategories of the productive wellbeing domain. As with many families, choices are governed by parental oversight and similarly at school the children's choices were restricted within the school structure and overseen by the teacher.

Each of the children made some choices in their lives, e.g., they chose what to buy with their pocket money and what activities they wanted to do in their spare time at home, like watching television or playing on the computer. At school the children were able to choose which library book they wanted to borrow. However, none of the children chose where they sat in the classroom. The teachers made this decision to ensure the children were all placed where they could best learn.

Parents concurred that their children with a disability needed opportunities to learn how to make choices but overall the parents made decisions about the boundaries of those choices. Parental perception and respect for their child, coupled with the demonstration of negotiating skills was empowering for the children. In all of the families the parents expressed that their children knew how to be assertive – a skill that they valued – but there were times when their children understood parental authority too. For example, when one child was asked if it upset her when she did not get to choose, she gently replied, "No, I know about [mum and dad] saying no." The mutual respect expressed by both the children for their parents and by the parents for their children's growing development and independence was important to these children's Quality of Life. The way in which children are viewed by their parents influences not only their self-esteem but the opportunities that are presented to them, and consequently the way they develop.

Individual *productivity* and *contribution* were also part of the productive wellbeing domain. When considering this aspect of life quality for children with a disability, it is important to note that their primary occupation outside of the family home is obtaining an education. The children's level of productivity and contribution at school was highly varied. However, the parents of one child were able to distinguish when their child had been appropriately stimulated or motivated by the learning environment at school and when she had not because of the way she would behave at home. This perceptiveness offers an alternative to parents who only see the deficits in their child's learning, possibly without considering the environmental stimulation that their child may or may not be receiving. The teacher seemed to make all the difference.

Aside from the academic aspects of school, some of the children were involved with school-based activities like sports, the end of year concert, special assemblies, and the local pageant at Christmas – transferring their inclusion from school into their community environment.

In addition to school activities, each of the children was also involved in leisure and community activities outside of school hours. One family were active members of a church group and as a family they contributed to mission work for the church in the community. Their daughter with a disability was involved in this activity as part of the family's contribution. Another child was involved with a sailing club over the summer and, yet again, a different child had participated in three weddings, as flower girl.

Aside from these organized activities and events, all of the children were visible participants in their local communities. They went to the shops, to the movies and socialized with family and friends. Some of the children also talked about their contribution to home life – washing the dishes, collecting wood and putting the meals on the table at dinner time.

Material Wellbeing

The material wellbeing of these children with a disability was intrinsically linked to the material wellbeing of their families. This is typical for children in this age group. The children did not have a separate income nor did they have a routine for earning money on a regular basis, and although some of the children were provided with pocket money, most of their additional money came from other incidental sources like the "tooth fairy," birthdays and so forth. Most of the children were involved with money handling to various degrees and were developing basic financial management skills. They bought things they liked and could afford to buy, such as videos, books, ornaments, toys and treat foods (e.g., chips and candies).

This study's families functioned similarly with regard to their children's possessions. Parents provided for their children and the children were able to access family assets such as computers, videos, television, transportation vehicles, etc. Family meals were provided and housing quality varied. But each family had a single unit home with a yard and two forms of private transportation. Two of the family homes had a swimming pool in the back yard. As mentioned these children with a disability had access to their families' provisions and their financial security was linked to that of their family's.

Social Wellbeing

The quality of life framework divides social wellbeing into two major dimensions – interpersonal *relationships* and *community involvement – both* of which interrelate at times. The children of this study had extensive interpersonal relationships through their friends and family and all were involved in with community activities. They had many friends and spoke of their friends at school with enthusiasm. One of the children mentioned numerous friends during her interview and her parents went on to explain that she goes to school like everyone else and everyone knows her, probably more than they know her brother and sister. The children also spoke eagerly of family relationships, activities they did with their parents or siblings and mentioned extended family members such as grandparents and cousins. All of the families reflected a philosophy that valued family involvement and the child with disability benefited from this aspect of their family's lifestyle. These children were included in community-oriented family activities, like going out for dinner once a week or attending church.

Overall, the social relationships of these children with a disability were a positive aspect of their lives. However, some of the parents expressed concerns that the inclusion of their daughters into their peers groups may wane in the future. The parents of the eldest child commented on the reduction in the number of friends' names being discussed at home by their daughter, as she grew older, suggesting a reduction in the number of friends that she had at school.

Some instances of negative interactions were discussed, but mostly this was raised by the parents – the children did not respond negatively about their social lives. Some parents mentioned teasing at school but emphasized that these were isolated incidents and were not an enduring problem. Sometimes, the relationship between their child and a particular teacher had not been very good, and at these times the parents had taken steps to remedy the situation.

The parents supported their children's relationships, and the children were encouraged to visit a friend's home to play or to have a friend over to their house to play. Two families spoke of inviting the child's teacher to their home to share a meal at the end of the school year, as a way of thanking them for their effort and a way to nurture this relationship positively.

In addition to family and school life, the children were involved in community activities – playing sport, attending dance or gymnastics class (just to name a few). Each child had a blend of both mainstream group activities and specialized activates for children with a disability, depending on the availability of the activity and the needs of the child. This level of inclusive involvement for children with a disability within their home and community life supported the inclusive aspect of their school lives, and provided a foundation for continued community inclusion as the children aged.

Emotional Wellbeing

The parents all showed a level of respect for their children with a disability, which supported the child's status and enhanced their self-esteem. The children were not only respected, loved, and supported by their parents in multiple areas of their lives but extended family members also showed this support; grandparents, siblings, aunties and cousins. This level of social support assists families to cope and represents a very positive attribute of these family's lives. *Respect* was not an aspect of emotional wellbeing explicitly listed in the quality of life framework but would also seem to be an important inclusion.

Certain aspects of the children's lives had definite emotional effects, e.g., poor health appeared to reduce the children's confidence. However, when their parents intervened to look after their interests, this demonstration of love and support was seen to contribute to the emotional security of the children with a disability and enhanced their sense of self-worth.

Parents also commented that their children were beginning to understand that they were somehow different from their peers. The affect of this awareness was not clear and varied between families. One father expressed his concern by saying, "it's very soul destroying to point out to your child that she is different." However, another family had been very up front with their child about her disability from an early age. They commented that she seemed to enjoy her difference. Yet, in contrast, another child showed sensitivity and an awareness of her disability by not wanting to discuss how she received extra help.

There were no indications of adverse mental health conditions among the children of this study, although there were indicators of distress. For example, one mother spoke of her daughter crying a lot when she was younger. This same child had previously demonstrated behavior that was difficult for the school staff to manage like hiding under tables and wandering out of the school grounds. Her parents commented that these issues had settled down, now she was older.

"Spirituality," "Faith," and "Sexuality" were also subcategories of emotional wellbeing in the quality of life framework. However, questions directly related to these aspects of life were not asked. Three of the families indicated an association with the Christian faith and their children were actively involved in this aspect of family life, but to varying degrees. Sexuality was not discussed as an issue for the children because the children were prepubescent.

Physical Wellbeing

Each of the children appeared to have major health difficulties when younger. Three of the children with Down syndrome had heart conditions which required specialist attention and in some instances surgery as a baby. The child with cerebral palsy also had epilepsy, which at the time of the interview was under control but had had adverse affects on her wellbeing in the past. Another child had a sleep disorder that required specialist attention.

It was found that physical competence and health had a significant impact on children's quality of life both negatively and positively. These children were all physically capable of independent mobility, although three of the children were not as physically capable as their peers and required some modification of activities.

Safety was also considered an important issue for the children with a disability Specific issues regarding safety were mainly to do with an undeveloped sense of boundaries, and this factor, although commonly associated to children with Down syndrome (Stratford, 1989) was also a concern for the parents whose daughter had cerebral palsy.

Planning for the Future

It was considered important to discuss with the children their views, aspirations, and images for their future, because these provided insight for adult planning, decision-making, and the management of future opportunities. Mitchell (1993) emphasized that the decisions which are made on behalf of a child in the early stages of their lifetime, together with the values that influence these decisions, are critical foundations for the children's quality of life. The children of this study often expressed a vision for their future. Their parents also expressed a vision for their child, which was not dissimilar to their child's vision, but in addition they expressed a degree of concern for their child's future because of their increasing difficulty over academic achievement. Also, there was awareness by some parents that the number of friendships was diminishing and the maturity levels of their children and that of their peers grew further apart as the child aged. The parents wanted to minimize the negative effects of this phenomenon.

The children with a disability were encouraged in their abilities and were provided with opportunities to explore their potential further. Their lives were valued highly by their parents and other family members who supported them to achieve their best. Monitoring the children's desires and ambitions would be important if they were to continue to achieve high quality of life outcomes. Understanding their perceptions as they grow, develop, and become increasingly independent, was encouraged, so the children could be appropriately supported in areas that held value for them. The way in which parents accommodate their child's choices in the future, for example, their desire for relationships, employment, or leisure activities, would either stimulate or dispel their aspirations, and, in turn, have implications for their quality of life.

The children themselves were not focused on their more distant future and did not recall events of the distant past. When asked what they would like to do when they left school and became adults, some just did not know – others wanted to be a bride, a dancer, or a hairdresser. It was evident that the responsibility for future planning for children of this age rests with their parents.

Conclusions

Overall, this study was able to demonstrate how the Felce and Perry (1997) framework of quality of life domains, together with the major principles associated with the conceptualization of quality of life, could be applied to provide a reliable and sensitive basis for in-depth qualitative inquiry into the quality of life of children with an intellectual disability. The research method of face-to-face interviews provided voluminous and rich information from each child, complemented by elaboration from both their mother and father.

During analysis it was possible to extract major themes across the group, which directly related to the context and framework of a quality of life approach. Many issues relating to disability in each of the families, not just in terms of family intervention but in terms of the families interface with other organizations such as school, community groups, and disability agencies were present. The results also included a focus on children's perceptions, which had not yet been explored in any detail within the disability field. These children were equipped with skills for effective participation in the social and practical aspects of their lives – skills which were likely to develop further, allowing them to continue to participate in life in an inclusive manner.

The children's academic competencies were delayed but a negotiated curriculum at school had been provided to address this difference, and the schools were able to provide some level of one-on-one support through a special needs program. This specialized support was reserved for attention to particular skills within the areas of literacy and mathematics which was necessary to redress the children's skills delay and to develop their confidence in their abilities. This level of support should be maintained at a minimum, and possibly increased in future years, as the difference in competencies between these children and their non-disabled peers became greater.

The children had numerous friends and saw themselves as part of a social network. This had positive effects on their self-image and confidence, which transferred into their family lives and their participation in community activities. Each of the children displayed confidence when responding to questions during their interviews for this study. Their parents respected and nurtured these children in good relationships with friends and extended family, and with the school staff, in particular with their child's teacher, the school support officer and the principal.

Professional in-service training of school staff on disability topics and liaison with specialist disability organizations were considered to be advantageous. Comprehensive knowledge of the child's disability and of their unique personality and functioning were positive elements of inclusive schooling. Such knowledge dispelled any myths or negative assumptions that may have existed prior. The level to which these families went to help their children was insightful. This needs to be understood and acknowledged by the professionals working in partnership with such families. The study underscores the importance of a wide range of variables for children with a disability, such as opportunities for choice, adult knowledge of the child and their level of development, social relationships, inclusiveness, the importance of home structure to school, and the necessity for collaboration between interacting environments.

A limitation of this study was that is only collected subjective data. While it has been argued that the perceptions of the individuals are perhaps the most important elements of quality of life measurement (Andrews & Withey, 1976; Brown 1996), an objective assessment of life conditions would have added even greater depth and context to the study. To have observed the physical environment of the child's school would have been particularly valuable. In addition, qualitative interviews with siblings, extended family, friends, teachers and other participants in the child's life may also have broadened the depth of understanding. These are areas which remain to be explored and further research is warranted.

Although this study was not intended to be comparative, it would also be of interest to examine and discuss the findings of similar research, which explores the quality of life of children with a disability of similar age, but in different circumstances such as the nature of their disability or the environment in which their live (e.g., rural). It may be necessary to develop a collaborative approach to this type of quality of life research for children with a disability, where the findings of various studies can be linked, to present a holistic, lifespan view of quality of life across ages. Alternatively, this study provides a sound baseline for longitudinal research of the same children and their families.

Information collected about the quality of life of children with a disability can serve as valuable information for families, government, and service providers in understanding the role of professional practice and intervention. Of interest is whether services understand individual's perceptions and are able to accommodate choices. The challenge for researchers is to reliably collect information on children and their families, to generate descriptors of wellbeing and then, to see how this information can be generalized to the broader population to inform policies and professional practice.

References

Andrews, F. M., & Withey, S. B. (1976). *Social indicators of well-being: American's perceptions of life quality*. New York: Plenum Press.

Brown, R. I. (1997). *Quality of life for people with disabilities: Models research and practice*. Cheltenham: Stanley Thornes.

Brown, R. I. (1996). People with developmental disabilities: Applying Quality of Life to assessment and intervention. In R. Renwick, I. Brown, & M. Nagler (Eds.), *Quality of life in health promotion and rehabilitation* (pp. 253–267). Thousand Oaks: Sage.

Brown, R. I., Bayer, M. B., & Brown, P. M. (1992). *Empowerment and developmental handicaps: Choices and quality of life*. North York, ON: Captus University Press.

Brown, R. I., Bayer, M. B., & MacFarlane, C. (1989). *Rehabilitation programmes: Performance and quality of life of adults with developmental handicaps*. Toronto, ON: Lugus Productions Ltd.

Brown, I., & Brown, R. I. (2003). *Quality of life and disability: An approach for community practitioners*. London: Jessica Kingsley.

Brown, I., & Brown, R. I. (Eds.). (2000). Inclusion and quality of life: Special theme issue. *Exceptionality Education Canada*, *9*(1&2), 1–171.

Brown, I., Brown, R., Cummins, R. A., Felce, D., Mattika, L., Keith, K., et al. (2000). *Quality of life: Its conceptualization, measurement, and application*. A consensus document. International Association for the Scientific Study of Intellectual Disabilities.

Cummins, R. (1991). The comprehensive quality of life scale – intellectual disability: An instrument under development. *Australia and New Zealand Journal of Developmental Disabilities*, *17*(2), 259–264.

Felce, D., & Perry, J. (1993). *Quality of life: A contribution to its definition and measurement*. Cardiff: Mental Handicap in Wales Applied Research Unit.

Felce, D., & Perry, J. (1997). Quality of Life: The scope of the term and its breadth of measurement. In R. L. Brown (Ed.), *Quality of life for people with disabilities: Models research and practice* (pp. 49–62). Cheltenham: Stanley Thornes.

Goode, D. (1994a). The national quality of life for persons with disabilities project: A quality of life agenda for the United States. In D. Goode (Ed.), *Quality of life for persons with disabilities: International perspectives and issues* (pp. 139–161). Cambridge, MA: Brookline Books.

Goode, D. (1994b). *Quality of life for persons with disabilities: International perspectives and issues*. Cambridge, MA: Brookline Books.

Isaacs, B. J., Brown, I., Brown, R. I., Baum, N., Myerscough, T., Neikrug, S., et al. (2007). The international family quality of life project: Goals and description of a survey tool. *Journal of Policy and Practice in Intellectual Disabilities*, *4*(3), 177–185.

McKenzie, S. (2000). Using quality of life as the focus for investigating the lives of people who have children with disabilities. *International Journal of Practical Approaches to Disability, 23*(2), 9–16.

Mitchell, D. (1993). Quality of life for infants and toddlers. *Australia and New Zealand Journal of Developmental Disabilities, 18*(4), 229–234.

Parmenter, T. R. (1994). Quality of life as a concept and measurable entity. In D. M. Romney, R. I. Brown, & P. S. Fry (Eds.), *Improving the quality of life: Recommendations for people with and without disabilities* (pp. 8–46). Dordrecht: Kluwer.

Renwick, R., Brown, I., & Nagler, M. (1996). *Quality of life in health promotion and rehabilitation.* Thousand Oaks, CA: Sage.

Renwick, R., Brown, I., & Raphael, D. (1994). Quality of life: Linking a conceptual approach to service provision. *Journal on Developmental Disabilities, 3*(2), 32–44.

Schalock, R. L. (1996). *Quality of life: Conceptualisation and measurement.* Washington, DC: American Association on Mental Retardation.

Schalock, R. L., Brown, I., Brown, R., Cummins, R. A., Felce, D., Matikka, L., et al. (2002). Conceptualization, measurement, and application of quality of life for persons with intellectual disabilities: Report of an international panel of experts. *Mental Retardation, 40*(6), 457–470.

Schalock, R. L., Gardner, J. F., & Bradley, V. J. (2007). *Quality of life for people with intellectual and other developmental disabilities: Applications across individuals organizations, communities, and systems.* Washington, DC: American Association on Intellectual and Developmental Disabilities.

Schalock, R. L., Keith, K. D., Hoffman, K., & Karan, O. C. (1989). Quality of life: Its measurement and use. *Mental Retardation, 27*(1), 25–31.

Shalock, R. L., & Verdugo, M. (2002). *Handbook on quality of life for human service practitioners.* Washington, DC: American Association on Mental Retardation.

Stratford, B. (1989). *Down's syndrome: Past, present and future.* London: Penguin.

Taylor, S. J. (1994). In support of research of quality of life, but against QOL. In D. Goode (Ed.), *Quality of life for persons with disabilities: International perspectives and issues* (pp. 260–265). Cambridge, MA: Brookline Books.

Timmons, V. (1993). *Quality of life of teenagers with special needs.* Unpublished doctoral thesis, University of Calgary, Calgary.

Timmons, V., & Brown, R. L. (1997). Quality of life: Issues for children with handicaps. In R. L. Brown (Ed.), *Quality of life for people with disabilities: Models research and practice* (pp. 183–200). Cheltenham: Stanley Thornes.

Turnbull, A. P., Brown, I., & Turnbull, R. (Eds.). (2004). *Families and people with mental retardation and quality of life: International perspectives.* Washington, DC: American Association on Mental Retardation.

Chapter 14
The Quality of Life of Disabled Children

Eric Emerson

Introduction

One of the main purposes of attempting to measure 'quality of life' or 'well-being' is to monitor social progress, including reductions in avoidable inequalities (or injustices) in the life experiences of marginalized or vulnerable groups or populations. Populations of interest may be defined by global region, nation or national regions (e.g. people living in the world's low-income countries). Specific groups within these areas may be defined by gender, age, ethnicity, migrant status or disability. For example, the annual series of *World Development Reports* and *Human Development Reports* seek to describe and compare important aspects of the conditions under which people in different global regions and countries live out their lives (United Nations Development Program, 2006, 2007; World Bank, 2005, 2006, 2007). The annual report on the *State of the World's Children* undertakes a similar task for children (UNICEF, 2005b, 2006, 2007c). Other global reports focus on the situation of youth (United Nations, 2007) or health (World Health Organization, 2005, 2006, 2007).

In this chapter I will explore some aspects of measuring 'quality of life' to monitor trends in inequalities in the life experiences of disabled children. This information is critical for evaluating the impact of local, regional, national or global policies that seek to support the equalization of opportunities for disabled children. As noted in the preamble to the 2007 UN Convention on the Rights of Persons with Disabilities, 'persons with disabilities continue to face barriers in their participation as equal members of society and violations of their human rights in all parts of the world'. There is much evidence to support such an assertion when applied to

---

E. Emerson (✉)
Centre for Disability Research, Lancaster University, Lancaster, UK; Australian Family and Disability Studies Research Collaboration, University of Sydney, Sydney, Australia
e-mail: eric.emerson@lancaster.ac.uk

A note on terminology: Throughout this chapter I will use the term 'disabled children' in preference to the alternative term 'children with disability/ies'. This choice reflects the emphasis placed within social models of disability on the ways in which social structures and practices actively make people disabled.

R. Kober (ed.), *Enhancing the Quality of Life of People with Intellectual Disabilities*, Social Indicators Research Series 41, DOI 10.1007/978-90-481-9650-0_14,

disabled children (Elwan, 1999; Emerson, Fujiura, & Hatton, 2007; Groce, 2003; UNICEF, 2005a 2007b).

How best can we measure quality of life? There are two quite different answers to that question that reflect two very distinct conceptual traditions (Sirgy et al., 2006). The first of these uses 'objective' *social indicators* to characterize the social and material conditions under which people live their lives (e.g. the percentage of the population exposed to income poverty) and/or the consequences these conditions may have for human capabilities and functioning (e.g. the percentage of the adult population who are literate, the number of children per 1,000 live births who die before their fifth birthday, the percentage of working age adults in full-time employment). This is the strategy adopted by the global-monitoring reports mentioned above. The strength of this approach is that it is often possible to identify social indicators that are relatively easy to collect over time across and within countries. It is an approach that focuses very clearly on documenting the material and social conditions under which people live out their lives.

The validity of this approach is dependent, however, on there being a degree of consensus on: (1) what constitutes a 'good life' or a 'good society'; and (2) which are the most important resources and conditions that enable people to pursue a 'good life'(Diener & Suh, 1997; Grasso & Canova, 2008). In recent years much attention has been paid to the use of more explicit conceptual frameworks to guide the selection of social indicators. Foremost among these are the 'capabilities' frameworks of Sen and Nussbaum (Anand, Hunter, & Smth, 2005; Headey, 2006a; Nussbaum & Sen, 1993; Sen, 2001; The Equalities Review, 2007). As has been argued, these frameworks overlap with and have the potential to enrich social models of disability (Burchardt, 2004).

In a parallel development, others have used frameworks based on human rights instruments to define the freedoms that people should enjoy in a 'good society' (Bradshaw, Hoelscher, & Richardson, 2007; Emerson, Honey, & Llewellyn, 2008; UNICEF, 2007a). For example, UNICEF used the framework provided by the UN Convention on the Rights of the Child to select social indicators to characterize the well-being of children in the World's richer countries (Bradshaw et al., 2007; UNICEF, 2007a). More recently, my colleagues and I used the UN Convention on the Rights of Persons with Disabilities to select social indicators to characterize the well-being of Australian adolescents and young adults with long-term health conditions, impairments or disabilities (Emerson et al., 2008; Emerson, Honey, Madden, & Llewellyn, 2009).

The main alternative to this approach is to consider quality of life as a psychological state of 'well-being' and then to measure the quality of life of groups or populations in terms of average levels of expressed life-satisfaction or happiness (Kahneman, Diener, & Schwarz, 1999; Sirgy et al., 2006). This approach to conceptualizing and measuring quality of life has become increasingly influential over the past decade (Edwards & Imrie, 2008; Sointu, 2005). Indeed, it has recently been argued that subjective well-being or happiness should be *the* yardstick with which to measure social progress (Layard, 2005; Marks & Shah, 2005). Similarly, the World Health Organization defines quality of life in terms of 'an individual's *perception* of their position in life' (World Health Organization, 1995). And within the field of disability it has been argued that quality of life 'remains a notion rooted in individual *perceptions* and values' and that it is '... *primarily the perception* of the individual that reflects the quality of life he/she experiences' (Schalock et al., 2002).

As we shall see, these two approaches lead to quite different conclusions with regard to the extent and nature of disadvantage experienced by 'vulnerable' or 'at risk' groups, including disabled children. The 'problem' is that there appears to be little relationship between 'objective' indicators of a person's living conditions and how satisfied they report themselves to be about their life (Argyle, 1999; Diener, Suh, Lucas, & Smith, 1999; Easterlin, 2003; Kahneman et al., 1999; Layard, 2005; Ryan & Deci, 2001; Sirgy et al., 2006). This is particularly true with regard to *changes* in the living conditions of populations and changes (or the lack of) in the average measured subjective well-being (SWB) of members of the population. These, and other, observations led to the development of 'set point' models of SWB (Brickman & Campbell, 1971; Carver & Scheier, 1990; Cummins, 2003; Frederick & Loewenstein, 1999; Headey & Wearing, 1989; Lykken & Tellegen, 1996). These models emphasized the role of: (1) genetic, personality and cognitive variables in establishing a set point for an individual's SWB (some people are persistently happier than others, regardless of their life experiences); and (2) adaptive processes which ensure that unless *temporarily* overwhelmed by external events (positive or negative), SWB remains close to that set point. In short, such models argue that people adapt to their circumstances.

However, recent research using longitudinal data suggests that SWB may be more sensitive to objective life conditions than was originally thought, that long-term levels of SWB *do* change and that adaptation to changing situations is not inevitable (Diener, Lucas, & Scollon, 2006; Headey, 2006b, 2008; Headey, Muffels, & Wooden, 2008; Lucas, 2007a, b). For example, recent data suggest that the onset of disability in adulthood may be associated with marked declines in SWB with no evidence of adaptation over a follow-up period of up to 7 years (Krause, 1997; Lucas, 2007a, b), although wealth may play an important role in buffering (or moderating) the impact of the onset of disability (Smith, Langa, Kabeto, & Ubel, 2005). There is also increasing evidence that disabled adolescents and adults do have lower SWB than their non-disabled peers although the effect is often not large (Albrecht & Devlieger, 1999; Dijkers, 1997; Emerson & Hatton, 2008; Lucas, 2007b; Mehnert, Krauss, Nadler, & Boyd, 1990), and again maybe moderated by wealth and social connectedness (Emerson et al., 2009). While this evidence has forced a re-evaluation of these models, process of adaptation to changing circumstances does remain central to our understanding of the relationship between living conditions and subjective 'well-being' (Diener et al., 2006).

The relative insensitivity of SWB to external living conditions (and in particular to changes in them) presents some major problems for using SWB to evaluate the quality of life of marginalized or disadvantaged groups. As the Nobel Laureate Amartya Sen has argued 'Concentrating exclusively on mental characteristics (such as pleasure, happiness or desires) can be particularly restrictive when making interpersonal comparisons of well-being. ... Our desires and pleasure-taking abilities adjust to circumstances, especially to make life bearable to adverse situations.... deprived people tend to come to terms with their deprivation because of the sheer necessity of survival, [as such]... the deprivation of the persistently deprived may look muffled and muted' (Sen, 2001).

The current emphasis placed on SWB may be *particularly* problematic when used to characterize the quality of life of disabled children. First, children may be even more adaptable than adults. Second, given that such an approach is based on complex cognitive appraisals, it would effectively disenfranchize young disabled children and disabled children with more severe cognitive impairments.[1] These difficulties are illustrated in a recent pan-European study of more than 800 children (aged 8–12) with cerebral palsy (Dickinson et al., 2007). First, the researchers were only able to collect self-report data on SWB for less than two thirds (61%) of the participating children. Second, there were no differences in SWB between the children with cerebral palsy and reference data on non-disabled children (Dickinson et al., 2007). Similar results have been reported from Hong Kong (Chow, Lo, & Cummins, 2005). In this case, however, information was also collected on objective indicators of quality of life. These results indicated that while there were no between-group differences with regard to SWB, children with physical disabilities did have a significantly poorer 'objective' quality of life.

If would appear then that if one thinks about quality of life in terms of a psychological state, it is necessary to conclude that children with cerebral palsy or other physical disabilities experience the same overall quality of life as their non-disabled peers. Such a conclusion sits uneasily with evidence that such children are at significantly increased risk of poverty, social exclusion and human rights abuses (Elwan, 1999; Groce, 2003; UNICEF, 2005a 2007b). In Sen's terms, the focus on SWB 'muffles and mutes' the disadvantage faced by such children.

As a result, it would appear more appropriate to adopt a social indicators approach to characterizing and monitor the quality of life of disabled children. In the following sections I will present three examples of the use of social indicators to compare the quality of life of disabled children and their non-disabled peers. These examples focus on: (1) changes in the quality of life of disabled Australian children (age 0–14); (2) the quality of life of very young children in the UK who are at risk of disability; (3) the quality of life of young disabled children in Bangladesh, Macedonia, Mongolia and Thailand.

In each of these examples I have attempted to use the framework provided by Bradshaw and colleagues (itself based on the UN Convention on the Rights of the Child) to, wherever possible, identify social indicators based on: (1) material situation; (2) housing; (3) health; (4) subjective well-being; (5) education; (6) children's relationships; (7) civic participation; (8) risk and safety. In each example indicators were selected from existing nationally representative datasets of disabled children and their non-disabled peers (Bradshaw et al., 2007; UNICEF, 2007a).

[1] One option in such circumstances would be to collect information from proxy respondents (e.g. a parent or a sibling). Unfortunately, however, the existing research suggests that there is very poor agreement indeed between self-report and information collected from proxy respondents on such matters as happiness or life-satisfaction (Cummins, 2002; Eiser & Morse, 2001).

The Quality of Life of Disabled Australian Children in 2001 and 2006

The first example illustrates the possible use of social indicators to monitor trends in the differences in the quality of life of disabled and non-disabled children over time. This type of information is essential to evaluating progress (or otherwise) towards the equalization of opportunity for disabled children.

The Data

Data were extracted from Waves 1 and 6 of the survey of *Household Income and Labor Dynamics in Australia* (HILDA). Full details of HILDA are available in a series of technical and annual reports (Headey, Warren, & Harding, 2006; HILDA, 2006; Watson, 2008). Briefly, HILDA is a non-refreshed annual panel survey originating from a national probability sample of approximately 7,500 Australian households in 2001 (Wave 1). Continuing panel members include all panel members of Wave 1 households, any children subsequently born to or adopted by panel members and all new entrants to a household who have a child with an existing panel member. All household members aged 15 or above are invited to participate in a personal interview. Brief information is collected on younger children from the primary respondent for the household.

Children (age 0–14) were identified as being disabled if the primary respondent answered in the positive to a question 'Look at these [show cards] does anyone living here have *any, long-term health condition, disability or impairment such as these?* The show card, which listed a variety of health conditions and disabilities included the additional information that the condition should: (1) have lasted, or are likely to last, 6 months or more; (2) restricts everyday activity and (3) cannot be corrected by medication or medical aids.

Wave 1 data (collected in 2001) included interviews with 2,235 households containing one or more child aged 0–14. Of the 4,111 children living in these households, 297 (7%) were identified as disabled. 245 (11%) of households contained one or more disabled child aged 0–14. All analyses were undertaken on data weighted to correct for cross sectional unit non-response. Wave 6 data (collected in 2006) included interviews with 1,972 households containing one or more child aged 0–14. Of the 3,553 children living in these households, 254 (7%) were identified as disabled. One hundred and ninty-six (10%) of households contained one or more disabled child aged 0–14.

Results

It was only possible from the available data top extract social indicators related to the domains of material situation and housing. These were: (1) income poverty

Table 14.1 Quality of life of disabled Australian children (age 0–14) in 2001 and 2006

	2001			2006		
	HH with disabled child (%)	Other HH with children (%)	OR, p	HH with disabled child (%)	Other HH with children (%)	OR, p
Material situation						
Income poverty	29	20	1.61*	26	19	1.53*
Material hardship	62	48	1.73**	40	26	1.88**
Housing						
Bedroom overcrowding	31	21	1.70**	28	18	1.50*
Neighbourhood deprivation	26	20	1.38***	23	19	1.31

Note: OR = Odds ratio $^{*}p < 0.05$, $^{**}p < 0.01$, $^{***}p < 0.001$

(household equivalized income lower than 60% of the total sample median); (2) material hardship (within the last year an adult member of the household had *as a result of shortage of money* done one of the following: could not pay electricity, gas or telephone bills on time; could not pay the mortgage or rent on time; pawned or sold something; went without meals; was unable to heat home; asked for financial help from friends or family; asked for help from welfare/community organization); (3) bedroom overcrowding (average of 1.5 or more persons per bedroom); (4) neighbourhood deprivation (lives in area in bottom quintile of SEIFA 2001 index of relative socio-economic disadvantage). The results of cross-sectional analyses of data from 2001 and 2006 are summarized in Table 14.1.

The results indicate that: (1) in both 2001 and 2006 disabled children were significantly more likely than their non-disabled peers to be living in households characterized by income poverty, material hardship and overcrowding; and (2) while absolute scores on each of these items improved between 2001 and 2006, the extent of relative disadvantage experienced by disabled children remained constant. In 2001, but not in 2006, disabled children were significantly more likely than their non-disabled peers to be living in deprived areas. However, the change in relative disadvantage between these two dates is not itself statistically significant.

The main conclusion that can be drawn from these results is that disabled children in Australia, who are already at risk of social exclusion, are significantly more likely than non-disabled children to be exposed to the types of material living conditions that are known to reduce the child's life chances and opportunities, both in childhood and in later life (Fabian Commission on Life Chances and Child Poverty, 2006; Graham, 2007). Furthermore, there is little evidence that even in a time of generally increasing living standards, the extent of the relative deprivation experienced by disabled children has changed at all. Similar data have been reported for disabled adolescents and young adults in Australia over the same time period (Emerson et al., 2009).

The Quality of Life of Pre-school Children at Risk of Disability in the UK

The second example illustrates the use of social indicators to explore in more depth the quality of life of disabled and non-disabled children at a critical point in their development, the pre-school years. Given the importance of early childhood experiences for later educational attainment, employment opportunities, health and well-being (Graham & Power, 2004; Graham, 2007; Kuh, Power, Blane, & Bartley, 2003), such information helps inform us of the likely futures of very young children at risk of disability.

The Data

Data were extracted from the first two waves of the UK's Millennium Cohort Study [MCS] (Dex & Joshi, 2005; Hansen & Joshi, 2007; Hansen, 2006). Full details of the sampling procedure, response rates and procedure are available in a series of technical reports (Hansen, 2006; Plewis & Ketende, 2006; Plewis, 2003). Briefly, the MCS is designed to follow through life a sample of children born between 2000 and 2002 who at age 9 months were alive and living in the UK. The attained sample at Wave 1 (in 2000/01 when most children were 9 months old) was 18,819 children in 18,552 families. The attained sample at Wave 2 (in 2003/4 when children were 3 years old) was 15,808 children in 15,590 families.

Children were identified as disabled (or more accurately as being at risk of being disabled) at age 3 if they met one of three criteria: (1) they scored in the lowest 3% on a test of general cognitive functioning (Bracken, 2002); (2) they scored in the top 3% on a measure of behavioral difficulties (Goodman, 1999); (3) they were reported by their main carer to have a long-term health condition that restricted their activities. Given that cognitive tests were administered in English, the sample used in the present analyses was restricted to children living in monolingual English speaking households. Use of this definition identified 11% of children as being 'at risk' of disability. All analyses were undertaken on data weighted to take account of sample design (oversampling in particular areas) and non-participation at Waves 1 and 2.

Results

The results of cross-sectional analyses of data collected when the children were 3 years old are summarized in Table 14.2.

Table 14.2 Quality of life of 3-year-old children 'at risk' of disability in the UK

	Child at risk of disability (%)	Child not at risk of disability (%)	OR, p
Material situation			
Income poverty[a]	50	24	3.10*
Material hardship[b]	56	32	2.69*
Housing			
Lives in rented accommodation	54	27	3.13*
Neighbourhood deprivation[c]	34	17	2.40*
Health			
Child obese	7	5	1.45**
Vaccination record incomplete[d]	4	3	1.61**
Education			
Read to daily	48	63	0.53*
Medium/high intensity of in-home education[e]	62	69	0.74*
Children's relationships			
Highly pro-social[f]	15	16	0.89
Been visited by friends with young children	87	93	0.49*
Risk & safety			
Accidental injury resulting in hospital attendance	36	32	1.21**
Main carer reports local area to be 'unsafe'	12	5	2.56*

Note: OR = Odds ratio $*p < 0.05$, $**p < 0.01$, $***p < 0.001$
[a]Equivalized household income less than 60% of total sample median.
[b]Wanting, but being unable to afford, one or more items of a list of nine 'essentials'.
[c]Living in area in lowest quintile of national local area indices of multiple deprivation.
[d]Missing at least one vaccination for polio, diphtheria, tetanus, whooping cough, Hib, meningitis.
[e]Within sample terciles of frequency with which child: (1) is taught the alphabet; (2) is taught songs; (3) paints/draws; (4) is taught to count.
[f]Scores in top 15% on pro-social scale of the *Strengths and Difficulties Questionnaire*.

The results indicate that 3-year-old children at risk of disability had a significantly lower quality of life than their not 'at risk' peers on 11 of the 12 indicators. The extent of relative disadvantage was particularly high for exposure to poverty, material hardship and poor housing conditions. These results are particularly worrying, given the importance of early childhood experiences in shaping future well-being (Graham & Power, 2004; Graham, 2007; Kuh et al., 2003).

The Quality of Life of Young Disabled Children in Bangladesh, Macedonia, Mongolia and Thailand

The vast majority of research investigating quality of life is undertaken in the world's richer countries. However, only 16% of the world's population live in high-income countries (World Bank, 2007). Over twice as many (37%) live in low-income countries (the remaining 47% living in middle-income countries). The final example focuses on the quality of life of young disabled children in two lower-middle income countries (Thailand and Macedonia) and two low-income countries (Bangladesh and Mongolia).

The Data

Data were extracted from the round three of UNICEF's Multiple Indicator Cluster Surveys (MICS3: http://childinfo.org/mics3_background.html). MICS is a household survey methodology designed for use in low- and middle-income countries, the results from MICS are used to measure progress towards the achievement of the Millennium Development Goals and in the compilation of the annual UNICEF reports on the *State of the World's Children* (UNICEF, 2006, 2007c). An optional module on child disability for children aged 2–9 years of age was introduced in round two of MICS (Loaiza & Cappa, 2005). In this example, I have used data from MICS3 surveys undertaken in 2005 in Bangladesh, Macedonia, Mongolia and Thailand (four of the earliest countries that included the disability module to release their data).

In each country children were identified as disabled on the basis of primary informant report that *any* of the following conditions were met: (1) the child has serious delay in sitting, standing or walking; (2) the child has difficulty seeing in the daytime or nighttime; (3) the child has difficulty hearing; (4) the child does not understand when asked to do something; (5) the child has difficulty walking or moving; (6) the child has fits or loss of consciousness; (7) the child does not learn to do things like other children; (8) the child cannot say recognizable words; (9) the child's speech is different from normal; (10) compared to other children the child appears mentally slow or backward. Indicators were extracted from other MICS3 items in relation to: (1) material situation; (2) housing; (3) health; (4) education; and, for Bangladesh only, (5) risk and safety.

In Bangladesh the disability module was applied to 58,441 children, with 19% being identified as disabled. In Macedonia the disability module was applied to 5,917 children, with 23% being identified as disabled. In Mongolia the disability module was applied to 4,912 children, with 26% being identified as disabled. In Thailand the disability module was applied to 16,564 children, with 13% being identified as disabled.

Results

The results of cross-sectional analyses of data collected when the children were 3 years old are summarized in Table 14.3.

Table 14.3 Quality of life of disabled children in Bangladesh, Macedonia, Mongolia and Thailand

	Bangladesh			Macedonia			Mongolia			Thailand		
Indicator	DC (%)	NDC (%)	OR, p (%)	DC (%)	NDC (%)	OR, p (%)	DC (%)	NDC (%)	OR, p (%)	DC (%)	NDC (%)	OR, p (%)
Material situation												
Poor[a]	28	25	1.16*	31	24	1.39**	28	23	1.32*	25	23	1.16*
Housing												
Use of flush toilet	17	19	0.83*	97	98	0.87	16	19	0.78**	99	99	1.06
Water piped into house	3	3	0.81*	86	88	0.81	13	16	0.74**	17	20	0.86*
Health												
Has received some vaccinations	98	98	0.71***	88	86	1.26	88	95	0.42***	92	92	0.94
Severe to moderate stunting	n/a			8	8	0.93	28	24	1.24	16	10	1.57*
Education												
Child attends early education programme	16	15	1.10	10	12	0.82	34	40	0.82	57	62	0.82*
Currently attending formal school	84	86	0.88**	76	83	0.67***	93	94	0.81	96	95	1.17
Risk and safety												
Accidental injury	13	9	1.55*					n/a				
Living in environmentally hazardous area	25	23	1.14*									

Note: OR = Odds ratio; n/a Data not available.
$^{*}p < 0.05$, $^{**}p < 0.01$, $^{***}p < 0.001$
[a]Household in lowest wealth quintile for total sample

The results indicate that: (1) in all four countries disabled children were significantly more likely to be living in poverty (household assets in lowest 20% of total sample) than non-disabled children; (2) on the remaining six indicators that were collected across the four countries, disabled children had a poorer quality of life in 18 of 25 comparisons (statistically significant in 10); (3) on no indicator in any country did disabled children have a significantly better quality of life than their peers.

Concluding Comments

The three examples presented above illustrate the some of the potential value of using social indicators to: (1) monitor change in the quality of life of disabled children relative to that of their non-disabled peers; (2) describe the quality of life of disabled children at a critical stage in the life course; and (3) compare the relative quality of life of disabled children across regional and national boundaries in some of the world's poorer countries. The examples varied in terms of the wealth and culture of the countries in which they were undertaken, the ages of the children who participated, the operational definitions of disability used, the specific indicators employed and the sampling frames used.

Some of the findings, however, were remarkably consistent. First, in all six countries disabled children were significantly more likely than their non-disabled peers to be living in poverty. While not surprising (Elwan, 1999), these data do illustrate the point that around the world disabled children (who are already vulnerable to social exclusion, poorer health and restricted life chances) are at increased risk of living under material conditions that will further increase their risk of social exclusion and poor health and further restrict their life opportunities. Second, on none of the 49 comparisons made did disabled children have a significantly better quality of life than their peers. On 35 (71%) they had a significantly poorer quality of life. These observations stand in stark contrast to those of studies who have conceptualized quality of life in terms of subjective well-being, where in Sen's words, their disadvantage does indeed look 'muffled and muted' (Chow et al., 2005; Dickinson et al., 2007).

The use of this approach does raise some difficult technical issues. First, the available data commonly rely on carer (typically maternal) report of child disability. Such reports are likely to be influenced by maternal knowledge regarding typical or normative development and by linguistic and cultural differences. The former are likely to underestimate the prevalence of disability in highly deprived communities. The latter create marked difficulties in making comparisons across different cultural or linguistic groups (Loaiza & Cappa, 2005). They are likely to be less problematic, however, in making comparisons regarding relative differences in quality of life. Second, by counting (and comparing) disabled people, such approaches may reinforce the notion that disability is a characteristic of people, rather than the result of the interaction between variations in bodily structures and social structures and practices (Fujiura & Rutkowski-Kmitta, 2001; Soder, 2004; Tossebro & Kittelsaa, 2004; World Health Organization, 2001)

More important, however, are the implications associated with choosing between the two dominant approaches to thinking about 'quality of life'; living conditions that influence peoples' capabilities and functioning or psychological state of well-being. At a pragmatic level the two approaches lead to quite different conclusions. Social indicators document the poorer social conditions under which disabled children grow up. Psychological indicators suggest that disabled children experience a quality of life comparable to their peers. The latter approach gives no support to social policies that seek to improve the life chances of disabled children. Indeed, the results arising from such an approach are consistent with paternalistic social policies that view disabled as being different, but 'happy with their lot in life'.

At a more general level, defining quality of life in terms of psychological state is consistent with the emerging 'politics of well-being' (Edwards & Imrie, 2008; Sointu, 2005). As Edwards and Imrie argue, the emphasis of the well-being agenda on 'biologism, personality and character traits, and a policy prognosis that revolves around self-help and therapy, or individuated actions and (self) responsibilities' (p. 339) involves significant risks for disabled people and other marginal groups. The increasing focus on biological and psychological states and processes can all too easily drive concerns with social conditions and processes into the background. It could, quite simply, feed into a view that disabled people are only marginally disadvantaged and, to the extent that they are, are in need of therapy or support in personal development.

References

Albrecht, G. L., & Devlieger, P. J. (1999). The disability paradox: High quality of life against all odds. *Social Science & Medicine*, *48*, 977–988.

Anand, P., Hunter, G., & Smth, R. (2005). Capabilities and well-being: Evidence based on the Sen-Nussbaum approach to welfare. *Social Indicators Research*, *74*, 9–55.

Argyle, M. (1999). Causes and correlates of happiness. In D. Kahneman, E. Deiner, & N. Schwarz (Eds.), *Well-Being: The Foundations of Hedonic Psychology* (pp. 353–373). New York: Russell Sage Foundation.

Bank., W. (2005). *World Development Report 2006: Equity & Development*. Oxford: Oxford University Press.

Bank., W. (2006). *World Development Report 2007: Development & the Next Generation*. Washington: World Bank.

Bank., W. (2007). *World Development Report 2008: Agriculture for Development*. Washington, DC: World Bank.

Bracken, B. A. (2002). *Bracken School Readiness Assessment*. London: Harcourt Assessment.

Bradshaw, J., Hoelscher, P., & Richardson, D. (2007). An index of child well-being in the European Union. *Social Indicators Research*, *80*, 133–177.

Brickman, P., & Campbell, D. T. (1971). Hedonic relativism and planning the good society. In M. H. Apley (Ed.), *Adaptation-Level Theory: A Symposium* (pp. 287–302). New York: Academic Press.

Burchardt, T. (2004). Capabilities and disability: The capabilities framework and the social model of disability. *Disability and Society*, *19*(7), 735–751.

Carver, C., & Scheier, M. (1990). Origins and functions of positive and negative affect: A control-process view. *Psychological Review*, *97*, 19–35.

Chow, S., Lo, S., & Cummins, R. (2005). Self-perceived quality of life of children and adolescents with physical disabilities in Hong Kong. *Quality of Life Research*, *14*, 415–423.

Cummins, R. (2002). Proxy responding for subjective well-being: A review. In L. M. Glidden (Ed.), *International Review of Research in Mental Retardation* (Vol. 25, pp. 183–207). San Diego, CA: Academic Press.

Cummins, R. (2003). Normative life satisfaction: Measurement issues and a homeostatic model. *Social Indicators Research*, *64*(2), 225–256.

Dex, S., & Joshi, H. (Eds.). (2005). *Children of the 21st Century: From birth to nine months*. Bristol: Policy Press.

Dickinson, H., Parkinson, K., Ravens-Sieberer, U., Schirripa, G., Thyen, U., Arnaud, C., et al. (2007). Self-reported quality of life of 8–12-year-old children with cerebral palsy: A crosssectional European study. *Lancet, 369*, 2171–2178.

Diener, E., Lucas, R. E., & Scollon, C. (2006). Beyond the hedonic treadmill: Revising the adaptation theory of well-being. *American Psychologist, 61*, 305–314.

Diener, E., & Suh, E. (1997). Measuring quality of life: Economic, social and subjective indicators. *Social Indicators Research, 40*, 189–216.

Diener, E., Suh, E. M., Lucas, R. E., & Smith, H. L. (1999). Subjective well-being: Three decades of progress. *Psychological Bulletin, 125*, 276–302.

Dijkers, M. P. (1997). Quality of life after spinal cord injury: A meta analysis of the effects of disablement components. *Spinal Cord, 35*, 829–840.

Easterlin, R. A. (2003). Explaining happiness. *Proceedings of the National Academy of Sciences, 100*, 11176–11183.

Edwards, C., & Imrie, R. (2008). Disability and the implications of the wellbeing agenda: Some reflections from the United Kingdom. *Journal of Social Policy, 37*(3), 337–355.

Eiser, C., & Morse, R. (2001). Can parents rate their child's healthrelated quality of life? Results of a systemic review. *Quality of Life Research, 10*, 347–357.

Elwan, A. (1999). *Poverty and Disability: A survey of the literature*. Washington, DC: World Bank.

Emerson, E., Fujiura, G. T., & Hatton, C. (2007). International perspectives. In S. L. Odom, R. H. Horner, M. Snell, & J. Blacher (Eds.), *Handbook on Developmental Disabilities*. New York: Guilford Press.

Emerson, E., & Hatton, C. (2008). The self-reported well-being of women and men with intellectual disabilities in England. *American Journal on Mental Retardation, 113*(2), 143–155.

Emerson, E., Honey, A., & Llewellyn, G. (2008). *The Well-Being and Aspirations of Australian Adolescents and Young Adults with a Long-term Health Condition, Disability or Impairment*. Canberra: Australian Research Alliance for Children and Youth.

Emerson, E., Honey, A., Madden, R., & Llewellyn, G. (2009). The well-being of Australian adolescents and young adults with self-reported long-term health conditions, impairments or disabilities: 2001 and 2006. *Australian Journal of Social Issues, 44*, 37–51.

Fabian Commission on Life Chances and Child Poverty. (2006). *Narrowing the Gap: The Final Report of the Fabian Commission on Life Chances and Child Poverty*. London: Fabian Society.

Frederick, S., & Loewenstein, G. (1999). Hedonic adaptation. In D. Kahneman, E. Deiner, & N. Schwartz (Eds.), *Well-Being: The Foundations of Hedonic Psychology* (pp. 302–329). New York: Sage.

Fujiura, G. T., & Rutkowski-Kmitta, V. (2001). Counting disability. In G. L. Albrecht, K. D. Seelman, & M. Bury (Eds.), *Handbook of Disabilities Studies* (pp. 69–96). Thousand Oaks: Sage.

Goodman, R. (1999). The extended version of the strengths and difficulties questionnaire as a guide to child psychiatric caseness and consequent burden. *Journal of Child Psychology and Psychiatry, 40*, 791–801.

Graham, H. (2007). *Unequal Lives: Health and Socioeconomic Inequalities*. Maidenhead: Open University Press.

Graham, H., & Power, C. (2004). Childhood disadvantage and health inequalities: A framework for policy based on lifecourse research. *Child: Care, Health & Development, 30*, 671–678.

Grasso, M., & Canova, L. (2008). An assessment of the quality of life in the European Union based on the social indicators approach. *Social Indicators Research, 87*, 1–25.

Groce, N. E. (2003). *Adolescents and Youth with Disabilities: Issues & Challenges*. Washington: World Bank.

Hansen, K. (2006). *Millennium Cohort Study: First and Second Surveys – A Guide to the Datasets*. London: Centre for Longitudinal Studies, University of London.

Hansen, K., & Joshi, H. (2007). *Millennium Cohort Study Second Survey: A User's Guide to Initial Findings*. London: Centre for Longitudinal Studies, University of London.

Headey, B. (2006a). *A framework for assessing poverty, disadvantage and low capabilities in Australia*. Melbourne: Melbourne Institute of Applied Economic and Social Research, University of Melbourne.

Headey, B. (2006b). Subjective well-being: Revisions to dynamic equilibrium theory using national panel data and panel regression methods. *Social Indicators Research, 79*, 369–403.

Headey, B. (2008). the set-point theory of well-being: Negative results and consequent revisions. *Social Indicators Research, 85*, 389–403.

Headey, B., Muffels, R., & Wooden, M. (2008). Money does not buy happiness: Or does it? A reassessment based on the combined effects of wealth, income and consumption. *Social Indicators Research, 87*, 65–82.

Headey, B., Warren, D., & Harding, G. (2006). *Families, Incomes and Jobs: A Statistical Report of the HILDA Survey*. Melbourne: Melbourne Institute of Applied Economic and Social Research, The University of Melbourne.

Headey, B., & Wearing, A. (1989). Personality, life events and subjective well-being: Toward a dynamic equilibrium model. *Journal of Personality and Social Psychology, 57*, 731–739.

HILDA. (2006). *HILDA Survey Annual Report 2006*. Melbourne: Melbourne Institute of Applied Economic and Social Research, University of Melbourne.

Kahneman, D., Diener, E., & Schwarz, N. (Eds.). (1999). *Well-Being: The Foundations of Hedonic Psychology*. New York: Russel Sage Foundation.

Krause, J. (1997). Adjustment after spinal cord injury: A 9 year longitudinal study. *Archives of Physical Medicine & Rehabilitation, 78*, 651–657.

Kuh, D., Power, C., Blane, D., & Bartley, M. (2003). Socioeconomic pathways between childhood and adult health. In D. L. Kuh & Y. Ben-Shlomo (Eds.), *A lifecourse approach to chronic disease epidemiology: Tracing the origins of ill-health from early to adult life* (2 ed., pp. 371–395). Oxford: Oxford University Press.

Layard, R. (2005). *Happiness: Lessons from a New Science*. London: Penguin.

Loaiza, E., & Cappa, C. (2005). *Measuring Children's Disability via Household Surveys: The MICS Experience*. New York: Unicef.

Lucas, R. E. (2007a). Adaptation and the set-point model of subjective well-being. *Current Directions in Psychological Science, 16*(2), 75–79.

Lucas, R. E. (2007b). Long-term disability is associated with lasting changes in subjective well-being: Evidence from two nationally representative longitudinal studies. *Journal of Personality and Social Psychology, 92*(4), 717–730.

Lykken, D., & Tellegen, A. (1996). Happiness is a stochastic phenomenon. *Psychological Science, 7*, 186–189.

Marks, N., & Shah, H. (2005). A well-being manifesto for a flourishing society. In F. Huppert, N. Baylis, & B. Keverne (Eds.), *The Science of Well-being*. Oxford: Oxford University Press.

Mehnert, T., Krauss, H., Nadler, R., & Boyd, M. (1990). Correlates of life satisfaction in those with disabling conditions. *Rehabilitation Psychology, 35*(1), 3–17.

Nussbaum, M., & Sen, A. (Eds.). (1993). *The Quality of Life*. Oxford: Oxford University Press.

Plewis, I. (2003). *Millennium Cohort Study: First Survey. Technical Report on Sampling* (2nd ed.). London: Centre for Longitudinal Studies, Institute of Education, University of London.

Plewis, I., & Ketende, S. (2006). *Millennium Cohort Study: Technical Report on Response*. London: Centre for Longitudinal Studies, Institute of Education, University of London.

Ryan, R. M., & Deci, E. L. (2001). On happiness and human potentials: A review of research on hedonic and eudaimonic well-being. *Annual Review of Psychology, 52*, 141–166.

Schalock, R. L., Brown, I., Brown, R., Cummins, R., Felce, D., Matikka, L., et al. (2002). Conceptualization, measurement and application of quality of life for persons with intellectual disabilities: Report of an international panel of experts. *Mental Retardation, 40*(6), 457–470.

Sen, A. (2001). *Development as Freedom*. Oxford: Oxford University Press.

Sirgy, M. J., Michalos, A. C., Ferriss, A. L., Easterlin, R. A., Patrick, D., & Pavot, W. (2006). The quality of life research movement: Past, present and future. *Social Indicators Research, 76*, 343–466.

Smith, D. M., Langa, K. M., Kabeto, M. U., & Ubel, P. A. (2005). Health, wealth, and happiness: Financial resources buffer subjective well-being after the onset of a disability. *Psychological Science, 19*(9), 663–666.

Soder, M. (2004). Why head counting? In J. Tossebro & A. Kittelsaa (Eds.), *Exploring the Living Conditions of Disabled People* (pp. 211–228). Lund, Sweden: Studentlitteratur.

Sointu, E. (2005). The rise of an ideal: Tracing changing discourses of well-being. *Sociological Review, 53*(2), 255–274.

The Equalities Review. (2007). *Fairness and Freedom: The Final Report of the Equalities Review*. London: The Equalities Review.

Tossebro, J., & Kittelsaa, A. (2004). Studying the living conditions of disabled people: Approaches and problems. In J. Tossebro & A. Kittelsaa (Eds.), *Exploring the Living Conditions of Disabled People* (pp. 17–44). Lund, Sweden: Studentlitteratur.

UNICEF. (2005a). *Children and Disability in Transition in the CEE/CIS and Baltic States*. Florence: Unicef Innocenti Research Centre.

UNICEF. (2005b). *The State of the World's Children 2006: Excluded and Invisable*. New York: Unicef.

UNICEF. (2006). *The State of the World's Children 2007: Women and Children. The Double Dividend of Gender Equality*. New York: Unicef.

UNICEF. (2007a). *Child Poverty in Perspective: An overview of child well-being in rich countries*. Florence: Unicef Innocenti Research Centre.

UNICEF. (2007b). *Promoting the Rights of Children with Disabilities*. Florence: Unicef Innocenti Research Centre.

UNICEF. (2007c). *The State of the World's Children 2008:Child Survival*. New York: Unicef.

United Nations. (2007). *World Youth Report 2007: Young People's Transition into Adulthood*. New York: Department of Economic and Social Affairs, United Nations.

United Nations Development Program. (2006). *Human Development Report 2006: Beyond scarcity: Power, poverty and the global water crisis*. New York: United Nations.

United Nations Development Program. (2007). *Human Development Report 2007: Fighting Climate Change. Human Solidarity in a Divided World*. New York: United Nations Development Program.

Watson, N. (Ed.). (2008). *HILDA User Manual – Release 6*. Melbourne: Melbourne Institute of Applied Economic and Social Research, University of Melbourne.

World Health Organization. (1995). The World Health Organization Quality of Life assessment (WHOQOL): Position paper from the World Health Organization. *Social Science & Medicine, 41*, 1403–1409.

World Health Organization. (2001). *International Classification of Functioning, Disability and Health*. Geneva: World Health Organization.

World Health Organization. (2005). *The World Health Report 2005: Make Every Mother and Child Count*. Geneva: World Health Organization.

World Health Organization. (2006). *World Health Report 2006: Working Together for Health*. Geneva: World Health Organization.

World Health Organization. (2007). *World Health Report 2007: A safer future, global public health security in the 21st Century*. Geneva: World Health Organization.

Part V
Family Quality of Life

Chapter 15
Theorizing About Family Quality of Life

Nina Zuna, Jean Ann Summers, Ann P. Turnbull, Xiaoyi Hu, and S. Xu

Theorizing About Family Quality of Life

Value of a Theory of Family Quality of Life

In the past two decades, research and scholarship have led to greater advancements in the conceptualization and measurement of quality of life (QOL) for individuals with intellectual disabilities (Cummins, 2005; Schalock et al., 2002; Verdugo, Schalock, Keith, & Stancliffe, 2005). More recently, researchers in the international disability field have begun a similar process of conceptualization and measurement of family quality of life (FQOL) in families of individuals with intellectual disabilities (Isaacs et al., 2007; Turnbull, Brown, & Turnbull, 2004; Turnbull, Summers, Lee, & Kyzar, 2007). Despite these advancements, several critical issues remain unresolved. Several conceptual frameworks proposing domains of FQOL circulate the field (Brown, MacAdam-Crisp, Wang, & Iarocci, 2006; Hoffman, Marquis, Poston, Summers, & Turnbull, 2006; Verdugo, Cordoba, & Gomez, 2005). This diversity is reflected in a range of measurement indicators and response stems proposed to assess FQOL. The accumulated research also reveals varying stages of psychometric development of the current FQOL assessment tools (Turnbull et al., 2007). Finally, with FQOL researchers primarily directing their attention toward the identification of indicators of FQOL and development of measures to assess FQOL as an outcome, little attention has been devoted to theory development to propose critical elements both within and outside the family that may explain variations in that outcome. To date, no theory of FQOL has been explicated in the literature.

Given research conducted to date, it is an opportune time to engage in the theorizing process to guide future FQOL research. As we will note in this chapter, a theory requires (a) definitions of concepts, (b) a set of propositions hypothesizing the relationships among variables, and (c) an overarching premise that provides an explanation for an outcome of interest. We will demonstrate that current research on

N. Zuna (✉)
Beach Center on Disability, University of Kansas, Lawrence, KS 66045, USA
e-mail: nzuna@ku.edu

R. Kober (ed.), *Enhancing the Quality of Life of People with Intellectual Disabilities*, Social Indicators Research Series 41, DOI 10.1007/978-90-481-9650-0_15,

FQOL in the disability field has provided sufficient evidence to enable us to propose a unified theoretical framework to depict relationships among multiple variables impacting FQOL in families who have a member with a disability. Theory guides research; research informs policy and practice. Therefore, we hope that research derived from a unified theoretical framework of FQOL would (a) inform systemic operations across education, health, and social service agencies to effectively and efficiently serve families who have a child with a disability, (b) result in new and enhanced legislation and agency policy to address families' fundamental needs, and (c) demonstrate the necessity of a sufficient number of appropriately staffed programs to meet families' service and support needs.

Further, it is our aim to present a unified theory of FQOL that would help to inform and organize an interdisciplinary research agenda. As an area of research, FQOL for families who have children with intellectual disabilities does not reside within the disability field alone. Similar to person-first language for referring to an individual with a disability, families who have a member with a disability are a family first– a family that seeks to (a) access and enjoy all the benefits of their community, (b) reside in a safe home and neighborhood, (c) live, grow, and experience all the joys and sorrows a family encounters, and (d) remain emotionally, physically, and financially strong. Families are an integral part of every culture; understanding them and ensuring they remain the core unit of society is paramount. While our immediate aim is to understand families of children who have an intellectual disability, a theory of FQOL with respect to this population must still take into account factors that not only impact all families, but also all families who have children with a variety of disabilities. Meeting these comprehensive goals requires a collective research agenda – one that is guided by a unified theory.

This chapter has three primary purposes. First, we present a brief summary from methodologists and theorists to highlight the components of a theory and to illustrate the process of theory-building. Second, we review current FQOL definitions, conceptualizations, and models to determine if an emergent framework exists that may serve as a beginning step toward theorizing about family quality of life for families who have a member with a disability. Third, based on theory components and the findings from our review, we propose a unified theory illustrated by the theoretical linkage of multiple concepts to explain FQOL. As will be explained later, theories include unified (or grand) theories as well as less ambitious explanations of more narrow phenomena, in the form of middle-range or micro-theories. We will use our proposed unified theory to identify middle-range theories that have been previously tested in the literature to predict FQOL.

Components of a Theory

What Is a Theory?

The most simplistic definition of a theory is that it is an explanation of an observation or experience (Bengtson, Acock, Allen, Dilworth-Anderson, & Klein, 2005). Theories are often used to explain causal relationships. They are valued because they represent a "parsimonious way of summarizing knowledge" (Burr, Hill, Nye, & Reiss, 1979 p. 20). However, beneath this deceptively simple definition lies the fact that a true understanding of a theory encompasses its parts: concepts, variables, and propositions. To understand the proposed theories we will present in this chapter, we first provide brief explanations of each of these terms.

Concepts

Concepts are the most basic components of a theory. Concepts provide individuals with a way to "organize experience" (White & Klein, 2002, p. 10) that precludes the necessity to invent new terms to describe routinely occurring events. Researchers often refer to a concept as the summation of the essential characteristics of a phenomenon (Burr et al., 1979; Fawcett, 1999; Shoemaker, Tankard, & Lasorsa, 2004; White & Klein, 2002).

Variables

Shoemaker et al. (2004) define a variable as a concept which has measurable components assuming two or more values. Shoemaker et al. provide further clarification to distinguish between a concept and a variable, using female and sex as an example. Female is a concept which can be defined by biological characteristics; one typically would not measure femaleness, but instead would measure sex as a dichotomous variable with two outcomes: male or female. Similarly, family is a concept, but size of family is a variable.

Propositions

Fawcett (1999) defines propositions as "a statement about a concept or the relation between concepts" (p. 1). White and Klein (2002) similarly agree that propositions occur when concepts are meaningfully linked by a relation to another concept. These definitions of a proposition appear to have emanated from older research on theory in which propositions were restricted to only "identify relationships between variables" (Burr et al., 1979, p. 19). Concepts and variables represent the building blocks of a theory; propositions represent the link between variables, but a theory usually "comprises several propositions" (White & Klein, 2002, p. 12).

How Is a Theory Organized?

Theoretical and Operational Linkages

Theory organization begins with an explanation of the plausibility of the theory and the relationships therein. Theoretical linkages describe the plausibility – *why* the concepts are included in the theory and why they may be expected to have an impact on the outcome. The purpose of a theoretical linkage is "to give the theory explanatory power" (Shoemaker et al., 2004, p. 52). This can be accomplished in three ways: citing existing theory, using existing literature to illustrate results that are similar to the proposed hypothesis, and using a researcher's own logic to support hypothesis development (Shoemaker et al., 2004). While theoretical linkages explain the plausibility of a relationship among concepts, *operational linkages* explore the *testability* of the proposed relationships among variables which have been selected to represent those concepts. The relationship among variables may be depicted pictorially or statistically. Simple relationships among two–three variables are easily depicted in graphic format; more complex relationships are often illustrated using path diagrams. Statistical relationships may be stated a priori in the form of strength and direction of a correlation coefficient or other type of effect size.

Unified, Mid-Range, and Micro Theories

A theory may also be organized by its specificity. A grand theory attempts to explain an overall understanding of a phenomenon or provide a general structure of knowledge for a phenomenon (Peterson, 2004). Rather than the term *grand theory,* we prefer to use the term *unified theory* to describe the overarching conceptual theory of FQOL which we will propose in this chapter. Because a unified theory is by its nature intended to provide a broad overview of a phenomenon, it tends to be stated in terms of concepts rather than variables. However, this broadness serves a specific purpose in guiding theory development. The unified theory enables researchers to identify and define concepts as testable variables, to develop a set of propositions illustrating the operational linkages among the variables, and to propose a theory to explain the outcome, in our case, FQOL. Recognizing that no single study could test the broad scope of a unified theory, we will present our overarching conceptual theory as a framework upon which to build FQOL theory one study at a time.

In contrast, middle-range theories are much narrower than unified theories. They consist of "a limited number of concepts and propositions," are "generated and tested by means of empirical research," and are typically the type of theories presented within research proposals (Fawcett, 1999, p. 5). Because middle-range theories represent smaller sections of the mosaic of a unified theory, these are the tools for empirical testing through research. Thus, the concepts and propositions of middle-range theories may be translated to variables and testable hypotheses. The unified theory provides both a big picture perspective and an opportunity to place within this big picture a series of middle-range and micro-theories that will allow us to understand results of existing research and to propose next steps in the FQOL research agenda. Micro theories are "less abstract, more specific, and narrower in scope than middle range theory" (Peterson, 2004, p. 34). They are often referred to as practice theories or situation-specific theories. The main goal of a practice theory is to be action-oriented and to "shape reality to create a desired goal" (Peterson, 2004, p. 34). Due to space limitations, we will not address micro theories in this chapter.

Theory Development

Theory-building involves using a combination of sources: (a) existing theory, (b) existing literature, (c) researcher assumptions, and (d) logical reasoning (Shoemaker et al., 2004). Currently, no theory exists to explain FQOL for families of individuals with disabilities; therefore, we must draw upon (a) existing theories in the general family literature, (b) empirically based data from FQOL studies, and (c) our own assumptions to build logical relationships among theoretically important variables. This methodological approach will lead to the development of a logical, testable structure. The value of such a structure is that it presents a *set* of propositions describing relationships among variables which may be tested through individually designed repeated measures, single-subject methodology, and/or correlational research.

A theory of FQOL, like families themselves, should be dynamic, open to change, and based upon a continuous feedback loop which can be re-tested as the field develops a richer understanding of the variables impacting FQOL. It is this inherent flexibility that adds complexity to the development of a theory of FQOL. Borrowing from the more contemporary views of theory, we embrace multiple ways to approach theory development. Bengston and colleagues (2005) present three ways to utilize theories: scientific approach (e.g., explanation and prediction), interpretative approach (e.g., understanding), or critical approach (emancipation or empowerment of oppressed peoples or social groups). Each provides useful explanation "to view and understand the world of families . . ." (p. 13).

We seek to explain what causes FQOL to vary among families of children with intellectual and other disabilities, with a particular emphasis on understanding the variables that are amenable to change (i.e., policies, programs, services, and supports) and the role of static or unchanging characteristics or demographics (e.g., type of disability or family ethnicity) in predicting FQOL. While static traits should be included in the overall structure of a theory, they should primarily be used to describe interactions with various programs and services (e.g., ethnicity as a moderator variable) in order to create a model predicting optimal FQOL for families with different characteristics. For example, understanding how ethnicity interacts with different program and service variables in predicting FQOL provides useful information to administrators and practitioners to ensure the appropriate cultural adaptation of programs and services. Knowing which variables are responsive to change via supports and services provides an excellent opportunity to inform future research and is an impetus for advocacy at the policy and practice level. Thus, we believe a theory of FQOL should have value for *applications* by policymakers, practitioners, and researchers as well as families.

With these parameters in mind, we present a review of the literature on FQOL. After a brief description of our review methodology, we examine the literature related to the components of a possible theory (i.e., the definitions, concepts, variables, and relationships among variables) to explain FQOL. Based on this analysis, we will conclude by proposing a theory of FQOL, which we hope will be an impetus for intellectual interchange and consensus-building.

Literature Review Methodology

Article Location Methods

We conducted a key word search in 21 databases representing the categories of education, health, and social sciences. In line with our interest of studying FQOL in families of children with disabilities, we chose the following key words and combination of key words: (a) family quality of life, (b) quality of family life, (c) family well-being and disab* (*denotes disabled, disabling, disability, or disabilities), (d) family life and disab*, (e) famil* (denotes family or families) and quality of life, (f) famil* and disab* and impact, and (g) life satisfaction and famil* and disab*. Because the phrases, family quality of life and quality of family life often resulted in a return of a limited number of articles, in conjunction with the word "disability," the keyword *disability* (or more specifically, disab*) was not used as a pair word with these two phrases. We also chose to exclude the disability term for key phrases, family quality of life and quality of family life because we were interested in collecting articles on family quality of life and quality of family life outside of the disability field to enrich our understanding of the conceptualization of FQOL for all families.

Article Selection

While a larger key word scope was used to collect articles, the authors used a much narrower scope to select articles for inclusion in this review. Our literature search resulted in 113 articles. We used a two-tiered process to select articles. At the first tier, we selected articles if the title or abstract contained the following key phrases or key phrase and word combinations: "family quality of life," "quality of family life," or "quality of life" and famil*. This first-tier selection resulted in 37 articles. For the second-tier selection of articles, we selected articles for inclusion in this chapter review based on the criterion that the article provided insight to defining, conceptualizing, measuring, or theorizing about family quality of life (or a related term as long as the article addressed the quality of life of parents or all members of the family). We were primarily interested in quantitative studies that examined predictors of FQOL and selected our articles accordingly. The second-tier selection resulted in 24 articles. For purposes of theory-building, however, we must note that these 24 articles contain some redundancy due to the fact that two research teams are overrepresented. Of the 24 articles included in this review, two were related to the work of the International Quality of Life team (Brown, Anand, Fung, Isaacs, & Baum, 2003; Brown et al., 2006) and six emanated from the FQOL research generated at the Beach Center on Disability at the University of Kansas (Bayat, 2005; Hoffman et al., 2006; Summers et al., 2007; Verdugo et al., 2005; Wang et al., 2006; & Wang et al., 2004).

Table 15.1 presents a brief overview of each of the 24 selected articles, which we have analyzed to identify the essential components of a theory (i.e., the definitions, concepts, variables, and relationships among variables). The first column

Table 15.1 Review of family quality of life studies

Reference/sample	FQOL definition and concepts	Variables/methodology to assess FQOL relationships
1. Abbott et al. (2005) Professionals, families, and children/young people with a disability	FQOL Definition: none given FQOL Concepts: Qualitative interviews framed around seven areas: Individual needs: physical environment, financial well-being, social well-being, emotional well-being, skills and learning Family-level needs: daily family life Extra-familial supports: contact with services and professionals	Variables/Methodology: Qualitative Hypotheses proposed: How services are delivered has a positive impact on child health needs but may have a positive or no effect on child/family social and emotional needs. FQOL Relationships: Two thirds of families reported that their FQOL improved due to receiving multi-agency services (e.g., getting more sleep and reduction in number of appointments). Child health needs were met. Social/emotional needs were not addressed well; many families felt they had no one to turn to; young child with disability rarely had emotional support. Families still experienced major difficulties with daily routines (e.g., finding/organizing social activities for themselves and their child). Very little support to help families have short breaks or access to sitters. Very little support for claiming benefits entitlements. Families felt a lack of coordinated and flexible support from the multi-agency services to make home adaptations.

Table 15.1 (continued)

Reference/sample	FQOL definition and concepts	Variables/methodology to assess FQOL relationships
2. Anderson (1998) Patient with serious illness and patient designated family member to complete the surveys	FQOL Definition: None FQOL Concepts: Olson & Barnes (1982) – includes 12 subscales assessing satisfaction with: Individual needs: health, home, education, time, religion, employment, financial well-being Family-level needs: marriage and family life Extra-familial supports: friends, extended family, mass media, neighborhood/community	Variables/Methodology: Multiple regression analysis to investigate relationships between FQOL and: Family Characteristics: Family Sense of coherence (FSOC): explains the motivational and cognitive bases for transforming resources into actuality, to cope with stressors and promote health. Includes: (a) spouse agreement about perceptions of the family's ability to manage the demands of life and to see life as meaningful and comprehensible; (b) illness stress, (c) family system balance, (d) income; (e) length of relationship; (f) patient/family member employment status FQOL Relationships: Positive relationship between FSOC and FQOL (r =.55). FSOC as the largest predictor of FQOL (30% of the variance; the greater the FSOC, the greater FQOL). FSOC, illness stress, family system balance, length of family relationship, patient full-time job status, family income accounted for 57.6% of the variance that predicted FQOL. FSOC was a mediator in the impact of illness stress on the family, reducing the direct influence of illness stress on FQOL by half

Table 15.1 (continued)

Reference/sample	FQOL definition and concepts	Variables/methodology to assess FQOL relationships
3. Bayat, (2005) Families of children with autism. Primarily mothers (134), some fathers (30), and a few caregivers (11)	FQOL Definition: FQOL refers to the family's overall well-being and ability to meet the family's needs and enjoy life. FQOL Concepts: Use of Beach Center measure, see Hoffman et al. (2006) for a description.	Variables/Methodology: Multiple regression analysis using structural equation modeling (SEM) to investigate relationships among: Child Characteristics: Age of child, severity of autism Family Characteristics: Parental education, income Beck Depression Inventory, and coping strategies, defined through use of Kansas Inventory of Parental Perceptions (KIPP) (Behr, Murphy, & Ann, 1992), which included (a) parents' perceptions of positive contributions of child to family, and (b) parents' attributions of the cause of the autism System/Support Characteristics: Satisfaction with services FQOL Relationships: Structural model using KIPP Positive Contributions as a predictor of FQOL along with demographic variables: Significant predictors were: Income, depression, and child's age. After accounting for all demographic variables parental perceptions of positive effects of autism was a significant predictor of FQOL. Overall percent of variance explained in FQOL was 0.33. Structural Model using KIPP causal attributions as a predictor of FQOL along with demographic variables: Only age of child was a significant predictor of FQOL. After accounting for all demographic variables parental perceptions of the causes of autism was not significant predictor of FQOL. Overall percent of variance explained in FQOL was 0.25

Table 15.1 (continued)

Reference/sample	FQOL definition and concepts	Variables/methodology to assess FQOL relationships
4. Ben-Gashir, Seed, and Hay (2002) Families of children with childhood atopic dermatitis (AD). Primarily mothers (105 mothers and 1 father)	FQOL Definition: None FQOL Concepts: 10 items rated by parent; Individual needs: sleep of family members, leisure activities, time spent on shopping, cost of treatment or clothes, tiredness, emotional distress, caregiving impact Family-level needs: housework, food preparation, family relationships	Variables/Methodology: Regression model investigating relationship of FQOL and AD severity at two points in time. Child characteristics: symptom severity, skin color, sex, child's age Family characteristics: Family size and location FQOL Relationships: FQOL significantly correlated to symptom severity at two points in time, after controlling for child and family characteristics
5. Bowman (2001) Young children (0–3) and their families, i.e., mothers ($n = 228$)	FQOL Definition: none, but provides Schalock's, Brown's, and pediatric literature's definition of QOL, not FQOL. FQOL Concepts: Study developed a Quality of Life Interview (QOLI). 28 items in four subscales: Individual: Satisfaction Level, Behavior Problems, Developmental Level, and Psychiatric History	Variables/Methodology: Two analyses: (a) EFA for scale development and (b) MANOVA to examine group differences of QOL among parents whose children have different child characteristics: Child Characteristics: typically developing (TD), developmentally delayed (DD) or experiencing behavior problems (BP). Family Characteristics: race, religion, marital status, maternal education, income, city population FQOL Relationships: 4-factor solution with EFA for FQOL scale: Satisfaction Level, Behavior Problems, Developmental Level, and Psychiatric History MANOVA results: Differences were noted on all three factors of the QOL scale except for Satisfaction scale, which has items more typical of FQOL scales. Total QOL score differed for all three groups (e.g., TD, DD, and BP)

Table 15.1 (continued)

Reference/sample	FQOL definition and concepts	Variables/methodology to assess FQOL relationships
6. Brown et al. (2003) Mothers and fathers of children with intellectual disabilities; however, it was unclear if scores were averaged or scores were jointly agreed upon	FQOL Definition: None given FQOL Concepts: four concepts or dimensions: Opportunities–options available to families taking advantage of available opportunities Initiative-taking advantage of available opportunities Attainment-getting, having, or accomplishing those things that the family wants and needs. Satisfaction-overall perception of family members These four concepts were assessed for each of nine areas of FQOL as listed below; response stems included a mix of frequency and satisfaction Individual Needs: Health, financial well-being, careers and preparing for careers, spiritual and cultural life, leisure, community and civic involvement Family-level Needs: family relationships Extra-familial supports: support from others, support from services	Variables/Methodology: Bivariate correlations among families' assessment of opportunities, initiative, attainment, and satisfaction as related to the nine areas from the FQOL scale FQOL Relationships: Only selected correlations are displayed to conserve space. Positive correlation between attainment of health and satisfaction of health Positive correlation between attainment of financial well-being and satisfaction of financial well-being Opportunities: Lowest mean score was support from others, highest was spiritual/cultural beliefs Initiative: Lowest mean was support from others, highest was careers. Attainment: Lowest mean was support from others, highest was spiritual/cultural beliefs Satisfaction: Lowest mean was support from services, highest was spiritual/cultural beliefs
7. Brown et al. (2006) Primarily mothers of children ages 3–13 with Down syndrome, autism, and control group	FQOL Definition: None FQOL Concepts: Same as Brown et al. (2003)	Variables/Methodology: Correlation, analysis of variance, and descriptive data focusing on satisfaction with each of the nine domains; comparisons of families in three groups Child characteristics: Comparisons of families of typically developing children, Down syndrome, and autism Family characteristics: highest correlation of the combined groups between domains and FQOL include family relations, leisure/enjoyment of life, careers/preparing for careers, and health. FQOL Relationships: Families in the comparison group had the highest FQOL, followed by children with Down syndrome and then children with autism

Table 15.1 (continued)

Reference/sample	FQOL definition and concepts	Variables/methodology to assess FQOL relationships
8. Dunst et al. (2006) 801 parents of children with disabilities in early intervention	FQOL Definition: None FQOL Concepts: Global concept with a single-item assessment of respondent's FQOL, on a 10-point scale on the extent to which the "family had the worst or best life possible" (p. 241).	Variables/Methodology: A linear regression analysis focusing on the difference between two approaches to natural learning environments. Child Characteristics: Extent of delay/disability Family Characteristics: Parent age, ethnicity, education, marital, and employment status. Researchers also assessed parents' positive and negative well-being System/Support Characteristics: Implementation of early intervention in family and community activity settings, implemented by the practitioner versus by the parent FQOL Relationships: Using everyday family activities as learning opportunities was associated with enhanced parent well-being and family quality of life and decreased negative parent well-being; professionals implementing EI in activity settings was associated with reduced positive parent well-being and family quality of life and increased negative parent well-being
9. Feldman and Werner (2002) Families of children with DD and behavior disorders: 34 mothers, 1 father, 1 grandmother	FQOL Definition: None FQOL Concepts: Eight questions asking parents to rate the degree to which the child's behavior creates problems in the areas of: Individual Needs: daily activities/routines, learning Family-level needs: community integration, family social functions in home Extra-familial supports: participant's peer relationships, others' positive response toward participants	Variables/Methodology: MANOVA to identify differences among groups on variables. Child Characteristics: Degree of problem behaviors measured by Child Behavior Management Survey. Family Characteristics: Parental stress, depressive affect, self-efficacy, therapist rating of parental behavior management skills, and parent satisfaction with training System/Support Characteristics: Behavioral parent training, comparison of training with wait-listed group FQOL Relationships: Families receiving behavioral training had higher FQOL and self-efficacy

Table 15.1 (continued)

Reference/sample	FQOL definition and concepts	Variables/methodology to assess FQOL relationships
10. Gupta and Sharma (1998) 455 Indian working women	FQOL Definition: Enrichment of life, a socio-economical and socio-psychological process running through (a) social production of values concerning QOL, (b) social distribution of values concerning QOL, and (c) social perception of values concerning QOL. Scale adapted from Moos & Moos (1986) FQOL Concepts: Initial measure used 16 items including: Individual needs: intellectual enrichment, sharing problems, sharing day's happenings Family-level needs: Helpfulness, cooperation, caring, eating together, encouragement, team spirit, appreciate new ideas, emotional bond, communication, responsible, adjusting, relationship with other members. Other: criticizing habit	Variables/Methodology: Factor analysis of field test resulted in a 3-factor solution: Family Characteristics: (a) close-knit family environment, (b) cohesive–supportive family life, and (c) team spirit in family life FQOL Relationships: Three factor solution identified: Family cohesion (e.g., eating together, bonding), Helpfulness, and Team Spirit. Relationships not identified as this is an instrument development article
11. Hoffman et al. (2006) 208 families (Study 1) and 280 families (Study 2), of children with disabilities. Primary respondents were mothers	FQOL Definition: None given FQOL Concepts: Beach Center FQOL Scale: measured family perceptions of the importance and satisfaction of 25 questions in five domains: Individual needs: physical/material well-being, emotional well-being Family-level needs: family interaction, parenting Extra-familial supports: Disability-related supports	Variables/Methodology: Structural equation model depicting covariation of five lower order latent constructs (i.e., five FQOL domains) assessed by observable item indicators FQOL Relationships: SEM model supports five lower order latent constructs and FQOL as a higher-order construct; relationships not identified as this is an instrument development article

Table 15.1 (continued)

Reference/sample	FQOL definition and concepts	Variables/methodology to assess FQOL relationships
12. Hornstein and McWilliam (2007) 454 Parents, primarily mothers, of children with autism spectrum disorders, aged 0–6	FQOL Definition: none given FQOL Concepts: modification of an instrument previously used to measure FQOL in families of children who are deaf or hard of hearing (McWilliam, 2005, as cited in Hornstein and McWilliam, 2007). Parents rate satisfaction on 40 items, in five factors: Individual needs: Competence, knowledge, well-being Family-level needs: cohesion Extra-familial supports: alliances	Variables/Methodology: Exploratory-factor analysis to identify factors, correlations with family demographics: Family Characteristics: Family SES, ethnicity Service/Support Characteristics: Hours of services received FQOL Relationships: Variance explained in indicators by factors: Competence (15.57%); Knowledge (11.81%); Alliances (7.81%); Cohesion (7.69%); and Well-being (6.26%) Knowledge is lower in families with lower SES, and with fewer hours of service Cohesion is lower in nonwhite families Well-being is lower in families with lower SES
13. Mellon and Northouse (2001) 123 dyads: Cancer patient and family member; approximately half included spouse and another one third included adult children as a second respondent	FQOL Definition: None FQOL Concepts: Uses Olson & Barnes (1991) measure – see Anderson (1998) in this table.	Variables/Methodology: Model testing involving correlational analysis, hierarchical multiple regression, and regression equation testing for mediation Individual characteristics: Illness survival stressors – concurrent stressors from family, fear of recurrence, and somatic concerns, patient employment Family characteristics: Family hardiness, family meaning of cancer illness System/support characteristics: Family social support FQOL Relationships: 63% of variance in FQOL was explained by the model; FQOL was impacted by patient employment status, concurrent family stressors, family member fear of recurrence, family social supports, and family meaning.

Table 15.1 (continued)

Reference/sample	FQOL definition and concepts	Variables/methodology to assess FQOL relationships
14. Poston et al. (2003) Qualitative study to identify indicators and meaning of FQOL; 78 family members, 50 professionals	FQOL Definition: None FQOL Concepts: Framework presented as a result of qualitative, grounded theory research study. Domains include: Individual needs: Advocacy, Emotional Well-Being, Health, Environmental Well-Being Family-level needs: Daily Family Life, Family Interaction, Financial Well-Being, Parenting	Variables/Methodology: Qualitative study using a combination of focus groups and individual interviews of non-English-speaking family members; sampling plan includes a diversity of SES and ethnicity, as well as both family members and professionals FQOL Relationships: FQOL framework is the outcome of the study. No relationships were reported as this is an exploratory study intended to identify dimensions of FQOL
15. Rettig & Bubolz (1983) A study of 250 couples to validate perceptual indicators of family well-being	FQOL Definition: Integration of human needs, economic and psychological resources, and interpersonal satisfaction as a basis for development of perceptual indicators of family well-being FQOL Concepts: Structure of resources are based on two coordinates: concrete-symbolic, and universalistic–particularistic (higher value when resource is provided by a specific other individual) for six resources: Individual needs: Love, status, services, information, money, goods FQOL is measured with a global item – "how do you feel about your own family life" on the 7-point "delighted to terrible" scale	Variables/Methodology: Cluster analysis to identify hierarchical clustering of the six resources, and predictive contributions to global rating of FQOL. Satisfaction with resources received on a 7-point "delighted-terrible scale," and frequency with which resources are received on an 8-point scale, from "never" to "2–3 times a day" FQOL Relationships: Social–psychological and economic resources are important to FQOL. More particularistic resources (love, status) make stronger contributions to FQOL

Table 15.1 (continued)

Reference/sample	FQOL definition and concepts	Variables/methodology to assess FQOL relationships
16. Rettig and Leichtentritt (1999)	FQOL Definition: An individual's experience of family life will depend upon the extent to which personal needs are met, as judged by the personal values, standards, and aspirations one has for an ideal family life Framework/Theoretical orientation: Three "nested" theories: Human ecological systems theory, resource theory, and facet theory FQOL Measure: See Rettig and Bubolz (1983), this table	Variables/Methodology: Results analyzed using Multidimensional Scaling analysis to determine underlying structure, using scatter diagrams to learn proximities Using this mapping strategy, the purpose was to determine whether the six resources would cluster in the hypothesized circular pattern FQOL Relationships: The results confirmed the model. Items representing love and money are on the vertical axis (e.g., OK to get money from many sources, need love from specific people), and on the concrete-symbolic horizontal axis (money is concrete, expressions of love may be symbolic)
17. Ricci, Bendandi, Bellini, Patrizi, and Masi (2007) A study of 45 Italian parents of children with atopic dermatitis (AD)	FQOL Definition: None FQOL Concepts: 10 questions, same as Ben-Gashir et al. (2002), this table	Methodology/Variables: Descriptive correlation between three levels of severity and FQOL questions Child Characteristics: Mild, moderate, and severe AD FQOL Relationships: FQOL appeared to be moderately altered in families of children with more severe AD with greatest problem being disrupted sleep
18. Summers et al. (2007) A study of 180 parents (Primarily mothers) of young children 0–5 with disabilities	FQOL Definition: none given FQOL Concepts: Beach Center FQOL Scale. See Hoffman et al. (2006), this table	Methodology/Variables: Structural equation model examining the mediating effect of family–professional partnerships on the relationship between service adequacy and FQOL. Variables: System/Support Characteristics: (a) parents' ratings of adequacy of services received for child and family; (b) parents' ratings of satisfaction with the quality of partnership with the early childhood professional FQOL Relationships: Service adequacy significantly predicted FQOL. Family–professional partnerships was a partial mediator of the effects of service adequacy on FQOL

Table 15.1 (continued)

Reference/sample	FQOL definition and concepts	Variables/methodology to assess FQOL relationships
19. Verdugo, Cordoba, & Gomez (2005) 385 parents (primarily mothers) of children with disabilities in Cali, Columbia	FQOL Definition: none given FQOL Concepts: Spanish version of Beach Center FQOL Scale, see Hoffman et al. (2006), this table	Methodology/Variables: Structural equation modeling to assess the fit of the 5-factor measurement model of the Spanish version of the Beach Center FQOL Scale. Participants rated both importance and satisfaction with all items FQOL Relationships: All item factor loadings were greater than 0.50. Model fit was excellent: Importance: GFI = 0.99; NFI = 0.99; RFI = 0.99 Satisfaction: GFI = 0.98; NFI = 0.97; RFI = 0.97
20. Voydanoff et al. (1994) Study of stepfamilies and first marriage families. N = 3,120 in sample where both spouses participated	FQOL Definition: Not defined FQOL Concepts: Global construct questions rating: Individual Needs: none Family-level needs: (a) happiness with marriage, (b) satisfaction with quality of relationship of parent with each child Extra-familial supports: None	Methodology/Variables: Data were drawn from a large National Survey of Families and Households. Analysis involved multiple regression models to determine contributions of: Family-level characteristics: Family demographics (education, income, race), family structure (first marriage versus stepfamilies), role organization (task/role divisions in work and household tasks), disagreements over household tasks, sense of equity about role divisions FQOL Relationships: Parents in stepfamilies report lower quality of parent–child relationships; no clear relationship to marital quality. Role organization satisfaction was related to marital happiness

Table 15.1 (continued)

Reference/sample	FQOL definition and concepts	Variables/methodology to assess FQOL relationships
21. Wang et al. (2004) 130 fathers and 234 mothers of young children (0–5) with disabilities	FQOL Definition: none given FQOL Concepts: Beach Center FQOL Scale, see Hoffman et al. (2006), this table	Variables/Methodology: Structural equation modeling to predict relationships of variables to FQOL: Child Characteristics: level of severity of child's disability based on parent report Family characteristics: Family income defined as total household income FQOL Relationships: Mothers: income was a weak but significant positive predictor of FQOL. Severity of disability was a strong negative predictor of FQOL Fathers: income, while a positive predictor of FQOL was not significant. Severity of disability was a strong negative predictor of FQOL For both mothers and fathers, the interaction effect was not significant. The final SEM model explained 17% of the variance in FQOL for mothers and 16% for fathers
22. Wang et al. (2006) Mothers and Fathers from 107 families of young children (0–5) with disabilities	FQOL Definition: none given FQOL Concepts: Beach Center FQOL Scale, see Hoffman et al. (2006), this table	Variables/Methodology: Structural equation model testing measurement invariance across mothers and fathers on FQOL, in addition to examining differences in means, variances, and correlations for the two latent FQOL constructs: importance and satisfaction FQOL Relationships: Measurement invariance held for mothers and fathers in terms of importance and satisfaction; there were no significant differences between mothers and fathers for importance and satisfaction in terms of FQOL means, variances, or correlation between importance and satisfaction

Table 15.1 (continued)

Reference/sample	FQOL definition and concepts	Variables/methodology to assess FQOL relationships
23. Weigel et al. (1995) 328 mothers and 187 fathers who were State-classified employees at land grant universities who had children under the age of 18	FQOL Definition: Authors proposed three variables to represent FQOL: family satisfaction, family cohesion, and family decision-making. Predictor variables were used for each of these three outcomes FQOL Concepts: Adapted from Bloom's (1985) revised Self-Report of Family Functioning. The measure includes five statements rated on a 4-point scale (very untrue to very true for my family) in three areas: Individual needs: None Family-level needs: Cohesion (emotional bonding and contact among family members), decision-making style process of evaluation in choosing or resolving alternatives, family satisfaction (positive or negative assessment of family life)	Variables/Methodology: Path analysis by gender (mothers/fathers but not in same family) examining mediating role between seven work family characteristics (e.g., job quality, job value, housework, age of youngest child) and Work-Family Conflicts and Stress in predicting Quality of Family Life Parent characteristics: job type, hours worked, stress, work–family conflict Family characteristics: composition and structure of family (age of youngest child, division of household labor) FQOL Relationships Mothers: Stress was a significant direct negative predictor of FQOL for family satisfaction (F.S.); family cohesion (F.C); and family decision-making (F.DM). Age of youngest child was also a significant negative predictor for all three FQOL variables. Variance accounted for in overall model for the three FQOL indicators: $R^2 = 0.45$ (F.S.), $R^2 = 0.37$ (F.C.), and $R^2 = 0.23$ (F.DM) Fathers: Stress was a significant negative predictor for two of the FQOL variables for fathers: family satisfaction (F.S.) and family cohesion (F.C.); there was not direct path between stress and family decision-making (F DM). There was no direct path between age of youngest child and F.S.; a negative relationship was reported between stress and F.C.; and a positive relationship was reported between stress and F.DM. Variance accounted for in the overall model for the three FQOL indicators: $R^2 = 0.32$ (F.S), $R^2 = 0.28$ (F.C.) $R^2 = 0.21$ (F.DM).

Table 15.1 (continued)

Reference/sample	FQOL definition and concepts	Variables/methodology to assess FQOL relationships
24. Zabriskie and McCormick (2003) Relationships between family leisure involvement and FQOL in 179 families including 1 parent and 1 youth aged 12–15 from each family	FQOL Definition: None FQOL Concepts: Modified version of Satisfaction with Family Life Scale (SWFL) (Diener et al., 1985), including five statements about family life rated on a 7-point scale from strongly disagree to strongly agree (specific items are not described in this chapter), therefore we are treating the construct for our purposes as a global indicator of FQOL	Variables/Methodology: Regression model to predict FQOL: Family Characteristics: Satisfaction and involvement with leisure activities using Family Leisure Activity Profile (FLAP); family demographics including age, gender, ethnicity, marital status, family size, and income FQOL Relationships: Data analyzed three ways: youth only, parents only, and combined parent/youth means Youth: Demographic block ($R^2 = 0.103$, $p<0.05$) Family Leisure block did not result in a statistically significant change in variance. (R^2 change = 0.016, $p>0.05$) Parents: Demographic block did not account for a significant proportion of variance in SWFL. ($R^2 = 0.08$, $p>0.05$) Family Leisure block did result in a statistically significant change in variance. (R^2 change = 0.083, $p<0.05$) Combined: Demographic block did not account for a significant proportion of variance in SWFL ($R^2 = 0.099$, $p>0.05$) Family Leisure block did account for a significant additional amount of variance in explaining SWFL (R^2 change = 0.052, $p = 0.01$)

includes the reference and a brief description of the sample. The second column includes a description of the FQOL definitions and concepts described in the chapter. The third column includes a description of the specific variables, methodology, and results as depicted through the relationships among the variables to predict FQOL. To construct a unified theoretical framework of FQOL, we focused primarily on the concepts, variables, and relationships among the variables shown in Table 15.1.

A Proposed Unified Theory of Family Quality of Life

Defining FQOL – The Outcome

A first step in building a theory is to clearly identify and define the concepts used. Logically, the first concept to define is the outcome, in this case FQOL. We begin by reviewing the definitions of FQOL identified in the literature, which we listed in the second column of Table 15.1. Consistent with a similar review of family outcomes in the disability literature (Turnbull et al., 2007), we also observed that only 6 of these 24 articles provided an explicit definition of FQOL. We hasten to say that this does not mean these research teams do not have a definition; rather, the definitions were not articulated in the articles. In attempting to determine how these researchers were defining FQOL, we made some inferences from the measures they used as well as any explicit definitions provided.

We identified several common themes among the FQOL definitions. First, satisfaction as a concept was mentioned explicitly in three definitions. Family sense of well-being, perceptual indicators, and judgment by personal values were also mentioned as definitional components. Collectively, these components suggest a principle: The nature or quality of family life is not to be judged by outsiders but rather is dependent on the *subjective* impressions of family members' satisfaction with their quality of life. Family satisfaction, in short, is "one's positive or negative assessment of family life" (Weigel, Weigel, Berger, Cook, & DelCampo, 1995, p. 10). In terms of measurement, satisfaction as an explicit concept was operationalized as all or part of the dependent variable (i.e., satisfaction used as the response stem in measurement of the respondent's ratings across a variety of items) in 15 of the 24 articles in this review.

A second theme emerging from these definitions is the notion of *meeting individual family member needs.* For example, Rettig and Leichtentritt (1999) note: An individual's experience of family life will . . . "depend upon the extent to which personal needs are met, as judged by the personal values, standards, and aspirations one has for an ideal family life" (p. 310). Thus, the idea of FQOL reflects the belief that the family as a unit has a responsibility to meet the individual needs of each of its family members. This idea may or may not be true across all cultures, as in some cultures there is a much stronger collectivist as contrasted to individualistic orientation (Lynch & Hanson, 2004; McGoldrick, Giordano, & Pearce, 1996). However, five of the six available definitions mention the notion of meeting individual family member needs. In terms of measurement, the theme of meeting individual family needs resulted in the creation of a series of domains or factors which the researchers used to categorize aspects of individual need. These included, for example, daily family life (Abbott, Watson, & Townsley, 2005); emotional, physical, and social well-being (Brown et al., 2003; Hoffman et al., 2006); and satisfaction with resources (Rettig & Bubolz, 1983).

Finally, a third theme is that the family as a *unit* has characteristics of its own that cannot be described simply by understanding its individual members. The Weigel et al.'s (1995) definition refers to family cohesion, family decision-making, and family satisfaction as components of FQOL, suggesting that different knowledge may be gained by considering the family as a unit as opposed to assessing and aggregating the satisfaction of individual needs of each family member. In terms of measurement, only a few researchers measured FQOL as a collective or summative construct using multiple family members' perspectives (Anderson, 1998; Rettig & Bubolz, 1983; Rettig & Leichtentritt, 1999; Zabriskie & McCormick, 2003) or at a minimum assessed FQOL by considering multiple family sub-systems (e.g., marital, parental) (Voydanoff, Fine, & Donnelly, 1994). Anderson (1998), using the Olson and Barnes QOL measure (1982), calculated a family mean score to "represent the behavior of the family as a unit" (p. 177). Both Rettig and Bubolz (1983) and Rettig and Leichtentritt (1999) assessed FQOL as a collective average of husband and wife scores across six areas of family life (e.g., love, goods, money) using a scale ranging from 1 (terrible) to 7 (delighted). Zabriskie and McCormick (2003) collected FQOL scores from parents, as well as youth, using a revised version of the Satisfaction with Family Life Scale (SWFL) (Diener, Emmons, Larsen, & Griffin, 1985). The revised SWFL scale measures individual family members' satisfaction of their collective family life on a scale from 1 (strongly disagree) to 7 (strongly agree). Finally, Voydanoff et al. (1994) conceptualized FQOL as overall satisfaction within two family sub-systems: marital relationships and child–parent relationships.

Based on the three themes, we have identified as common across the articles we reviewed, we offer the following definition of FQOL as an *outcome* for purposes of theorizing about FQOL:

Family quality of life is a dynamic sense of well-being of the family, collectively and subjectively defined and informed by its members, in which individual and family-level needs interact.

FQOL Concepts – Explanatory or Influencing Concepts

Consistent with theory-building principles, we now turn to identifying and defining the specific concepts within the overall FQOL model. In a later section, we provide examples of how the variables are used within the selected research studies to predict FQOL. In reviewing the studies, we chose concepts that were directly or indirectly related to FQOL as an outcome. To build our unified theory, we identified the concepts represented by the variables used as predictor, independent, or mediator variables in the studies we reviewed (see the third column of Table 15.1). While we primarily included quantitative studies ($n = 22$) to develop our theoretical model, we also included two qualitative studies that provided additional theoretical insight (Abbott et al., 2005; Poston et al., 2003). Across all of the studies, four clusters of concepts emerged: (a) family-unit concepts, (b) individual family-member concepts, (c) performance concepts (e.g., services, practices, and supports), and (d) systemic concepts (e.g., systems, policies, and programs). To clarify, the individual and family-unit explanatory concepts described in this section are different concepts than individual and family-level *needs* previously discussed and defined as part of FQOL as an outcome. The concepts described herein represent the broad categories from which variables are selected as predictors of FQOL, not defining components of an FQOL measure. These four concepts, together with their theoretical linkages to each other and to the FQOL outcome, form our proposed unified theory.

Before attempting a parsimonious statement of our unified theory, we first present an in-depth explanation of the four concepts, each of which encompasses a large number of potential variables. Because FQOL as a field of study is still in its infancy (as compared to individual quality of life), sufficient empirical data are not available across all four concepts. In fact, much of the available research assesses the impact of individual and family-unit performance concepts (e.g., services or practices) on FQOL. However, the lack of empirical data across the four concepts should not preclude theory development. On the contrary, it provides an opportunity for *theorizing*. In this manner, we incorporate both tested and untested hypotheses within one theoretical model and use evidenced-based data from empirical studies and novel ideas and assumptions from researchers to build a theoretical model. Interjection of researcher assumptions within theory-building is in line with contemporary views of theory-building (Bengtson et al., 2005; Fawcett, 1999; Shoemaker et al., 2004) which encourage creativity and curiosity as an input to inform science.

Family-Unit Concepts

The family-unit is defined as the collective number of individuals who consider themselves to be part of a family and who engage in some form of family activities together on a regular basis (e.g., eating, social gatherings, school/sporting events). A family-unit describes a family as a whole. Two family-unit concepts consistently reported in the FQOL literature were family characteristics and family dynamics (Fig. 15.1). We define family-level *characteristics* as traits or descriptors of the family as a whole, including, for example, family income, size of family, family geographic location, religious preference, ethnicity, or family form (e.g., stepfamily versus first marriage family). We define family *dynamics* as aspects of interactions and ongoing relationships among two or more family members. Examples of family dynamic concepts typically assessed include family sense of coherence, adaptability, hardiness, and decision-making. Of the 24 articles we reviewed, nine studies included one or more family characteristic or family dynamic concept which were operationalized as variables and then used either as a predictor or as a mediator related to the FQOL outcome.

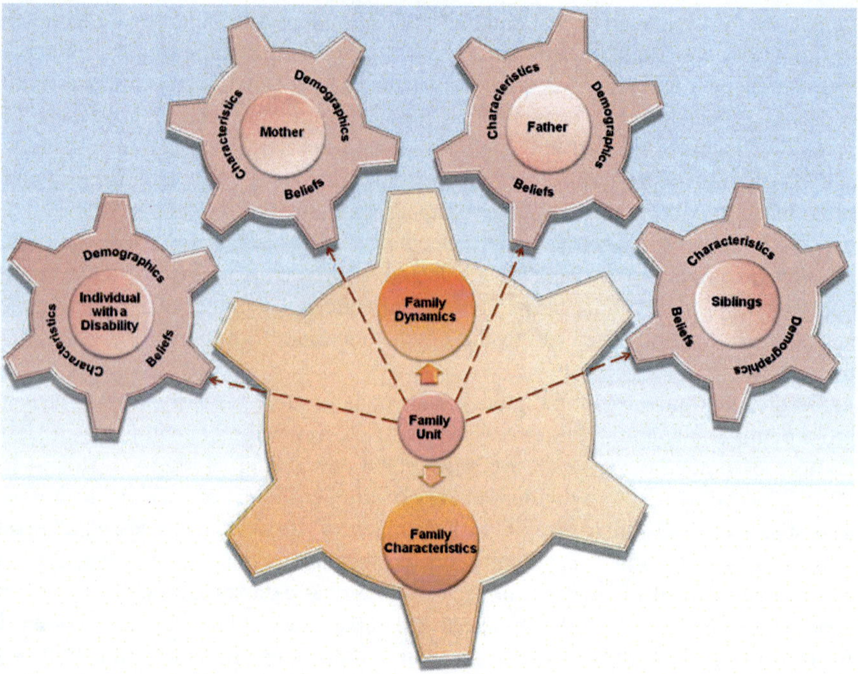

Fig. 15.1 Family-unit and individual family member interaction

Individual Family Member Concepts

In contrast to family-unit concepts, individual family member concepts refer to aspects of the person with a disability, parent, siblings, or other individual family member. Individual family member concepts, especially those related to the child with the disability, were frequently operationalized as variables and used as predictors in many of the FQOL studies included in this review. We identified three types of individual family member concepts: individual family-member characteristics, demographics, and beliefs (Fig. 15.1). We define *individual demographics* as basic traits such as the child's age, type of disability, or gender; or parent's education level, ethnicity, or employment status; or sibling's age or gender. We define *individual characteristics* as more complex and multidimensional traits which might vary over time, such as child behavior, parent depression, or sibling health status. We define *beliefs* as an individual family member's attributions of meaning, expectations, or understanding about a phenomenon, such as the meaning of the child's disability for the family, expectations about the child's future, or understanding/expectations about parental roles in partnership with professionals. We found that 11 of the 24 articles included one or more individual characteristics and/or demographic concepts articulated as variables and used in the research. However, only two studies (Bayat, 2005; Mellon & Northouse, 2001) utilized beliefs as a variable.

Performance Concepts

The three performance concepts include services, supports, and practices. The performance concepts represent the crux of the FQOL theory and are represented at the individual (Fig. 15.2) and the family (Fig. 15.3) level. As the name suggests, performance concepts imply an action – something that is delivered or acted upon on behalf of individuals with intellectual disabilities and their families. In our unified theory, these are the formal services, supports, and practices developed and offered to individuals with intellectual disabilities and their families. *Services* are a range of educational, social, and health-related activities expected to improve outcomes for the individual or of the family as a whole. Examples include respite care, counseling, medical/dental care, or therapies such as speech-language therapy. *Supports* are more difficult to define, and we recognize that the distinction between services and supports is not always clear. For purposes of our theory, we suggest that supports are less tangible resources provided to the individual or to the whole family which are expected to improve outcomes for the individual or family. Examples of supports include the emotional supports provided through a parent's interaction with an early intervention service provider, knowledge and information

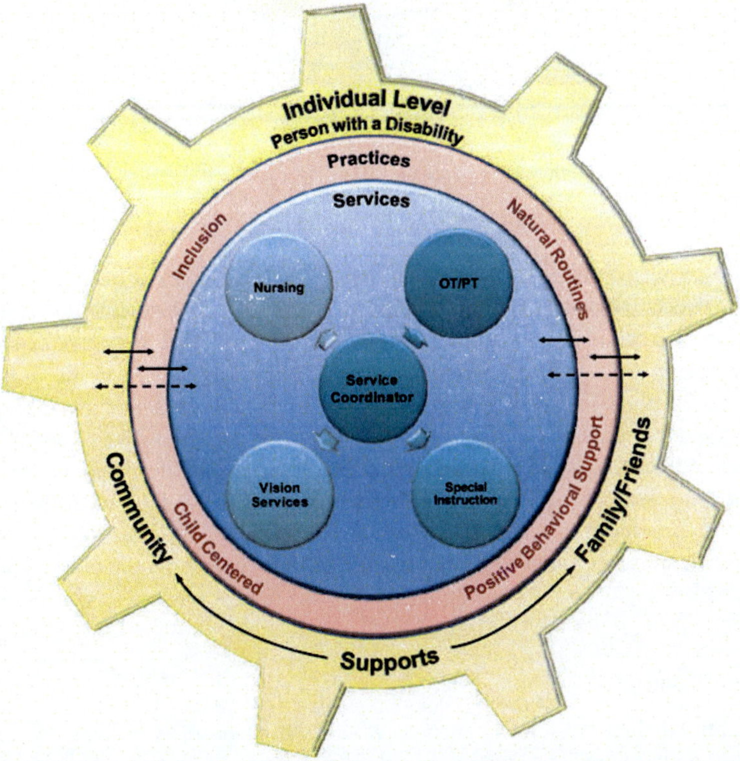

Fig. 15.2 Individual level performance concepts

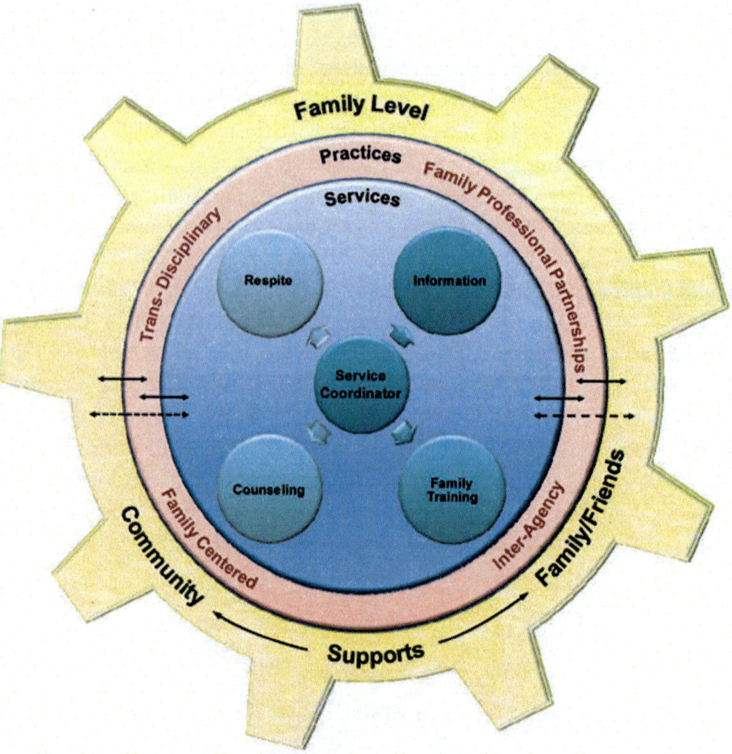

Fig. 15.3 Family-level performance concepts

received through participation in a parenting class on positive behavior support, or self-advocacy skills achieved by an individual with a disability through participation in a self-determination training. Finally, we define *practices* as specific procedures or processes through which services and supports may be delivered. Examples of practices include routines-based early intervention (i.e., incorporating interventions such as range of motion or language activities in the family's daily routine) and positive behavior support (i.e., describing a set of procedures to assess behavior and rearranging the environment to reduce the individual's challenging behavior). Among the 24 articles we reviewed, only eight utilized some aspect of services, supports, or practices, with services and supports being the most frequently researched.

Systemic Concepts

We identified three systemic concepts which we propose as influencing FQOL: systems, policies, and programs. We define *systems* as a collection of interrelated networks organized to meet the various needs of society, such as health care, education, and legal systems. These systems are present in all industrialized nations and have often been linked to quality-of-life issues (Phillips, 2006). *Policies* are guidelines establishing, organizing, and regulating the procedures for implementing programs and systems. Policies differ by country. With respect to the United States, a few policies relevant to FQOL theory include: Individuals with Disabilities Education Act (IDEA), Americans with Disabilities Act (ADA), and Family Opportunities Act (FOA). Policies might also be established to encourage cross-systems cooperation. An example of this policy would be a government regulation requiring the creation of inter-agency (across systems) agreements to ensure services provided to families are coordinated across programs and systems. We define *programs* as formally or informally organized entities that provide services and supports to an identified population. Examples include early intervention agencies serving young children with disabilities and their families, developmental disabilities agencies that provide supports and services to children and adults with disabilities, or family support programs such as Parent to Parent (Santelli, Turnbull, Marquis, & Lerner, 2000), providing supports to families by matching a veteran parent with a parent needing supports. Programs, in other words, are located within systems or networks, and are regulated by policies. None of the 24 articles examined the impact of programs, systems, or policies on FQOL using a quantitative predictive model; however, one article qualitatively examined the impact of multi-agency systems on families' quality of life (Abbott et al., 2005).

Variables and Propositions – A Unified Theory of Family Quality of Life

Figure 15.4 is a graphic representation of our unified theory of family quality of life. It depicts the complex interactions (i.e., their theoretical linkages) among the concepts which we propose as explaining variations in FQOL outcomes. Figures 15.1, 15.2, and 15.3 are subsumed within the larger theoretical framework represented in Fig. 15.4. Following is a description of a few relational linkages drawn from our proposed unified theory that researchers could use to develop middle-range theories:

- Family characteristics and dynamics interact with individual characteristics to influence FQOL outcomes.
- Family and individual performance factors (i.e., supports, services, and practices) act as mediating or moderating variables on the effects of family-unit or individual family member factors to predict FQOL.
- Program quality predicts implementation of best practices; implementation of best practices impacts an individual child factor (e.g., reduction in tantrums), which in turn impacts FQOL.

In Fig. 15.1, the family-unit and individual family member cogs illustrate the interaction among family dynamics and family characteristics with each individual member's characteristics, demographics, and beliefs. Figures 15.2 and 15.3 illustrate the performance factors for the individual and family-unit, respectively. The inner

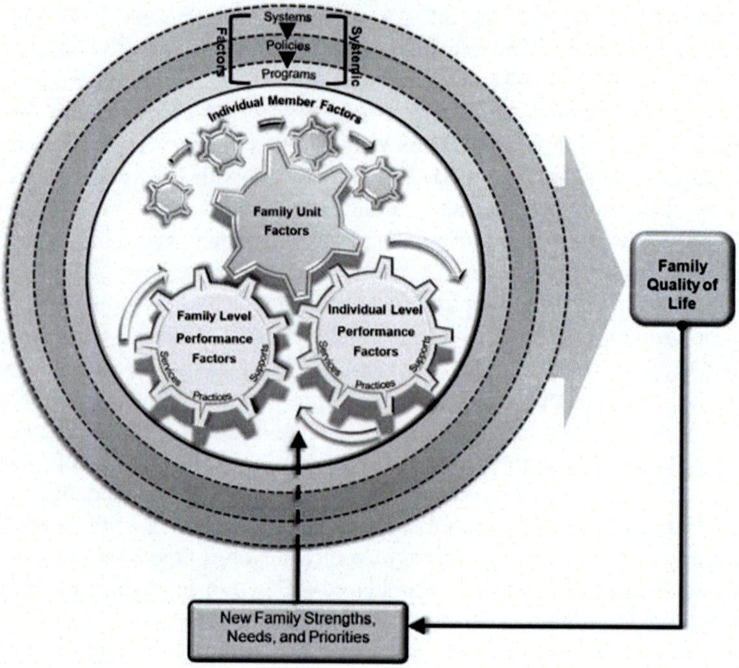

Fig. 15.4 Unified theory of FQOL

circle of Fig. 15.4 illustrates the multiple interactive operational linkages between the family-level and individual-level performance factors, between family-unit and individual member factors, and among all seven inner cogs. Figure 15.4 also illustrates the distal impacts of systems, polices, and programs; these are represented by the outer circles. We placed the systemic factors as circles with dashed lines around the edge of the interactive cogs to emphasize their role as indirect influences on the directly interactive elements within the inner circle of the theoretical model.

If one of the system factors changes (i.e., elimination of a program or policy), this will disrupt the smoothly running "cogs," leading to changes in FQOL until adaptation or homeostasis occurs within the individual or family. For example, if a service is denied or a support falls through, this impacts FQOL. If a parent suddenly loses his or her job or becomes chronically or terminally ill, this again impacts FQOL. If a child "ages out" of the educational system and needs to be served by an adult service system, FQOL will be impacted while a whole new set of performance factors, with new services, practices, and supports, is activated. Each factor addresses the complexity of families' lives at the unit and individual level. The model is complex because families are complex. Using our theoretical model (Fig. 15.4), we now present our unified theory. A unified (or grand theory) is the most abstract of the three levels of theory (i.e., grand, middle-range, and micro theory) (Peterson, 2004).

A grand theory is often viewed as a way to organize knowledge using a conceptual framework and serves as the "starting point for middle-range theory development" (Fawcett, 1999, p. 5). We state our unified FQOL theory as:

> Systems, policies, and programs indirectly impact individual and family-level supports, services, and practices; individual demographics, characteristics, and beliefs and family-unit dynamics and characteristics are direct predictors of FQOL and also interact with individual and family-level supports, services, and practices to predict FQOL. Singly or combined, the model predictors result in a FQOL outcome that produces new family strengths, needs, and priorities which re-enter the model as new input resulting in a continuous feedback loop throughout the life course.

If nothing has changed, then FQOL will be relatively stable; if, as indicated earlier, services are dropped, policies are changed, or new practices are implemented, this may result in new levels of FQOL. Our theoretical model represents FQOL as an outcome of a dynamic process consisting of multiple interactive factors – an outcome to be individually experienced and defined by the family and its members. It is the innermost framework of the model (Figs. 15.1, 15.2, and 15.3) that is unique to each family resulting in unique FQOL outcomes. Each individual and family will have different characteristics and beliefs that interact with the provision of services, supports, and practices leading them to make unique decisions about their life and their family's life.

Current FQOL assessment tools have typically measured FQOL at one point in time, not throughout the lifespan. Further, researchers have represented FQOL as a relatively stable trait; however, this is yet to be determined. Because the goal of FQOL researchers is to lead to improvements in FQOL, we can not avoid that which is difficult to measure or complex to articulate. Disability is one aspect of families; a theory of FQOL of families who have a member with a disability must address multiple aspects of families' lives. Our model aims to meet this goal.

Our general theoretical framework enables us to proceed in two steps. First, our unified theory enables us to present a "thoughtful and insightful appraisal of existing ideas or creative intellectual leaps beyond existing knowledge rather than by means of empirical research" (Fawcett, 1999, p. 4). Second, it provides us with a useful unified theoretical model to present and generate middle-range theories with the explicit purpose of validating empirical research. Recognizing that no single study could test the broad scope of the unified theory, we present it as a framework and a procedure to build FQOL theory one study at a time. Next, we present examples of propositional statements that are supported by the current literature on FQOL. We will situate these research findings within the unified theory to illustrate how they contribute to explaining FQOL.

Middle-Range Theories of Family Quality of Life

The unified theory we propose in Fig. 15.4 not only summarizes the many components involved in predicting or explaining variations in FQOL, but it also presents a useable model for researchers to generate multiple testable theoretical statements.

Shoemaker et al. (2004) note that using models is an excellent method to "suggest new theoretical statements," to recognize subsets of variables that "represent chains of causes or effects," and to eliminate nonsensical relationships through the use of "time ordering of variables" (p. 135). Our unified theoretical model clearly illustrates that the systemic concepts are distal inputs, while the family-unit, individual family member factors, and performance factors are the key or direct predictors of FQOL, both singly and interactively, as mediators and moderators.

Much of the available research on FQOL is characterized by simpler propositional statements using a limited number of variables – statements which are logically and statistically capable of being tested. As we noted earlier in the chapter in defining elements of theories, middle-range theories provide testable propositions through the use of a more manageable subset of a larger, unified theory. This unified theory serves as an organizing theoretical framework from which researchers can draw down specific testable middle-range theories based upon their own research interests. Additionally, researchers can work collaboratively from a unified theoretical framework to understand FQOL. In this section, we present middle-range theories identified from our literature review that fit within our unified theoretical model. At this juncture, we also transition our use of terminology from concepts to variables to illustrate the variables arising from individual member concepts, family-unit concepts, and systemic concepts, and how they are used in a predictive model. For example, an individual child characteristic is a concept, but the severity of the child's disability is a variable that might be used to predict FQOL.

Individual Family Member Variables

Eight of the 24 articles used some type of child characteristic or demographic as a predictor variable in the research design. In general, severity of the disability and presence of behavior problems were negatively related to FQOL. Similarly, families of typically developing children tended to have higher FQOL than families of children with disabilities. For example, Brown et al. (2006) found significant differences in overall FQOL scores among families who have children with Down syndrome, families who have children with autism, and families of typically developing children. Wang et al. (2004) also demonstrated that for both mothers and fathers, the severity of the child's disability was a strong negative predictor of FQOL.

Other family member demographics, characteristics, and beliefs were also investigated as predictors of FQOL. For example, Wang et al. (2006) examined

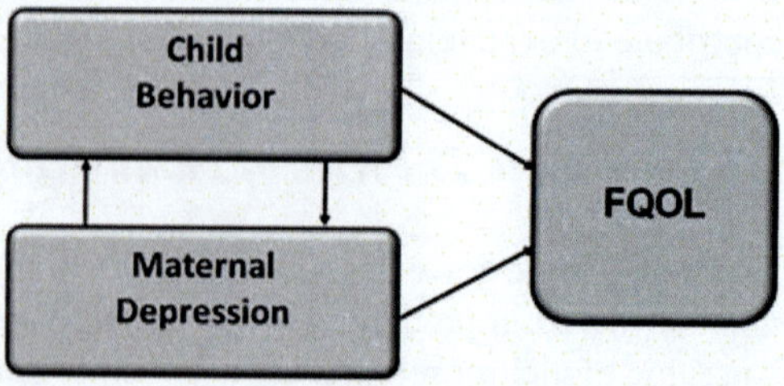

Fig. 15.5 Individual member relationship with FQOL

differences in FQOL conceptualization by parent gender and found no differences. Similarly Zabriskie and McCormick (2003) found no relationship between parent gender and family satisfaction. Individual family member characteristics may also impact FQOL. Mellon and Northouse (2001), in their examination of family member illness, found that family member's fear of recurrence (designated a "belief" in our FQOL theory) contributed to the variance of FQOL. Four studies included a measure of stress, depression, or negative well-being in parents (Bayat, 2005; Dunst, Trivette, Hamby, & Bruder, 2006; Feldman & Werner, 2002; Weigel et al., 1995). In general, higher levels of depression and/or stress had a negative relationship with FQOL. Collectively, these results are consistent with family research utilizing other outcomes variables such as stress or depression (i.e., disability tends to create challenges in families) (Turnbull et al., 2007). Figure 15.5 depicts how these individual family factors may be expected to predict FQOL.

Family-Unit Variables

The propositional relationships identified across the studies examining family-unit characteristics suggested that FQOL was lower in families with low incomes (Hornstein & McWilliam, 2007; Wang et al., 2004), from backgrounds other than European American (Hornstein & McWilliam, 2007), and in stepfamilies (Voydanoff et al., 1994).

Family dynamics identified within our article review included such variables as family sense of coherence (Anderson, 1998), family hardiness (Mellon & Northouse, 2001), satisfaction with division of family labor (Voydanoff et al., 1994), and work–family conflict (Weigel et al., 1995). Higher scores on all of these variables had a significant relationship with higher levels of FQOL, with the exception of work–family conflict, which had an inverse relationship. Figure 15.6 depicts these relationships.

The individual concepts (e.g., demographics, characteristics, and beliefs) and family-unit concepts (e.g., characteristics and family dynamics) are abstract enough to allow for multiple theories to be generated from these broad concepts; yet, they also are narrow enough to identify variables for a testable theory. At a more abstract level, one example of a middle-range theory of FQOL could state that the interaction of individual and family-unit factors together predict FQOL. A finer distinction of a middle-range theory may simply propose that individual factors

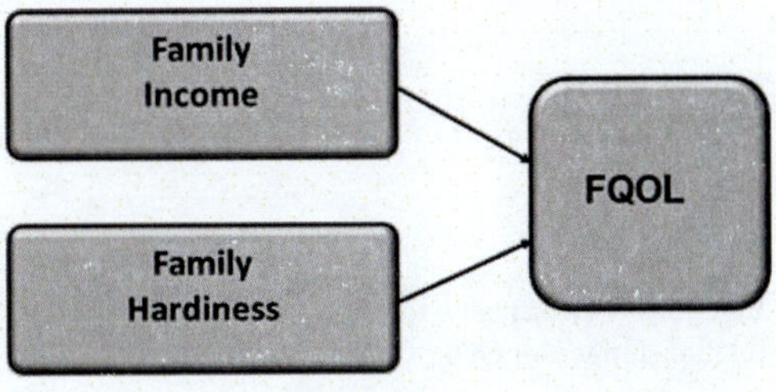

Fig. 15.6 Family-unit relationship with FQOL

predict FQOL, while another middle-range theory might state that family-unit factors predict FQOL. Both Figs. 15.5 and 15.6 provided examples of what might be considered smaller testable components within the larger middle-range theories of individual and family-unit factors predicting FQOL.

Performance Variables

One example was found in the FQOL literature illustrating the relationship between how a service was delivered (i.e., practice) and FQOL. Dunst et al. (2006) reported that parents who used everyday family activities as learning opportunities to enhance their child's development experienced higher FQOL; however, when professionals implemented early intervention within everyday activities, FQOL was reduced. This finding was consistent with the work of Rettig and Bubolz (1983) and Rettig and Leichtentritt (1999) whose work suggests that satisfaction of some types of individual and family needs (e.g., emotional needs) varies depending on *who* addresses the needs.

Much more commonly observed and measured in the FQOL literature and consistent with our review was the impact of services and supports on FQOL within programs. Seven of the 24 articles in our review included a variable related to services or supports from formal and/or informal sources. In all cases there were some positive associations between services and supports and FQOL, but in some cases the results were equivocal. For example, Abbott et al. (2005) investigated the relationship of multi-agency coordinated services and found that families experienced improved sleep but other factors (e.g., daily routines) were not affected. Other relationships were more clear-cut, such as the relationship between type of service and FQOL. For example, Feldman and Werner (2002) found higher FQOL in families receiving behavioral training than those who did not receive training or received a reduced number of hours of training. Similarly, Mellon and Northouse (2001) found higher FQOL in families who had positive family social supports. Both amount of and satisfaction with services was also related to FQOL. Hornstein and McWilliam (2007) found FQOL to be lower with fewer hours of service, while Summers et al. (2007) observed higher scores on parents' ratings of service adequacy for themselves and their child related to higher levels of FQOL. Figure 15.7 illustrates the testable theory of the impact of services and supports on FQOL.

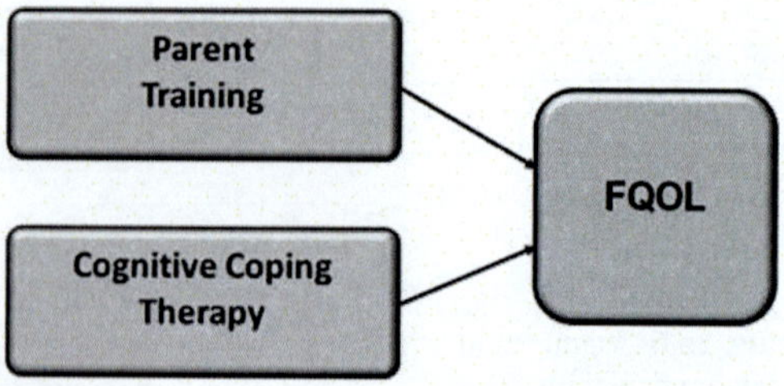

Fig. 15.7 Performance factor relationship with FQOL

Systemic Variables

None of the 24 studies in our literature review attempted to assess quantitatively the impact of these large and distal entities (e.g., systems, policies, and programs), and a comprehensive research effort to do so would be necessarily multifaceted and cumbersome. However, historical trends exist that provide insight into the impact of systems, policies, and programs on FQOL. For example, the passage of IDEA, affording rights to a free and appropriate education to children with disabilities (Turnbull, Stowe, & Huerta, 2007) likely freed many parents who previously had been required to stay at home with their children to enter the job market when their children were allowed to go to school and, thus, did not require daily care during school hours. Parent first-person accounts of raising children without the current array of policies provides compelling testimony to the impact of policies on FQOL (Turnbull & Turnbull, 1978, 1985). Without policies in place, very few programs, services, and supports for families of children with disabilities would exist. It is this reason that we include systems, policies, and programs as the backdrop for our FQOL theory. While the proximal variables are more easily measurable, the distal variables still have a rightful place in a FQOL theory. Currently, the only way to assess the distal variables is through state and national data. In the United States this includes federal agency reporting requirements assessing programs (e.g., early intervention programs) within agencies (Department of Education). Figure 15.8 illustrates the hypothesized relationship of US early intervention policy and FQOL. In Fig. 15.8, Variable 1, parents know their rights, is a federal reporting requirement for all states as well as variable 2, the child's use of appropriate behavior to meet their needs (Hebbeler, Kahn, Barton, & Greenwood, 2007). The mediator model in Fig. 15.8 illustrates the direct effect of parents' knowing their rights (e.g., parents' knowledge about the right to request a functional behavioral assessment for their child) on the child's use of appropriate behavior and the direct effect of the child's behavior on FQOL. This model also illustrates the indirect effect of parents' knowing their rights on FQOL.

Research Limitations

Before considering the implications of these findings for theory-building, we should insert a caveat about the quality of the research we reviewed. There were a number of limitations that warrant caution in the interpretation of these findings across all the

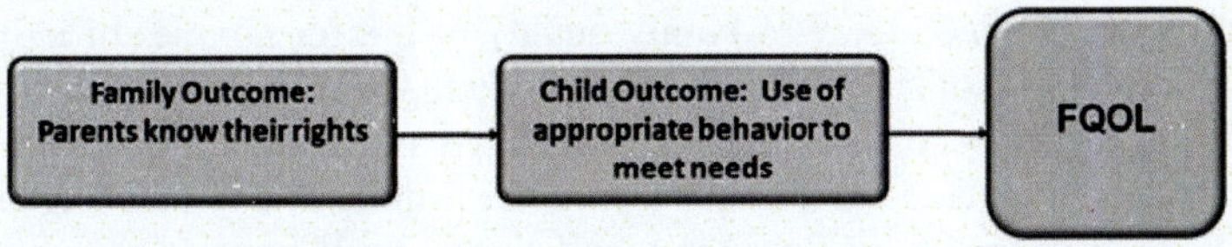

Fig. 15.8 Systemic factor relationship with FQOL

studies. First, limitations from a design point of view include the fact that the majority of studies utilized convenience samples; in fact, many did not include a control or comparison group, and still others were qualitative studies and as such should be considered primarily exploratory. Second, limitations to generalizability are raised due to the lack of diversity of study respondents across the pool of available literature. For example, the majority of these studies purporting to report family data focused on responses from one family member (i.e., the mother). Also, while many of these articles did not report the ethnicity or income level of study participants, those that did so reported a predominance of European American and middle-income families. Finally, the research is limited by the fairly small community of researchers represented by this literature. Much of the FQOL research from which the empirical data were drawn to develop this theory (eight of the 24 studies) comes from two of the most active FQOL research agendas: the International Quality of Life Research Project (Brown et al., 2003; Brown et al., 2006) and the Beach Center on Disability (Bayat, 2005; Hoffman et al., 2006; Summers et al., 2007; Verdugo et al., 2005; Wang et al., 2006; & Wang et al., 2004).

Beyond these research limitations, we should note an important conceptual and operational limitation in our theory-building, and that is the unfinished business of the development of consensus about the nature and measurement of FQOL as an outcome. While we do not advocate that all FQOL researchers in the disability field should embrace one measure of FQOL over another, we do hope for continued dialogue and consensus-building about the purpose of measures and the multiple factors currently used to represent FQOL. We also need to closely examine the distinction between predictors and outcomes used within the domain structure of FQOL measures. For example, if FQOL is an outcome and the purpose of the research is to explore the impact of services and supports (as we present in our theory), then measures of the FQOL outcome cannot include assessments of the quality of services and supports as a domain factor. A further issue is the lack of variability in response when satisfaction is the primary construct for measuring FQOL. The tendency of families to report fairly high levels of satisfaction (see, e.g., Hoffman et al., 2006) means that the data are negatively skewed, creating a number of problems both statistically and conceptually. These and other conceptual and measurement issues should be addressed to enable more meaningful exploration of an FQOL theory.

Conclusion: Recommendations for a Research Agenda

In our proposed unified theory of family quality of life for families of individuals with intellectual and other disabilities, we presented a larger theory than what is currently supported by research data. Thus, many parts of the theory require additional research to validate the theory we propose. Similar to a research agenda, our unified theoretical framework lays the foundation to build upon FQOL theory one proposition at a time. We hope our contribution provides researchers with a road map to guide their research – a place to fit their particular research agenda into the model, whether it is research on an individual family-member factor (i.e., impact of parents' physical or emotional well-being on FQOL), a performance factor (e.g., investigating the impact of a family-centered services on FQOL), or investigating a systemic factor (e.g., the impact of specific policies of FQOL). Particularly at the systemic level, a coherent theory forces us to think about different aspects of families' quality of life prior to implementing policies and also to consider how we would develop questions to investigate the impacts of policy implementation in terms of overall FQOL.

As we review those elements of our proposed theory that have empirical support, we note that the majority of research in the family literature focuses on the impacts of individual and family factors on outcomes such as FQOL. More recent research has begun to investigate the impacts of performance factors (e.g., practices, supports, and services) on family outcomes. Turnbull and colleagues (2007) make this observation as well, and call upon the field to move away from repeatedly investigating what is well-established (e.g., children's behavior problems negatively impact family well-being or FQOL) to investigating relationships that are less well-established and also amenable to change. For example, the work by Dunst et al. (2006, see Table 15.1) suggests that informal supports in everyday family activity settings are more effective in terms of family well-being, than supports or services implemented by early intervention professionals. More research is needed along these lines to determine the nature of specific performance factors (the *who*, *what*, *how*, and *where* of supports and services) that are most predictive of positive FQOL.

However, we cannot be so naive to assume the current FQOL assessment tools are sensitive enough to measure changes by the various predictors we present in our theoretical model. This is why continued work to refine the current FQOL measures is critically necessary. We also need to continue our work in middle-range and micro theory development to validate further our proposed FQOL theory. For example, research on the impact of parent training programs (e.g., performance factor) should investigate the impact of that intervention on family and individual characteristics such as parents' sense of empowerment and competence as a pathway to the FQOL outcome. Different aspects of FQOL may be impacted by different systemic and performance factors. We need to carefully construct follow-up assessments that are sensitive enough to detect these changes. However, this unified theory provides the opportunity for us (and others) to make recommendations for and implement future research in the inchoate field of FQOL.

Finally, as if our proposed FQOL theory were not complex enough, we must risk further complexity by pointing out the need to connect FQOL with outcomes for the individual. In our theory (see Fig. 15.4), we explicitly note that the performance factors (e.g., practices, services, and supports) impact both the family-unit and individual members. We try to show how the quality of life of individuals within the family (including the person with a disability) is intimately intertwined with the FQOL as a whole. But from the point of view of policymakers, this is not enough. Policymakers do not always accept families of people with disabilities as appropriate beneficiaries of programs enabled by their policies (Turnbull et al., 2005).

Advocates for families must, therefore, not only continue to justify the need for family supports on the rationale that all family members are affected by the disability of a family member, but also to justify family supports in terms of their critical link to effective outcomes for the child or adult with a disability. Our unified FQOL theory proposes a mechanism for why that is true (i.e., supports for the family affect the well-being of each of its members, including the person with a disability). Additionally, we need an explicit research agenda to continue strengthening the linkage between family and individual quality of life.

In conclusion, as we have engaged in theorizing about FQOL, we have embraced the idea of building theories as a "thoughtful and insightful appraisal of existing ideas or creative intellectual leaps beyond existing knowledge" (Fawcett, 1999, p. 4). Families and the world in which they live are extremely complex, and we have tried to articulate that complexity. Unified theories, such as the one we propose, are like a large-scale mural or other work of art. One must stand back to see how the parts fit together. But to truly understand it, one must look closely, piece-by-piece, to analyze the contributions of each part to the whole. It is a challenge. But it is one we hope you will agree is critical to the continued improvement of the quality of the lives of individuals with intellectual disabilities and their families.

References

Abbott, D., Watson, D., & Townsley, R. (2005). The proof of the pudding: What difference does multi-agency working make to families with disabled children with complex health care needs? *Child & Family Social Work, 10*(3), 229–238.

Anderson, K. H. (1998). The relationship between family sense of coherence and family quality of life after illness diagnosis: Collective and consensus views. In H. I. McCubbin, E. A. Thompson, A. I. Thompson, & J. E. Fromer (Eds.), *Stress, coping, and health in families: Sense of coherence and resiliency* (pp. 169–187). Thousand Oaks, CA: Sage.

Bayat, M. (2005). How family members' perceptions of influences and causes of autism may predict assessment of their family quality of life. *Dissertation Abstracts International: Section B: The Sciences and Engineering*, *66*(6–B).

Behr, S. K., Murphy, D. L., & Ann, S. J. (1992). *User's manual: Kansas inventory of parental perceptions (KIPP): Measures of perceptions of parents who have children with special needs.* Lawrence, Kansas: Beach Center on Families and Disability, University of Kansas.

Ben-Gashir, M. A., Seed, P. T., & Hay, R. J. (2002). Are quality of family life and disease severity related in childhood atopic dermatitis? *Journal of the European Academy of Dermatology and Venereology, 16*(5), 455–462.

Bengtson, V. L., Acock, A. C., Allen, K. R., Dilworth-Anderson, P., & Klein, D. M. (Eds.). (2005). *Sourcebook of family theory & research.* Thousand Oaks, CA: Sage Publications.

Bloom, B. L. (1985). A factor analysis of self-report measures of family functioning. *Family Process*, *24*(2), 225–239.

Bowman, R. A. (2001). Quality of life assessment for young children with developmental disabilities and their families: Development of a quality of life questionnaire. *Dissertation Abstracts International: Section B: The Sciences and Engineering*, *62*(7–B).

Brown, I., Anand, S., Fung, W. L. A., Isaacs, B., & Baum, N. (2003). Family quality of life: Canadian results from an international study. *Journal of Developmental and Physical Disabilities*, *15*(3), 207–230.

Brown, R. I., MacAdam-Crisp, J., Wang, M., & Iarocci, G. (2006). Family quality of life when there is a child with a developmental disability. *Journal of Policy and Practice in Intellectual Disabilities*, *3*(4), 238–245.

Burr, W. R., Hill, R., Nye, F. I., & Reiss, I. L. (Eds.). (1979). *Contemporary theories about the family*. New York: Free Press.

Cummins, R. A. (2005). Moving from the quality of life concept to a theory. *Journal of Intellectual Disability Research*, *49*(10), 699–706.

Diener, E., Emmons, R. A., Larsen, R. J., & Griffin, S. (1985). The satisfaction with life scale. *Journal of Personality Assessment*, *49*(1), 71–75.

Dunst, C., Trivette, C., Hamby, D., & Bruder, M. (2006). Influences of contrasting natural learning environment experiences on child, parent and family well-being. *Journal of Developmental and Physical Disabilities*, *18*(3), 235–250.

Fawcett, J. (1999). *The relationship of theory and research* (3rd ed.). Philadelphia, PA: F.A. Davis.

Feldman, M. A., & Werner, S. E. (2002). Collateral effects of behavioral parent training on families of children with developmental disabilities and behavior disorders. *Behavioral Interventions*, *17*(2), 75–83.

Gupta, S., & Sharma, A. (1998). Measuring quality of family life. *International Journal of Sociology of the Family*, *28*(1), 115.

Hebbeler, K., Kahn, L., Barton, L., & Greenwood, C. (2007). *National data on child and family outcome: Why? how? what next?* Paper presented at the 2007 Annual Conference of the Division for Early Childhood. Abstract retrieved March 22, 2008 from http://www.fpg.unc.edu/~ECO/pdfs/DEC2007_Data_on_%20Outcomes.pdf

Hoffman, L., Marquis, J., Poston, D., Summers, J. A., & Turnbull, A. (2006). Assessing family outcomes: Psychometric evaluation of the beach center family quality of life scale. *Journal of Marriage and Family*, *68*(4), 1069–1083.

Hornstein, S., & McWilliam, R. A. (2007). *Measuring Family Quality of Life in Families of children with autism spectrum disorders*. Paper presented at the 2007 Annual Conference of the Division for Early Childhood. Abstract retrieved December 15, 2007, from http://www.dec-sped.org/pdf/annualconference/FAM1177%20 Poster%20S27%20Measuring%20Family%20 Quality%20of%20Life.pdf

Isaacs, B. J., Brown, I., Brown, R. I., Baum, N., Myerscough, T., Neikrug, S., et al. (2007). The international family quality of life project: Goals and description of a survey tool. *Journal of Policy and Practice in Intellectual Disabilities*, *4*(3), 177–185.

Lynch, E. W., & Hanson, M. J. (2004). *Developing cross-cultural competence: A guide for working with children and their families* (3rd ed.). Baltimore, MD: Paul H. Brookes.

McGoldrick, M., Giordano, J., & Pearce, J. K.(Eds.). (1996). *Ethnicity and family therapy* (2nd ed.). New York: Guilford.

Mellon, S., & Northouse, L. L. (2001). Family survivorship and quality of life following a cancer diagnosis. *Research in Nursing & Health*, *24*(6), 446–459.

Moos, R. H., & B. S. (1986). *Family environment scale: A social climate scale manual*. Palo Alto, CA: Consulting Psychologists.

Olson, D. H., & Barnes, H. L. (1982). Quality of life. In D. H. Olson, H. I. McCubbin, H. Barnes, A. Larsen, M. Muxen, & M. Wilson (Eds.), *Family Inventories* (pp. 55–67). Minneapolis, MN: Life Innovations, Inc.

Peterson, S. J. (2004). Introduction to the nature of nursing knowledge. In S. J. Peterson & T. S. Bredow (Eds.), *Middle range theories: Application to nursing research*. Philadelphia, PA: Lippincott Williams & Wilkins.

Phillips, D. (2006). *Quality of life: Concept, policy and practice*. Abingdon, UK: Routledge.

Poston, D., Turnbull, A., Park, J., Mannan, H., Marquis, J., & Wang, M. (2003). Family quality of life: A qualitative inquiry. *Mental Retardation*, *41*(5), 313–328.

Rettig, K. D., & Bubolz, M. M. (1983). Perceptual indicators of family well-being. *Social Indicators Research*, *12*(4), 417–438.

Rettig, K. D., & Leichtentritt, R. D. (1999). A general theory for perceptual indicators of family life quality. *Social Indicators Research*, *47*(3), 307–342.

Ricci, G., Bendandi, B., Bellini, F., Patrizi, A., & Masi, M. (2007). Atopic dermatitis: Quality of life of young Italian children and their families and correlation with severity score. *Pediatric Allergy and Immunology, 18*(3), 245–249.

Santelli, B., Turnbull, A., Marquis, J., & Lerner, E. (2000). Statewide parent to parent programs: Partners in early intervention. *Infants and Young Children, 13*(1), 74–88.

Schalock, R. L., Brown, I., Brown, R., Cummins, R. A., Felce, D., Matikka, L., et al. (2002). Conceptualization, measurement, and application of quality of life for persons with intellectual disabilities: Report of an international panel of experts. *Mental Retardation, 40*(6), 457–470.

Shoemaker, P. J., Tankard, J. W., & Lasorsa, D. L. (2004). *How to build social science theories.* Thousand Oaks, CA: Sage Publications.

Summers, J. A., Marquis, J., Mannan, H., Turnbull, A. P., Fleming, K., Poston, D. J., et al. (2007). Relationship of perceived adequacy of services, family-professional partnerships, and family quality of life in early childhood service programmes. *International Journal of Disability, Development and Education, 54*(3), 319–338.

Turnbull, A. P., Brown, I., & Turnbull, H. R. (Eds.). (2004). *Families and persons with mental retardation and quality of life*. Washington, DC: American Association on Mental Retardation.

Turnbull, A. P., & Turnbull, H. R. (1978). *Parents speak out: Views from the other side of the two-way mirror*. Columbus, OH: Merrill.

Turnbull, A. P., & Turnbull, H. R. (1985). *Parents speak out: Then and now*. Columbus, OH: Merrill.

Turnbull, A. P., Turnbull, H. R., Agosta, J., Erwin, E., Fuijiura, G., Singer, G., et al. (2005). Support of families and family life across the life-span. In K. C. Lakin & A. P. Turnbull (Eds.), *National goals and research for people with intellectual disabilities and developmental disabilities* (pp. 217–256). Washington, DC: American Association on Mental Retardation.

Turnbull, A. P., Summers, J. A., Lee, S. H., & Kyzar, K. (2007). Conceptualization and measurement of family outcomes associated with families of individuals with intellectual disabilities. *Mental Retardation and Developmental Disabilities Research Reviews, 13*(4), 346–356.

Turnbull, H. R., Stowe, M., & Huerta, N. (2007). *Free appropriate public education: Law and the education of children with disabilities* (7th ed.). Denver: Love Publishing Co.

Verdugo, M., Schalock, R., Keith, K., & Stancliffe, R. (2005). Quality of life and its measurement: Important principles and guidelines. *Journal of Intellectual Disability Research, 49*(10), 707–717.

Verdugo, M. A., Cordoba, L., & Gomez, J. (2005). Spanish adaptation and validation of the family quality of life survey. *Journal of Intellectual Disability Research, 49*(10), 794–798.

Voydanoff, P., Fine, M. A., & Donnelly, B. W. (1994). Family structure, family organization, and quality of family life. *Journal of Family and Economic Issues, 15*(3), 175–200.

Wang, M., Summers, J. A., Little, T., Turnbull, A., Poston, D., & Mannan, H. (2006). Perspectives of fathers and mothers of children in early intervention programmes in assessing family quality of life. *Journal of Intellectual Disability Research, 50*(12), 977–988.

Wang, M., Turnbull, A. P., Summers, J. A., Little, T. D., Poston, D. J., Mannan, H., et al. (2004). Severity of disability and income as predictors of parents' satisfaction with their family quality of life during early childhood years. *Research and Practice for Persons with Severe Disabilities, 29*, 82–94.

Weigel, D. J., Weigel, R. R., Berger, P. S., Cook, A. S., & DelCampo, R. (1995). Work-family conflict and the quality of family life: Specifying linking mechanisms. *Family & Consumer Sciences Research Journal, 24*(1), 5–28.

White, J. M., & Klein, D. M. (2002). *Family theories* (2nd ed.). Thousand Oaks, CA: Sage Publications.

Zabriskie, R. B., & McCormick, B. P. (2003). Parent and child perspectives of family leisure involvement and satisfaction with family life. *Journal of Leisure Research, 35*(2), 163.

Chapter 16
Family Quality of Life and Older-Aged Families of Adults with an Intellectual Disability

Nancy S. Jokinen and Roy I. Brown

Introduction

Aging, family caregiving and quality of life have increasingly become integrated and important topic areas in public policy and service delivery. Aging demographics are a worldwide issue and have become a pressing challenge in both economically advanced and economically developing countries. Individually, aging is a process influenced by a number of biological and social factors and is expressed somewhat uniquely in each individual (McInnis-Dittrich, 2005). With increasing longevity, and this includes persons with an intellectual disability (Haveman, 2004; Kelly, Kelly, & Craig, 2007), older people commonly face inevitable transitions such as retirement, coping with death, and changes in health and family and personal living arrangements (Denton & Kusch, 2006). On a global level, there is also a call for communities and organisations to be more "age-friendly" to meet the needs of older people (Parke & Brand, 2004; World Health Organization, 2007).

The family context is vital in understanding the needs of older people as it should play a fundamental role in the provision of care for older-aged adults. In many countries, expectations of family caregiving have taken on greater significance due to demographic changes and social and health-care reforms (Bengtson, Lowenstein, Putney, & Gans, 2003). Familial care also reduces demand on publicly funded services (Fast, Keating, Otfinowski, & Derksen, 2004). Families are a fundamental feature of all societies yet various perceptions of family exist (Weigel, 2008) and the definition of family has changed over time. The Beach Center on Disability, for example, has defined family as a group of individuals related biologically and/or through marriage or significant relationship that are considered like family, all of whom nurture one another (Poston et al., 2003). Formal definitions used by government programs and service organisations often delineate who may be considered members of a family for the purposes of clarifying responsibilities and determining eligibility for benefits (Brown & Brown, 2003). For purposes of this chapter

N.S. Jokinen (✉)
School of Social Work, University of Northern British Columbia, Prince George, BC, Canada
e-mail: jokinnen@unbc.ca

R. Kober (ed.), *Enhancing the Quality of Life of People with Intellectual Disabilities*, Social Indicators Research Series 41, DOI 10.1007/978-90-481-9650-0_16,

and changes in our perception of families, it is appropriate to accept each family's own definition. In other words, it is who the family says they are (Brown & Brown).

Families are also significant in the lives of people with an intellectual disability. Previously, research involving families in the field of intellectual disability tended to focus on stress and burden associated with caregiving from a parental (maternal) perspective and the negative impact of disability on the family (Haley & Perkins, 2004; Hatton & Emerson, 2003). The research and literature particular to older-aged families spotlights co-resident parents and adults with an intellectual disability, and the need for futures planning (Bigby & Balandin, 2004; Bigby, 2004). As family members age, however, policies need to be developed that support a range of caregiving roles and respond to changing needs (Hogg, Lucchino, Wang, Janicki, & Group, 2000) for individuals in the developed and much of the developing world are living longer. Families may require support to adequately plan for and navigate transitions and events (Brown, Davey, Shearer, & Kyrkou, 2004) associated with later life that challenge both individual and overall family quality of life.

Enhancing or maintaining quality of life is often referred to in policy and practice statements. However, many empirical studies of individual quality of life and older adults in the general population lack a conceptual framework and use health-related quality of life synonymously with a holistic concept of quality of life. Furthermore, few methodological considerations for an aging populace are made (e.g. specific questions, print size on surveys) (Halvorsrud & Kalfoss, 2007). A qualitative study exploring perceptions of women aged 75+ identified several important dimensions of quality of life including holism, health, relationships, participation and activity (Berglund & Narum, 2007). Quality of life has also been linked with and may be considered an overarching goal of successful aging (Hilton, Kopera-Frye, & Krave, 2009). In the field of intellectual disability, significant contributions have been made to an understanding of individual quality of life (Schalock et al., 2002) although there are few references to the impact aging may have (see as exceptions Brown, 2000; McCallion & McCarron, 2007). More recently, the work on individual quality of life has expanded to explore the notion of family quality of life (Brown & Brown, 2004b) in response to a growing interest in the positive aspects of family life (Blacher & Baker, 2007), and family quality of life as a research and applied area is taking shape. Predominately, this work has focused on families of children and young adults (see as example Turnbull, Brown, & Turnbull, 2004).

Family quality of life, as an approach, offers opportunities for a more holistic picture of family life to emerge; to gain an understanding of both the benefits and the challenges of family life where there is a member of the family with an intellectual disability. It enables us to pinpoint where some of the major concerns arise and, as will be seen, these may vary remarkably. The questions are how and why this variability occurs. As a field of study, four fundamental premises guide family quality of life: (1) the research is directed to an holistic view of quality of life primarily through the perceptions of family members about family and individual functioning, (2) it is lifespan in orientation, (3) the purpose of family quality of life research is concerned with improving the lives of families and (4) the "voice" of family members is a vital component of research (Brown & Brown, 2004a).

Focus of This Chapter

This chapter explores family quality of life in the context of older-aged families of adults with an intellectual disability. It begins with three vignettes that illustrate the diverse circumstances of older-aged families. The names used in the vignettes have been changed. Next, background on family quality of life is provided including associated principles and concepts as well as highlights of three main initiatives. Family quality of life in relation to older-aged family members is then explored drawing predominately upon two studies (Jokinen & Brown, 2005; Jokinen, 2008). The chapter concludes with a discussion of the implications and benefits of a family quality of life approach to research, policy and practice in relation to later life families.

Vignettes

Parent

Mary, a widow in her late 70's has a daughter, Susan, in her early 50's. Twenty years ago, Mary arranged for Susan to move into a residential service despite opposition voiced by her other offspring. She did not want Susan to simultaneously face parental death and a move out of the family home. Members of the family have always maintained frequent contact with Susan and she is included in various family activities. A couple of years ago, Susan required surgery and experienced a lengthy recovery. Since then, Mary notices Susan "slowing down" and wonders if, for her age, Susan is involved in too many activities. She is always on the go, yet residential staff says she is otherwise bored.

Adult Sibling

Joan, aged 69, has a brother, Eric who is 68 years old. Both parents are deceased and an older sister lives out of town. Eric was institutionalised as a youth and familial contact was lost for a while. As an adult, he returned to his community and eventually married and worked part time. Contact between siblings was maintained on special occasions as Joan worked, raised children and cared for elderly relatives. Five years ago, Eric separated from his wife and Joan, now retired, began to help him more. Although he continues to live on his own with nominal help from intellectual disability services for money management, Eric has developed multiple and complex medical conditions. Joan finds it increasingly difficult to provide the daily help he needs and worries about her own health. She questions where else he might live that would better meet his needs without being an overly restrictive environment.

Adult with an Intellectual Disability

Paul is in his late 40's. He requires personal care assistance and uses a wheelchair to travel independently to and from a day program during the week. Paul's parents are separated and he lives with his mother in the family home. She recently had a stroke and they are managing at home on an interim basis with daily support from Paul's father and a home care service. Paul also has close sibling relationships although they work and have their own families; his siblings include him in various social activities and a sister helps Paul manage his money. Paul knows his mother will move into a nursing home as soon as a bed is available. He wants to stay in the family home, perhaps with a roommate, because he is familiar with the neighbourhood and people thereabouts. His family intends to help him maintain his living arrangement.

Quality of Life

Family quality of life is perhaps understood best from an historical perspective beginning with the concept of individual quality of life as developed in the field of intellectual disabilities. This conceptualisation of quality of life as expounded by Schalock et al. (2002) is based on an array of research from a variety of countries. One of the earliest studies is that of Brown, Bayer, & Macfarlane (1989). Furthermore, Brown, Bayer, and Brown (1992) looked at the development and behaviour of persons with intellectual disabilities over a 6-year period, which included assessments by parents on quality of life issues of their child with a disability. Gradually, this and other work (e.g. Taylor, Hogg, Felce and other colleagues) were integrated in a number of edited volumes (see Brown, 1997; Goode, 1994; Renwick, Brown, & Nagler, 1996). These provide a detailed background concerning research and practice as well as definition and conceptualisation in quality of life.

Key Concepts and Principles

Although there have been many definitions of quality of life put forward, most seem to contain similar ideas (Brown & Brown, 2003). These include social well-being, objective and subjective (perceptual) aspects of life, multidimensional aspects of life including friendship and family, the meeting of basic needs and ability to achieve personal goals, and a person's desired conditions of living (pp. 102–103). Some of the key concepts and principles include values, lifespan, holism, self-image, choice, personal control, empowerment, rights, anti-discrimination and domains. Domains are considered areas of living such as physical well-being, material well-being, social well-being, emotional well-being and productive well-being. These functioning areas of the individual lifestyle can be broken into different areas and sometimes differently labelled, but most authors appear agreed on these constructs and principles.

Brown and Brown (2003) believed that the conceptualisation should then be applied to practice and provided a text to illustrate, through research, application and professional practice, how this was not only possible but is now being applied in a number of services. The authors recognised that practice and policy need to go hand in hand, as without such links quality of life practice would likely fail due to conflicting standards and links between policy design, management direction and applications at the frontline. The authors went on to illustrate how, in practice, quality of life concepts could be applied to families. Indeed, to many of those working in the field, it appeared that a logical development of quality of life principles and concepts could be usefully applied to the field of families who have a relative with an intellectual disability. This last aspect was further developed in collaborative work between a variety of research and applied professionals (Turnbull, Brown et al., 2004).

Family Quality of Life

A number of different aspects needed to be considered in generalising this to family quality of life. Some of these ideas relate to the notion of family. What is family? As indicated earlier, any definition has to take into account variations within and between families, and has also to be culturally sensitive. Furthermore, in view of the quality of life construct of personal perception, any definition has to be suitable for each individual family, or at least the individual who is consulted and involved during either research or practice. The simplest and probably the most broadly acceptable definition is to accept the respondents' definition, i.e. family is whom the individual recognises under the rubric of family. This requires that an individual(s) identifies who, in their opinion, are members of their family. The description of family then varies including, for example, single-parent families (generally mother or father and their offspring), "blended" families (when single parents marry and merge families), and families headed by other relatives or significant others. The family may include step-children, foster or adopted children, and in some instances may encompass grandparents, nieces, nephews and other relatives, and possibly friends. An individual's concept of family is also likely to change over time and circumstance. To date, however, most family quality of life studies have unfortunately only interviewed mothers and, infrequently, fathers and this lack of paternal input has to be kept in mind. Also important are the views of siblings and other members in the family nucleus including, where possible the person with the disability, particularly as siblings in older-aged families often play an increasing and critical role. Such comprehensive accounting is not easily possible but the present chapter attempts to illustrate some of the different family perceptions and behaviours which occur and how they might be accommodated.

The notion of family quality of life has been taken on board by a number of researchers and some sharing and collaboration has ensued (see, for example, special issue of the Journal of Policy and Practice in Intellectual Disabilities (2006)) and includes work by members of the Special Interest Group on Quality of Life affiliated with the International Association for the Scientific Study of Intellectual Disabilities (IASSID). The challenge lies in attempting to integrate dimensions of family quality of life through its various domains and consider the major influences on the family. To date, as Turnbull et al. (2004) have indicated, attention in the family is frequently focused on the child with a disability thus slanting the family to a different way of life. This focus is often primarily dominated by the parents, particularly the mother, and impacts other children in the family. It may be expected that this is registered through the interactions between different domains and can be influenced by cultural concerns, neighbours and community as well as a host of other factors. Because of this, an attempt has been made to develop assessment procedures to at least evaluate the major impacts involved and the quality of life experienced by the family.

One of the characteristics of quality of life, however, is its attention to a lifespan approach to disability. As family members age, they all experience changes and are furthermore at risk of late onset disability that may frequently influence familial support and arrangements. There is some evidence to suggest the focus of older-aged families' attention, and therefore their efforts, change. For example, the needs of aging parents may become of equal concern or, indeed, supersede the needs of the relative with a disability and the family's main efforts are thus redirected (Jokinen, 2008).

Proactive thinking about issues at a family level over time is critical and has service implications. Indeed one of the present challenges is that though increase in longevity has been long forecast (Janicki and Ansello, 2000), its impact on individuals, families and service systems designed for the families and individuals with disabilities has been essentially overlooked on a practical level. For example, some families receive no appropriate services, older individuals with an intellectual disability may be placed in inappropriate facilities, and social and community resources to meet needs are in short supply. Aging both in terms of the numbers involved and diverse needs, including support needs, are critical issues. Policy and practice with younger-aged families tend to emphasise family integrity and family-centred services that aim to bolster family unity, respond to family needs and acknowledge the importance of family caregiving (Turnbull, Beegle, & Stowe, 2001). In contrast, these same notions are not necessarily applied when the person with a disability is middle-aged or older (Brown, Galambos, Poston, & Turnbull, 2007). Futures planning models, for example, tend to focus on the needs of the individual with a disability and not the family as a whole (see as examples Baxley, Janicki, McCallion, & Zendell, 2005; Heller & Caldwell, 2006).

Family Quality of Life Initiatives

To date three reasonably comprehensive family quality of life investigations have evolved and developed measurement tools. These are a Latin American initiative (Aznar & Castanon, 2005), efforts through the Beach Center on Disability at the University of Kansas (Turnbull, 2007) and the International Family Quality of Life Project (Isaacs et al., 2007). Though there are a number of other related measures, these tend to measure specific aspects of quality of life (e.g. satisfaction questionnaire) rather than the perceived domains of family quality of life and look in various

Table 16.1 Family quality of life initiatives

Initiative		Domains
Latin American[a]	Family-centred quality of life domains (Latin America)	Personal strength and development, rules of cohabitation, physical/material well-being, family life, interpersonal and community relations
Beach center[b]	Family quality of life scale	Family interaction, parenting, emotional well-being, physical/material well-being, disability-related support
International[c]	Family quality of life survey	Health, financial well-being, family relationships, support from other people, support from disability-related services, influence of values, careers and preparing for careers, leisure and recreation, community interaction

[a] Aznar and Castanon (2005).
[b] Beach Center on Disability (2008).
[c] Brown, Brown, Baum, et al. (2006).

depths to important but often isolated aspects of the family (e.g. support from services). Some, indeed, have restricted their measurement to special age groups (see as example summary by Mannan, Summers, Turnbull, & Poston, 2006) often making their data less useful for the ageing community. The three scales, which attempt to measure family quality of life more expansively attempt to assess overall domains. Table 16.1 identifies the domains used in each of these projects.

In the Latin American initiative (Aznar & Castanon, 2005), a research team worked with families from various locations in South America and identified six domains of family life with 42 corresponding indicators. The overall goal of this project was to develop a tool that was easily understood by family members, would empower families and be used as an intervention or program development guide. The tool may or may not have involved older-aged family members, however, it is apparently used with families of children and adults with an intellectual disability. From this work, the authors also proposed a topographic model of quality of life. Here quality of life is viewed as three interactive components; the "material (objective), personal (subjective) and social (contextual)" (p. 786). High values in all three components create a family landscape characterised by smooth gradual transitions. Thresholds, however, are thought to exist below which family quality of life is diminished. Shortcomings in any one component may be compensated by the other two, while concurrent low values in any two of the components likely impedes quality of life. The research team continues their work on this initiative with an overall goal to promote a better understanding of the cross-cultural nature of family quality of life.

The Beach Center's initiative is a family-centred model featuring a strengths perspective, family choice and support provided to the family as a unit (Hoffman, Marquis, Poston, Summers, & Turnbull, 2006; Summers et al., 2005; Turnbull et al., 2004). The impact of public policy and service provision is a major focus and the work involved focus group discussions with family members and service providers, policy analysis (Poston et al., 2003) and development of a quality of life scale (Park et al., 2003). This scale measures importance and satisfaction across five domains. An overall goal of the initiative is the development of the scale for use as a planning tool, assessment of family strengths and service evaluation. Few older-aged family members were, however, involved during the development of the scale (see for example Poston et al.) and it is apparently intended for use with families of children (Turnbull, 2007). The Beach Centre work has further proposed a family quality of life theory; defining key concepts (i.e. systemic, performance, individual member and family-unit) and use a composite family example to illustrate the application of theory to practice (Zuna, Turnbull, & Summers, 2009). Further details on this theoretical development can be found in Chapter 15.

The third initiative, an international project, *The Family Quality of Life Survey* was developed and recently revised (Brown, Brown, Baum, et al., 2006). Its development and characteristics are described in Isaacs et al. (2007). The survey has been developed through collaborative efforts of a team of researchers, practitioners and parents from various countries with a purpose to gain an in-depth understanding of quality of life from the perspective of families. It is being used in 18 countries and translated in several languages. This effort is the subject of considerable content in this chapter. Critical components of family quality of life encompass the three environmental levels (personal, community and societal) interacting with and on the family (e.g. family composition, critical appraisal of what is compared to what could be, social capital resources, legislation and legal structures). It consists of nine domains (see Table 16.1) and, within each domain, six dimensions are examined. Two dimensions, Attainment and Satisfaction, reflect outcome. The four remaining dimensions are: Importance, Opportunities, Initiative and Stability. It should be noted that each item is directed to the family as a whole, not just the person with a disability. Further, the tool can be used with any type of family and considered lifespan sensitive so it can be used with families of various ages. In this instance, it is critical as this chapter deals with families in the upper age brackets.

Aging and Quality of Life

In the field of intellectual disability, quality of life experienced by aging adults with a disability has received some attention (see as examples Brown, 2000; Janicki, 1997; McCallion & McCarron, 2007; Seltzer & Krauss, 2001) albeit there is continuing need to further explore this line of inquiry. Most family quality of life studies have focused on families of children and young adults (see as examples Brown, Anand, Fung, Isaacs, & Baum, 2003; Brown, MacAdam-Crisp, Wang, & Iarocci, 2006; Poston et al., 2003). Although various studies have included some older-aged participants, most studies do not distinguish younger from older-aged participants. One exception to this, an Australian study (see Brown et al., 2004), is detailed in Chapter 12.

Two Canadian studies have focused on older-aged families to better understand family beliefs, values, concerns and issues and factors that maintain or challenge family quality of life. One explored perceptions of family quality of life held by 15 parents (Jokinen & Brown, 2005) who represented 13 families. They ranged in age from 62 to 87 years with a mean age of 73.9 years. Their sons and daughters with a disability ranged in age from 41 to 52 years, mean age 47.1 years. The second study (Jokinen, 2008) involved 20 parents, 12 adult siblings and 12 adults with an intellectual disability. The parents ranged from 60 to 91 years with a mean age of 76.7 years. Siblings were aged 43 to 69 years; mean 54.4 years. Parents and siblings' relatives with an intellectual disability were 40–69 years in age. The adults with an intellectual disability who participated in this research were aged 40–60 years, mean age of 49.6 years. Parents and siblings that were involved also completed a *Family Quality of Life Survey* (revised Brown, Brown, Baum, et al., 2006). As far as we know, these are the first studies to take a family quality of life approach and use the survey exclusively with older-aged family members. This chapter now draws heavily on these original data, particularly the interview and focus group material, to illustrate quality of life in relation to older-aged families.

Family Quality of Life Survey

The *Family Quality of Life Survey* (Brown, Brown, Baum, et al., 2006) is one of three instruments being used with families of various ages in several English and non-English-speaking countries. The survey had a structured format and specific questions on six dimensions (i.e. Importance, Opportunity, Initiative, Attainment, Stability and Satisfaction) across nine domains. A rating scale is used for the questions in each domain. There is room on the questionnaire for qualitative commentary by respondents (Isaacs et al., 2007). The two Canadian studies with a focus on the perceptions of older-aged family members used this survey as a means to further explore perceptions of family quality of life. For the studies in question, the size and style of the font used in the survey was changed to accommodate potential age-related vision changes of respondents and some additional questions asked relevant to an aging population (e.g. are any family members living with a chronic medical condition?).

The following highlights survey findings in relation to older-aged parents and siblings' perceptions of importance and satisfaction across domains found in Jokinen (2008). The participants in this study that completed the survey included 17 parents (12 mothers and 5 fathers) representing 14 families. They ranged in age from 60 to 87 years; mean age 74.76. The parents' sons and daughters with a disability ranged in age from 40 to 55 years; mean age 47. Ten siblings (seven females and three males), representing eight families, also completed the survey and ranged in age from 46 to 69 years; mean 55.5.

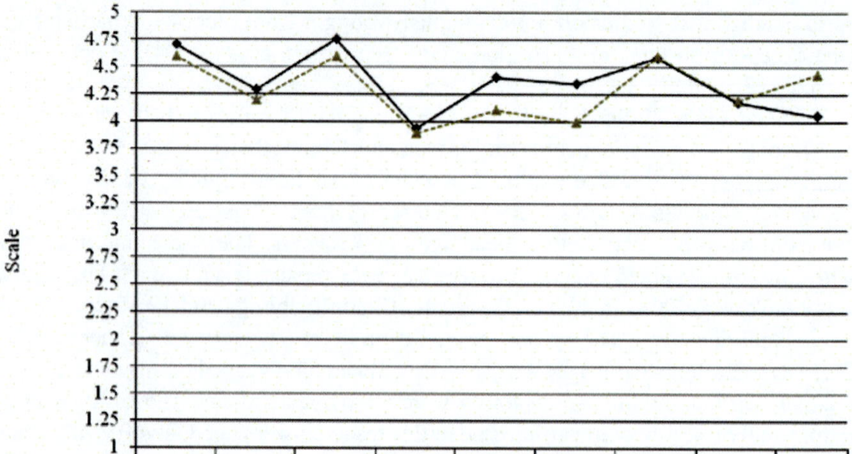

	Health	Financial	Family	Support Others	Services	Values	Work	Leisure	Comm Interact
Parent	4.71	4.29	4.76	3.94	4.41	4.35	4.59	4.18	4.06
Siblings	4.6	4.2	4.6	3.9	4.11	4	4.6	4.2	4.44

Fig. 16.1 Parent ($n = 17$) and sibling ($n = 10$) mean scores for importance across domains

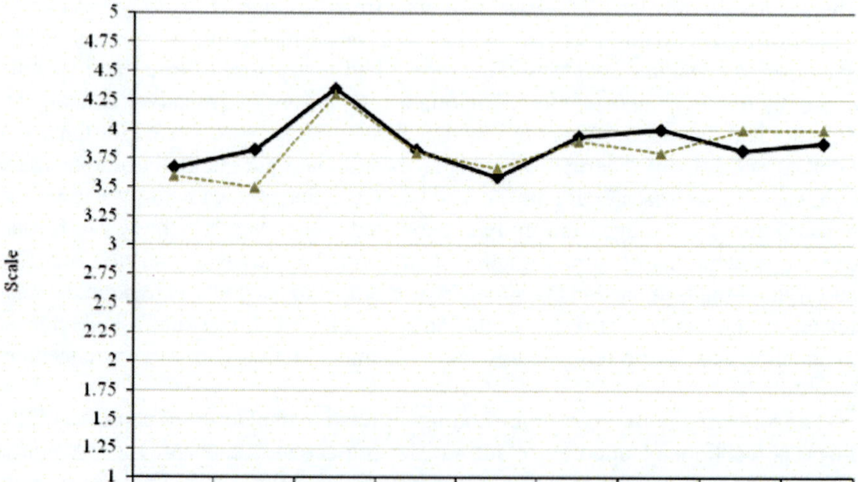

	Health	Financial	Family	Support Others	Services	Values	Work	Leisure	Comm Interact
Parent	3.67	3.82	4.35	3.82	3.59	3.94	4	3.82	3.88
Siblings	3.6	3.5	4.3	3.8	3.67	3.9	3.8	4	4

Fig. 16.2 Parent ($n = 17$) and sibling ($n = 10$) mean scores for satisfaction across domains

Figures 16.1 and 16.2 display the parent and sibling mean scores for Importance and Satisfaction, respectively, for each domain. Importance gives an indication of the respondent's assigned value or relevance of a domain. Satisfaction, a commonly used term in quality of life studies, refers to the respondent's perceived level of contentment associated with the domain.

As can be seen, the mean scores for Importance exceed those attributed to Satisfaction across all domains and similar type findings are beginning to appear in other studies (Brown, Brown, & Wang, 2006). A consistent discrepancy between these two dimensions could potentially support the development of policy and practice strategies that lead to enhanced family quality of life. For example, low importance would perhaps suggest one should not be too concerned with a lower satisfaction level than when there is dissatisfaction but a high level of importance.

As indicated in Fig. 16.1, parents rated the *Family Relationships* domain with the highest mean score for Importance (4.76, *SD* 0.44). The domains of *Health* (4.71, *SD* 0.47) and *Work* (4.59, *SD* 0.80) were rated second and third for Importance, respectively. Sibling's attributed the highest mean score (4.6, *SD* 0.70) to each of these three domains, suggesting both older-aged parents and siblings similarly value these particular domains. These results also confirmed interview and focus group findings discussed later in this chapter; family relations, health and work were important topics of the discussions. *Support from others*, as a domain, was rated the lowest mean score for Importance by both parents (3.94, *SD* 0.97) and siblings (3.90, *SD* 0.99), a finding consistent with other research including the study by Brown, MacAdam-Crisp, et al. (2006).

In Fig. 16.2, it can be seen that parents and siblings rated the highest mean scores for Satisfaction to the *Family Relationships* domain; 4.35 (*SD* 0.61) and 4.30 (*SD* 0.67), respectively, again consistent with interview and focus group findings of this research and other studies across ages. There was, however, some difference between parents and siblings' lowest mean scores for Satisfaction. Parents rated the *Support from Services* Domain with the lowest mean score (3.59, *SD* 0.94) and *Health* (3.67, *SD* 0.75) the second lowest. For siblings, the lowest mean for Satisfaction was in the *Financial* Domain (3.50, *SD* 0.85) and the second and third lowest means attributed to the *Health* (3.60, *SD* 0.97) and *Support from Services* (3.67, *SD* 0.87). Most of the data to date in a variety of studies has shown *Support from Services* the lowest or amongst the lowest of domain scores. The question then arises what is it that many parents need as supports from services for their families. Yet the mean scores appear to be numerically higher than in studies involving younger-aged parents (Brown, Brown, & Wang, 2006). There may be several reasons for this apparent difference. For example, older-aged family members may have had longer involvement with services, differing expectations and/or differences in service use as compared to younger-aged families. Stage in life may also be an influencing factor.

Overall, the pattern of the mean scores for Importance and Satisfaction reported here appears to be similar to results from other studies (e.g. high mean score for importance and satisfaction with *Family Relations*, low mean satisfaction score for *Support from Others*) (Brown et al., 2003; Brown, Brown, & Wang, 2006; Brown,

MacAdam-Crisp, et al., 2006). However, once again, the mean scores appear to be higher amongst older families than younger ones. There is some evidence that older families in the general population provide higher life satisfaction scores than younger families. Other possibilities arise. Older-aged parents and siblings completed the survey following their involvement in an interview or focus group and this may have sensitised them to notions of family quality of life and influenced their perceptions. The present sample is a small sample and caution and further research is needed. Nonetheless, these findings raise some interesting questions including the question as to whether or not some older-aged families perceive satisfaction in a different light. And, if so, what contributes to and insulates these more positive-oriented perceptions?

Maintaining Family Quality of Life

Family Relations

Family relations vary and change over the life course. These relationships may be an important source of support and provide a sense of belonging and inclusion in the most fundamental social unit, the family. Positive perceptions, familial support and routines are discussed as specific aspects of family relations that seem to have a positive influence on quality of life.

Older-aged family members often voice positive comments about the abilities and accomplishments of various individuals in their family, including the relative with a disability. Positive perceptions have also been noted in other research (see as examples Blacher & Baker, 2007; Carr, 2005) and are likely an important indicator of family quality of life. Family stories that bring to light a family's shared history are frequently conveyed with humour and/or a sense of pride or achievement. For example, one sibling and parent laughed together as they recalled male offspring in the family bringing new girlfriends home for dinner. At some point during dinner, inevitably the relative with disability would call the new girlfriend by an old girlfriend's name. While the family apparently anticipated this, it did present some awkward moments. In retrospect, these family members viewed the situation light-heartedly and without malice. Indeed, the relative with a disability was often perceived by older-aged family members as always being a part of the family. For many, there may be an underlying acceptance and accommodation of the disability within the family.

> " . . . she was just your sister, there wasn't a big deal made out of that she was different." Sibling

> "My family don't say much [about my disability], just say I need help. Yea it's ok with them. They, my family, understands." Adult with an intellectual disability

Familial support and routine is an integral part of family relations, although this unquestionably varies from family to family. Practical, emotional, and/or financial supports are provided by and to various family members. For instance, adult siblings provide emotional and practical support to aging parents. Many siblings will also likely carry on with familial support responsibilities for their brother or sister with a disability when parents are no longer able, as has been noted in other research (Bigby, 1997; Dew, Llewellyn, & Balandin, 2004). Reciprocal support between parents and offspring with a disability may also occur regardless of living arrangement, as has been found in research involving co-resident families (Heller, Miller, & Factor, 1997). Furthermore, some parents anticipate their offspring with a disability may be a source of support, as they themselves age and need help with daily living.

Examples of familial support that involve the relative with an intellectual disability include: (1) when a father had hip surgery, his son with Down syndrome helped him dress in the morning; (2) an adult with a disability who lived alone had an open invitation to stay overnight at her sister's home if she felt lonely; and (3) parents who lived separately from their son or daughter with a disability for many years provide financial support for special events, clothing and/or furniture. It is important to recognise that some older-aged family members may provide significant support to their relative with a disability, especially if there is minimal disability service involvement. For instance, a 79-year-old father regularly changed bedding for his son who lived alone.

> "... I didn't used to do that but I decided because I found half the time he wasn't he was sleeping on a mattress without any sheet on it or cover and I said enough of this ... I don't think they know the extent of the support that I give." Parent

In another family, a father in his mid 80's talked daily with his son who lived alone via telephone or face to face; the mother had difficulty understanding her son's speech. These parents also had their son for dinner frequently and he "shopped" free for groceries in their storage room. It was stocked with food the parents had purchased on sale. Familial support may also be extended to friends or roommates of the relative with a disability. Older-aged parents may also provide transportation to an activity for their son with a disability and include others with a disability living in the same neighbourhood. In yet another family, a sibling in her late 60's felt compelled to take on support responsibilities for her sister's roommate who also had an intellectual disability. The roommate's mother was unable to be actively involved. Unfortunately, this type of familial support may go unrecognised by services, although it can become a critical issue for both the adult with a disability and family members particularly when the level of support required can no longer be maintained.

Another important aspect of familial relations is routine. Regardless of living circumstance, routine seems to provide predictability and structure to familial contact and support. Many families have easily identifiable and specific routines that occur on a daily, weekly and seasonal basis. For instance, in the case of a co-resident parent and adult child, the parent shopped for groceries while her son attended a swim program. At home, they each had their own specific household chores and, together, dined at a friend's home on Saturday evenings. Another parent, living in an assisted living facility and separate from her offspring with a disability, arranged for a taxi every Sunday. The cab picked her son up first then the parent. The pair attended church and afterwards had lunch together. Her son then returned to his home via public transit. Other families have regular daily or weekly phone or face-to-face contact. Many parents and siblings also routinely have their relative with a disability visit on birthdays or during holidays.

> "He [son with disability] and John [roommate with disability] come up the day before Christmas ... When they're ready they call and I get them bring them up and they stay Christmas eve and Christmas night and go home Boxing day night." Parent

Knox and Bigby (2007) also found routine significant to older-aged families of adults with a disability. Family routines and rituals are, indeed, an important aspect of family life (Fiese et al., 2002) and maintaining some routines may better support families through various transitions (Zisberg, Young, Schepp, & Zysberg, 2007).

Activities Outside the Family

Engagement in activities outside the family also seems to have a positive impact on both individual and overall family quality of life. Opportunities to be involved in various outside activities appear to allow other family members to pursue individual interests (e.g. work, leisure). There are additional benefits to these activities including stimulating conversation between family members about associated events of the day and facilitating social support networks. While often portrayed as socially isolated and frail, many older-aged adults may be actively engaged in their communities. For instance, a parent in her late 80's indicated

> "I've had a lot of books published. ... Poetry mostly, but I have 4, 5 novels for children. ... We have all these wonderful, we have a poetry group that meets once a month." Parent

In the family quality of life studies that are the focus of this chapter, most of the older-aged parents and siblings were volunteers with local organisations or faith groups, actively involved in special interest groups (e.g. writer's guild), and/or gainfully employed. Siblings with children of their own were often active supporting their children's activities (e.g. in school or sports). Adults aging with an intellectual disability may also be active outside the family. Some attend day service programs, work part time and/or are involved in leisure activities (e.g. Special Olympics).

> "He [son with disability] goes swimming Monday night. Tuesday night he goes on a pop can run [for recycling] unless the weather is really bad ... Wednesday night is floor hockey ... Thursday night he has basketball ... Saturday afternoon he bowls ..." Parent

Work seems to be a particularly valued activity outside the home and perceived by family members to have both financial and social rewards. There is, however, a rather dismal record of employment for many middle-aged and older adults with an intellectual disability (see Hogg et al., 2000; Jokinen, 2003; Prosser & Moss, 1996). They may be the first to lose employment or have reduced hours when industry cutbacks occur or when technology is introduced at the worksite.

> "They [worksite] got a machine that does filing so she [daughter with a disability] was down to 3 days a week and then they got the Interact and so she's 2 days a week but anyway she still likes to go [to work]." Parent

In the absence of work, structured activities (e.g. volunteer, leisure) are important and provide occasions to connect with people as well as maintain friendships. Parents and siblings, however, often voice concerns about the limited opportunities for their relative with a disability to be active outside the family. Conversely, others may wonder about how their relative is involved in many activities, perhaps more than would be expected given age and stamina. Furthermore, although family members will indicate their relative may know a lot of people, they may also suggest their relative has few friends and a limited social life outside the family. This is particularly so if they are not involved in residential services. When adults with a disability live separate from family, certainly family members visit. Service staff may also be present. Yet few, if any, friends seem to visit. There seems to be a general reliance on structured activities (e.g. day services, Special Olympics) to maintain friendships as has been noted by others (Mahon & Mactavish, 2000).

Family Quality of Life Challenges

It is important not to romanticise family relations; some relationships are fraught with conflict and strife. Even when relations are positive, older-aged families have faced various family and individual challenges and conflicts over the years.

> "Yea, there are hard times but we always got through them all right." Parent

Some of these challenges are similar to those likely faced by many families, as has been noted in other commentary (Brown & Brown, 2003). Families, with and without a relative with an intellectual disability, may manage some of these challenges within the family while seeking help to resolve others. For example, like other families, a few families of adults with a disability have also experienced and struggled with alcohol abuse and domestic violence in the past. Mothers involved in such circumstances reported professional counselling and self-help groups alleviated their stress and anxieties. Older-aged families also increasingly endure the death of family members and friends. In death's wake, there is grief, loss and adjustments that often impact familial support and living arrangements.

Disability-Related Family Challenges

Disability does appear to add another layer of complexity to challenges, events or transitions that the family must manage. Sometimes there is strife in the family in how the disability is perceived or managed. Some adult siblings, for instance, may disagree with the parental stance towards their sister or brother with a disability (e.g. overprotection, provision of choice) or be overly critical of and want little involvement with their sibling with a disability. As older people go about their daily lives, they are also challenged by persistent negative public attitude towards disability.

> " . . . things like that don't even change. I mean even when they (adults with a disability) grow older, there are people who will say things. . . ." Parent

Estate planning, behavioural challenges associated with the disability and procurement of services to meet family needs are other common examples of challenges faced by older-aged families.

Some of these challenges represent significant, ongoing issues that have had impact across multiple domains of life. For example, parents and siblings of an adult with an intellectual disability face additional issues when their relative violates the law (e.g. judicial response and rehabilitative programs). For one family, repeated offences by the relative led to multiple jail terms. A therapeutic program, during one of these terms, suggested smoking as a means for their relative to relax. On subsequent release from jail, smoking has caused financial and other problems (e.g. selling off belongings to purchase cigarettes, health concerns). This compounded issues associated with what had led to conflict with the law in the first place. Although some help was attained from a smoking cessation program, years later, the family still struggles to provide support to prevent re-offending (i.e. daily check-ins by phone) and quell smoking behaviour.

Often times, family members will contact disability services for information and/or support when confronted with perplexing challenges or difficult transitions. Frequently, they may be frustrated about whom to contact and how to access supportive services. They are often unfamiliar with programs or the processes to access programs. Furthermore, they may be unaware of existing wait lists or suffer the effects of long waiting periods for support and respite.

In frontline work, it will be important to separate out the conflicts and challenges within families which can be normally expected from those that may exacerbate or be associated with an offspring or sibling's disability. This approach has been to a large degree ignored in studies of older-aged families and is only now beginning to be taken into account in younger families. Clear differences are being found across domains with families where there are no children with disabilities (see Brown, MacAdam-Crisp, et al., 2006) and it will be necessary to examine this with older families. Otherwise the domain and dimension effects between different types of families and ageing will be confused. It is also necessary in older-aged families to examine the differential effects of various types of disability particularly where these are multiple; although such research has commenced. See, for example, difference between families with a young child with Autism and families where there is a young child with Down syndrome (Brown, MacAdam-Crisp, et al., 2006).

Health

Older-aged family members recognise the importance of health and that changes in health can have impact across life domains. With advancing age, all adults may face challenges to maintaining their health. The impact aging has on individuals with a lifelong disability is just now beginning to be better understood yet little is known about age-related changes that may occur in some specific syndromes associated with intellectual disabilities (Janicki, Henderson, & Rubin, 2008). Ill health of any family member, however, appears to focus the family's attention on that relative and influence familial contact and support arrangements as well as their need for service. For example, in one older-aged family, a sibling had assumed familial responsibilities for her brother with a disability from her father who was in his late 70's. However, she was later diagnosed with cancer and had to undergo a treatment regime. The father resumed responsibilities for his son and the family, as a whole, focused efforts on supporting the sibling through her ordeal. This became their priority.

Many families may also rely on service staff to monitor the health of their relative with a disability and provide follow-up treatment support, particularly if they are involved in residential services. Adults with an intellectual may have only basic understanding of health (e.g. need to see doctor if sick) and rely on others (i.e. family or staff) for support. Some health-related needs may go unrecognised (e.g. dental care, nutrition, regular exercise). Apparently, there is a need for staff to be appropriately trained in age-related changes and have practice guidelines that promote good health and reduce the risk of preventable secondary conditions with advancing age. While other research has also documented many of health-related challenges (see as examples Davidson, Heller, Janicki, & Hyer, 2004; Ouellette-Kuntz, 2005), regrettably, application of research findings to practice seems lacking at least in some localities.

Despite the above commentary there are other issues associated with a lifetime of experiences which influence the families' perceptions. Older-aged family members report a myriad of changes over the lifetime of their relative with an intellectual disability and it is important to bear this in mind. When older-aged families were younger, social policy and practice were dominated by professional advice that encouraged institutionalisation. There were also limited education and employment opportunities for people with a disability as well as restrictions on individual rights (e.g. sterilisation without individual consent) (Parmenter, 2004). At the time, knowledge about disability and services were limited. These are all part of the experiences of older parents.

> "We spent quite a bit of energy trying to find out so that we might find help. ... We did the best we could. Oh the knowledge level is so different. Like autism is something people know something about today whereas one or two people in hundreds knew about it [then] ..." Parent

Many parents hold explicit memories of being told their son or daughter had a disability.

> "... when he was born, the nurse said he would never speak and would never walk and that was the worst part." Parent

As children, some older-aged adults with an intellectual disability were institutionalised.

> "When he was young like my mother had the other kids and he used to like to wander and she couldn't keep an eye on him and the other kids ... so the doctor recommended him going down to [an institution] ..." Sibling

Yet even when institutionalisation temporarily disrupted familial relations (e.g. geographic distance to visit), some families rekindled relations over time or with changed circumstances.

As children, older-aged adults with an intellectual disability may have attended only primary grades in a regular school for an extended period of time (e.g. 14 years old in grade 3) and were then excluded from the school system. Individuals in a slightly younger cohort may have had education provided exclusively or predominately in segregated school settings. Employment opportunities were also restricted to sheltered workshops and/or an array of part-time jobs over the years.

During the early years, family responses to these circumstances were diverse. Some families remained outside formal services and may, now, only come forward in older age with urgent need (see, for example, Janicki, McCallion, Force, Bishop, & LePore, 1998). Other parents became involved in grassroots efforts to develop a system of services and supports for their children. These same parents, however, now find themselves once again to be "pioneers" but with less stamina to advocate on behalf of their aging sons and daughters. Social context and life experiences shaped individual and family values, beliefs, concerns and issues related to disability and still continue to exert influence on older-aged family members.

From this research involving older-aged family members (i.e. parents, siblings and adults with an intellectual disability), common thoughts and issues have emerged. Fundamentally, family relations may be at the core of the quality of life experienced by families. Positive and supportive familial relations that are routine-oriented appear to have a positive impact on perceived family quality of life. Engagement in activities outside the family also appears to have a positive influence. Challenges to family quality of life include conflicts and issues that may be experienced by all families but layered with those that are disability-related (e.g. procuring services to meet needs). Maintaining health of older-aged members may also be a challenge; with advancing age, family members may experience ill health.

Over the coming years, we may expect that more severely disabled children will survive (see, for example, Kelly et al., 2007) and because of a strong inclusion movement in many countries they will be in the family home. On the other hand, more mildly disabled children will have benefited from an inclusive system but may as they age become more dependent on or return their parental family or on their siblings.

Discussion and Implications for Practice

A family quality of life approach provides some interesting advantages for work with older-aged families who have adult children with intellectual/developmental disabilities. One of the challenges found in the literature is that quite frequently research, and indeed clinical practice, focus on issues of stress and other challenges. Such work is important, but the advantage of a family quality of life approach is that it provides for a reasonably holistic examination of the feelings and views of family members. Admittedly, these are often the parents view, but as recounted in this chapter, both parents where possible were included, and separate accounts were also obtained from siblings and adults with an intellectual disability about their (parental) family life. The interactive nature at play between family, individual and social environment comes through in the perceptions held by participants and in what seems to maintain, enhance or challenge family quality of life.

The survey approach provides a more general examination of issues, concerns, advantages, challenges and disadvantages. The results from the survey in this chapter suggest some general thrusts in participant responses. While based on a small sample and caution should be taken in interpreting the data, they are not inconsistent with commentary from other families (Turnbull, Brown et al., 2004). To date the results and commentary begin to pinpoint areas of need and should enable services to better align their efforts with older-aged families and have a positive impact on quality of life.

The use of nine domains and questions relating to two of the dimensions, described earlier, also provides separate but integrated accounts of different aspects of life for the family. The advantage of this is that it can provide each member of the family with their own account and perceptions and, therefore, paves the way for more broad family data collection in terms of family members. It can also provide a forum for discussion, if required, and can highlight pluses and minuses in terms of perceived family life. In doing this, it enables the practitioner to examine carefully areas where support and help are most needed, and the types of support that family members think are most important. Where there is agreement or difference of opinion, this can be used, with consent, for discussion of the various issues that have arisen. The important point is that people's perceptions drive their behaviour and, where there are differences in a family, this can enrich outcomes if discussed and positive actions can follow. Alternatively, if ignored, these differences may cause dissention and ineffective or less-effective outcomes.

It is obvious that much more work needs to be done. Some of that work relates to the further standardisation of the *Family Quality of Life Survey* (Brown, Brown, Baum, et al., 2006) and its uses with older-aged families. For instance, based on the Canadian research reported in this chapter, the survey could incorporate a question or checklist that identifies key life events and transitions experienced within the past year (e.g. death of family member, retirement or change in living situation) that may impact quality of life (Denton & Kusch, 2006; Jokinen, 2008).

It is also important to see how effective this approach is with older-aged families in different cultures and countries. It is of interest that a previous edition of the family quality of life survey instrument shows similar results from different places where older families were involved (Brown et al., 2004). The combined results suggest that families where parents and the adult child with a disability are older may be more satisfied or happy than younger families. This may be due to changes in family life generally, and not simply due to ageing and disability, though it seems possible that both general factors and disability factors may be involved. For example, the present qualitative results suggest that in some families the presence of a child with a disability may be a comfort and a helper as parents become older, in poorer health and more lonely. In summary these changes may be due to different parent cohorts associated with variables over the lifespan, changing circumstances in older-aged families regardless of the presence of a relative with an intellectual disability and/or also change relating to variables associated with change as the person with a disability ages. Such challenges, and also the preservation of aspects of life which are positive, can be ascertained from the family quality of life approach.

Further Implications

What are the implications of such work? It underscores the importance of addressing the needs of families in a rather different way than we have done in the past. In coming to this conclusion it should also be noted that family quality of life is highly variable, that individuals who state that they have positive quality of life in some or all of the domains, still may have basic needs which need to be met by services, and importantly, it is worth stressing that the ability to meet those needs prior to stress and breakdown is an important precautionary approach and preventative measure to stabilise families so that they can continue to support their member with a disability. Older-aged families may also be accessing or need to access blended services from different systems of care. This may mean that the individual has residential accommodation through community services or similar agencies, but that the parents and siblings still continue to play a major role in the life of the individual, providing support whether that is in terms of familial affection, leisure time resources or actual support for practical needs which have to be met.

It should also be realised that one of the implications of the findings is that individuals with disability supply or provide supports for other family members; enriching their lives in many instances, and providing support and help which enables, particularly older parents, to continue functioning in their own homes. Obviously, this is not true in all instances but it should be recognised by government and agency services that this is important reciprocal aspect of the relationship between people with a disability and their family members, and, in fact, acts as a preventative measure in terms of promoting the general or overall health and well-being of family members both individually and as whole. As illustrated above, very often such older-aged children with disabilities provide company, support for physical activities. For example, they are often more able to carry items or carry out tasks such as bed making, which can become challenging or impossible for ageing parents. They also reduce the sense of isolation that many older people feel, and that is a source of stimulation both mentally and physically. There are many accounts where parents have come to see their son or daughter with a disability in a way that preserves or promotes family unison. This effect is not limited to parents, for there is clear evidence in a number of instances that the person with a disability, who may be an uncle or an aunt, provides broader family support to individuals within the family as a whole.

As indicated above, it is also important that we take data on quality of life on ageing into account when considering the responses from different age groups of families who have children with disabilities. It is therefore recommended that in future studies should also include contrast or control groups of families from similar cultural and economic backgrounds, and with similar numbers of children, who do not have children with disabilities, so that effective comparisons and if necessary partialling out the normal effects of family ageing. The rise in quality of life that we observe with older families could well be associated with ageing and/or cultural aspects associated with groups of people born at an earlier age. In future research such differences need to be fractioned out.

Conclusion

The family quality of life approach that we are recommending is one that provides for comprehensiveness both in terms of who provides information and the breadth of that information. It is an approach that orientates professionals to the family's perspective including their values, needs, concerns and expectations.

Not only should our response be proactive to an aging population, but it must now involve urgent and critical components. For example, in many developed countries, there are longstanding and extensive wait lists for intellectual disability services. Given this reality, there is an urgent need to support families to plan for inevitable transitions in living and support arrangements that impact all members of the family and help to avert crises. Services and their staff also need to understand and accommodate an aging population, including both adults and their family members, to better respond to changing needs. This requires education of personnel in tandem with effective government and agency policies. It calls for a redirection of services and supports to all family members in need, as much as is possible, in order that they can function effectively. It may include advice, counselling and practical interventions as well as support that are coordinated across various informal networks, service systems and agencies. For example, an 87-year-old widower lives with his 50-year-old son who has an intellectual disability. The son helps with household chores so the parent gains not only physical help but there is also reciprocal emotional support and companionship in the arrangement. This may reduce both physical and psychological stress on the parent and son thus helping to maintain their overall physical and mental health. The question then to be asked is whether this is a suitable arrangement in the eyes of any particular family. If so, what plans may need to be in place for services and/or supports to accommodate individual age-related change and maintain family integrity and unity through inevitable transition in the future. Other examples of this occur in the research reported in this chapter.

References

Aznar, A. S., & Castanon, D. G. (2005). Quality of life from the point of view of Latin American families: A participative research study. *Journal of Intellectual Disability Research, 49*(10), 784–788.

Baxley, D., Janicki, M. P., McCallion, P., & Zendell, A. (2005). *Aiding Older Caregivers of Persons with Intellectual and Developmental Disabilities: A Tool Kit for State and Local Aging Agencies*. Retrieved January 7, 2006, from http://www.uic.edu/orgs/rrtcamr/Aiding_older_caregivers.pdf

Beach Center on Disability. (2008). Beach center family quality of life scale. Retrieved July, 2008, from http://www.beachcenter.org/resource_library/beach_resource_detail_page.aspx?intResourceID=2391&Type=Tool

Bengtson, V., Lowenstein, A., Putney, N., & Gans, D. (2003). Global aging and the challenge to families. In V. Bengtson & A. Lowenstein (Eds.), *Global Aging and Challenges to Families* (pp. 1–26). New York: Walter de Gruyter.

Berglund, A., & Narum, I. (2007). Quality of life demands comprehension and further exploration. *Aging and Health, 19*(1), 39–61.

Bigby, C. (1997). Parental substitutes? The role of siblings in the lives of older people with intellectual disability. *Journal of Gerontological Social Work, 29*(1), 3–21.

Bigby, C. (2004). *Ageing with a Lifelong Disability: A Guide to Practice, Program and Policy Issues for Human Services Professionals*. London: Jessica Kingsley.

Bigby, C., & Balandin, S. (2004). Issues in researching the ageing of people with intellectual disability. In E. Emerson, C. Hatton, T. Thompson, & T. R. Parmenter (Eds.), *The International Handbook of Applied Research in Intellectual Disabilities* (pp. 221–236). West Sussex, England: Wiley.

Blacher, J., & Baker, B. (2007). Positive impact of intellectual disability on families. *American Journal on Mental Retardation, 112*(5), 330–348.

Brown, I., Anand, S., Fung, W., Isaacs, B., & Baum, N. (2003). Family quality of life: Canadian results from an international study. *Journal of Developmental & Physical Disabilities, 15*(3), 207–230.

Brown, I., & Brown, R. I. (2003). *Quality of Life and Disability an Approach for Community Practitioners*. London: Jessica Kingsley Publishers.

Brown, I., & Brown, R. I. (2004a). Concepts for beginning study in family quality of life. In A. P. Turnbull, I. Brown, & H. R. Turnbull (Eds.), *Families and People with Mental Retardation and Quality of Life: International Perspectives* (pp. 25–47). Washington: American Association on Mental Retardation.

Brown, I., & Brown, R. I. (2004b). Family quality of life as an area of study. In A. P. Turnbull, I. Brown, & R. Turnbull (Eds.), *Families and People with Mental Retardation and Quality of Life: International Perspectives* (pp. 3–10). Washington, D.C: American Association on Mental Retardation.

Brown, I., Brown, R. I., Baum, N., Isaacs, B., Myerscough, T., Neikrug, S., et al. (2006). *Family Quality of Life Survey: Main Caregivers of People with Intellectual Disabilities*. Toronto, ON: Surrey Place Centre.

Brown, I., Galambos, D., Poston, D., & Turnbull, A. (2007). Person-centered and family-centered support. In I. Brown & M. Percy (Eds.), *A Comprehensive Guide to Intellectual & Developmental Disabilities* (pp. 351–362). Baltimore: Paul Brookes.

Brown, R. I. (2000). Learning from quality of life models. In M. P. Janicki & E. F. Ansello (Eds.), *Community Supports for Aging Adults with Lifelong Disabilities* (pp. 19–40). Baltimore: Paul Brookes Publishing.

Brown, R. I. (Ed.). (1997). *Quality of Life for People with Disabilities* (2nd ed.). Cheltanham, England: Stanley Thornes.

Brown, R. I., Bayer, M., & Brown, P. M. (1992). *Empowerment and Developmental Handicaps: Choices and Quality of Life*. Toronto, Ontario: Captus Press.

Brown, R. I., Bayer, M. B., & MacFarlane, C. (Eds.). (1989). *Rehabilitation Programs: Performance and Quality of Life of Adults with Developmental Handicaps*. Toronto: Lugus Productions Ltd.

Brown, R. I., Brown, I., & Wang, M. (2006). *Conceptualizing and examining family quality of life: An international affair*. Paper presented at the International Summit for the Alliance on Social Inclusion, Montreal, Canada.

Brown, R. I., Davey, R., Shearer, J., & Kyrkou, M. (2004). Family quality of life in Australia. In A. P. Turnbull, I. Brown, & R. Turnbull (Eds.), *Families and Persons with Mental Retardation and Quality of Life: International Perspectives* (pp. 221–261). Washington, DC: American Association on Mental Retardation.

Brown, R. I., MacAdam-Crisp, J., Wang, M., & Iarocci, G. (2006). Family quality of life when there is a child with a developmental disability. *Journal of Policy and Practice in Intellectual Disabilities*, *3*(4), 238–245.

Carr, J. (2005). Families of 30–35-year olds with Down's syndrome. *Journal of Applied Research in Intellectual Disabilities*, *18*, 75–84.

Davidson, P., Heller, T., Janicki, M., & Hyer, K. (2004). Defining a national health research and practice agenda for older adults with intellectual disabilities. *Journal of Policy and Practice in Intellectual Disabilities*, *1*(1), 2–9.

Denton, M., & Kusch, K. (2006). *Well-Being Throughout the Senior Years: An Issues Paper on Key Events and Transitions in Later Life*. Retrieved 2009, January 15, from http://socserv.socsci.mcmaster.ca/sedap/p/sedap165.pdf

Dew, A., Llewellyn, G., & Balandin, S. (2004). Post-parental care: A new generation of sibling-carers. *Journal of Intellectual & Developmental Disability*, *29*(2), 176–179.

Fast, J., Keating, N., Otfinowski, P., & Derksen, L. (2004). Characteristics of family/friend care networks of frail seniors. *Canadian Journal on Aging*, *23*(1), 5–19.

Fiese, B., Tomcho, T., Douglas, M., Josephs, K., Poltrock, S., & Baker, T. (2002). A review of 50 years of research on naturally occurring family routines and rituals: Cause for celebration? *Journal of Family Psychology*, *16*(4), 381–390.

Goode, D. (Ed.). (1994). *Quality of Life for Persons with Disabilities: International Perspectiues and Issues*. Cambridge, MA: Brookline.

Haley, W., & Perkins, E. (2004). Current status and future directions in family caregiving and aging people with intellectual disabilities. *Journal of Policy and Practice in Intellectual Disabilities*, *1*(1), 24–30.

Halvorsrud, L., & Kalfoss, M. (2007). The conceptualization and measurement of quality of life in older adults: A review of empirical studies published during 1994–2006. *European Journal of Ageing*, *4*(4), 229–246.

Hatton, C., & Emerson, E. (2003). Families with a person with intellectual disabilities: Stress and impact. *Current Opinion in Psychiatry*, *16*(5), 497–501.

Haveman, M. J. (2004). Disease epidemiology and aging people with intellectual disabilities. *Journal of Policy and Practice in Intellectual Disabilities*, *1*(1), 16–23.

Heller, T., & Caldwell, J. (2006). Supporting aging caregivers and adults with developmental disabilities in future planning. *Mental Retardation*, *44*(3), 189–202.

Heller, T., Miller, A., & Factor, A. (1997). Adults with mental retardation as supports to their parents: Effects on parental caregiving appraisal. *Mental Retardation*, *35*(5), 338–346.

Hilton, J. M., Kopera-Frye, K., & Krave, A. (2009). Successful aging from the perspective of family caregivers. *The Family Journal*, *17*(1), 39–50.

Hoffman, L., Marquis, J., Poston, D., Summers, J., & Turnbull, A. (2006). Assessing family outcomes: Psychometric evaluation of the Beach Center Family Quality of Life Scale. *Journal of Marriage and Family*, *68*(4), 1069–1083.

Hogg, J., Lucchino, R., Wang, K., Janicki, M. P., & Group, W. (2000). *Healthy Ageing: Adults with Intellectual Disabilities: Ageing & Social Policy*. Geneva: World Health Organization.

Isaacs, B., Brown, I., Brown, R. I., Baum, N., Myerscough, T., Neikrug, S., et al. (2007). The International Family Quality of Life Project: Goals and description of a survey tool. *Journal of Policy and Practice in Intellectual Disabilities*, *4*(3), 177–185.

Janicki, M. P. (1997). Quality of life for older adults with mental retardation. In R. L. Schalock (Ed.), *Quality of Life Volume 11 Application to Persons with Disabilities* (pp. 105–115). Washington, D.C: American Association on Mental Retardation.

Janicki, M. P., & Ansello, E. F. (2000). Supports for community living, evolution of an aging with lifelong disabilities movement. In M. P. Janicki, & E. F. Ansello (Eds.), *Community Supports for Aging Adults with Lifelong Disabilities* (pp. 529–547. Baltimore: Paul Brookes Publishing.

Janicki, M., Henderson, C., & Rubin, L. (2008). Neurodevelopmental conditions and aging: Report on the Atlanta study group charrette on neurodevelopmental conditions and aging. *Disability and Health, 1*, 11–124.

Janicki, M. P., McCallion, P., Force, L., Bishop, K., & LePore, P. (1998). Area agency on aging outreach and assistance for households with older carers of an adult with a developmental disability. *Journal of Aging & Social Policy, 10*(1), 13–36.

Jokinen, N. S. (2003). Older adults with intellectual disability living in a community residential service. *International Journal of Disability, Community & Rehabilitation, 2*(1). Retrieved from www.ijdcr.ca

Jokinen, N. S. (2008). *Family Quality of Life in the Context of Aging and Intellectual Disability*. Doctoral Dissertation, University of Calgary.

Jokinen, N. S., & Brown, R. I. (2005). Family quality of life from the perspective of older parents. *Journal of Intellectual Disability Research, 49*(10), 789–793.

Journal of Policy and Practice in Intellectual Disabilities (2006). *Special Issue on Family Quality of Life Research, 3*(4), 209–270.

Kelly, F., Kelly, C., & Craig, S. (2007). *Annual Report of the National Intellectual Disability Database Committee 2007* (No. 2009 034X). Dublin, Ireland: Health Research Board.

Knox, M., & Bigby, C. (2007). Moving towards midlife careas negotiated family business: Accounts of people with intellectual disabilities and their families "Just getting along with their lives together". *International Journal of Disability, Development and Education, 54*(3), 287–304.

Mahon, M., & Mactavish, J. (2000). A sense of belonging older adults' perspectives on social integration. In M. P. Janicki & E. F. Ansello (Eds.), *Community Supports for Aging Adults with Lifelong Disabilities* (pp. 41–53). Baltimore: Paul Brookes Publishing.

Mannan, H., Summers, J. A., Turnbull, A., & Poston, D. (2006). A review of outcome measures in early childhood programs. *Journal of Policy and Practice in Intellectual Disabilities, 3*(4), 219–228.

McCallion, P., & McCarron, M. (2007). Perspective on quality of life in dementia care. *Intellectual and Developmental Disabilities, 45*(1), 59.

McInnis-Dittrich, K. (2005). *Social Work with Elders, A Biopsychosocial Approach to Assessment and Intervention* (2nd ed.). Boston, MA: Allyn and Bacon.

Ouellette-Kuntz, H. (2005). Understanding health disparities and inequities faced by individuals with intellectual disabilities. *Journal of Applied Research in Intellectual Disabilities, 18*(2), 113–121.

Park, J., Hoffman, L., Marquis, J., Turnbull, A. P., Poston, D., Mannan, H., et al. (2003). Toward assessing family outcomes of service delivery: Validation of a famiy quality of life survey. *Journal of Intellectual Disability Research, 47*(4/5), 367–384.

Parke, B., & Brand, P. (2004). An elder-friendly hospital: Translating a dream into reality. *Canadian Journal of Nursing Leadership, 17*(1), 62–77.

Parmenter, T. R. (2004). Family quality of life: Implications for policy. In A. P. Turnbull, I. Brown, & R. Turnbull (Eds.), *Families and Persons with Mental Retardation and Quality of Life: International Perspectives* (pp. 265–298). Washington D.C: American Association on Mental Retardation.

Poston, D., Turnbull, A. P., Park, J., Mannan, H., Marquis, J., & Wang, M. (2003). Family quality of life: A qualitative inquiry. *Mental Retardation, 41*, 313–328.

Prosser, H., & Moss, S. (1996). Informal care networks of older adults with an intellectual disability. *Journal of Applied Research in Intellectual Disabilities, 9*(1), 17–30.

Renwick, R., Brown, I., & Nagler, M. (Eds.). (1996). *Quality of Life in Health Promotion and Rehabilitation: Conceptual Approaches, Issues, and Applications*. Thousand Oaks, CA: Sage.

Schalock, R., Brown, I., Brown, R. I., Cummins, R., Felce, D., Matikka, L., et al. (2002). Conceptualization, measurement, and application of quality of life for persons with intellectual disabilities: Report of an international panel of experts. *Mental Retardation, 40*, 457–470.

Seltzer, M., & Krauss, M. (2001). Quality of life of adults with mental retardation/developmental disabilities who live with family. *Mental Retardation and Developmental Disabilities Research Reviews*, *7*(2), 105–114.

Summers, J. A., Poston, D. J., Turnbull, A. P., Marquis, J., Hoffman, L., Mannan, H., et al. (2005). Conceptualizing and measuring family quality of life. *Journal of Intellectual Disability Research*, *49*(10), 777–783.

Turnbull, A. (2007, December 6). *Discussion: Family quality of life. Where we are at and where we are going*. Paper presented at the IASSID Quality of Life Special Interest Research Group Meeting, ISQOLS, San Diego, CA.

Turnbull, A., Brown, I., & Turnbull, H. (Eds.). (2004). *Families and People with Mental Retardation and Quality of Life: International Perspectives*. Washington, DC: American Association on Mental Retardation.

Turnbull, A., Turnbull, R., Poston, D., Beegle, G., Blue-Banning, M., Frankland, C., et al. (2004). Enhancing quality of life of families of children and youth with disabilities in the United States. In A. P. Turnbull, I. Brown, & R. Turnbull (Eds.), *Families and Persons with Mental Retardation and Quality of Life: International Perspectives*. Washington, DC: American Association on Mental Retardation.

Turnbull, R., Beegle, G., & Stowe, M. (2001). The core concepts of disability policy affecting families who have children with disabilities. *Journal of Disability Policy Studies*, *12*(3), 133–144.

Weigel, D. (2008). The concept of family: An analysis of laypeople's views of family. *Journal of Family Issues*, *29*, 1426–1447.

World Health Organization. (2007). *Global Age-friendly Cities: A Guide*. Retrieved September 22, 2008, from http://www.who.int/ageing/publications/Global_age_friendly_cities_Guide_English.pdf

Zisberg, A., Young, H., Schepp, K., & Zysberg, L. (2007). A concept analysis of routine: Relevance to nursing. *Journal of Advanced Nursing*, *57*(4), 442–453.

Zuna, N., Turnbull, A., & Summers, J. (2009). Family quality of life: Moving from measurement to application. *Journal of Policy and Practice in Intellectual Disabilities*, *6*(1), 25–31.

Chapter 17
A Comparison of Two Family Quality of Life Measures: An Australian Study

Fiona Rillotta, Neil Kirby, and Joanne Shearer

Background

From the 1970s, widespread acceptance of deinstitutionalization together with growing demands for government sponsored community-based services, and rising costs for these services, led to an increase in the number of people with an intellectual disability living quasi-independently in the community or at home, with their families taking responsibility for their primary care throughout their lifespan (I. Brown, Anand, Fung, Isaacs, & Baum, 2003; R. I. Brown, Davey, Shearer, & Kyrkou, 2004; Llewellyn, Gething, Kendig, & Cant, 2003). Given that many families have not been prepared for the duration and intensity of this caregiving role (Isaacs et al., 2007), a multitude of issues and concerns have arisen for these families and for the services that support them. These issues and concerns have led to the need for research in how they affect Family Quality of Life (FQOL).

Quality of Life (QOL) has been a concept studied and developed within the field of disability since the mid-1980s (e.g., I. Browne & Bramston, 1996; Brown, Brown, et al., 2000; R. I. Brown, 1988; Cummins, 1991; Dennis, Williams, Giangreco, & Cloninger, 1993; Goode, 1994; Rapley, 2003; Schalock, 2004a; Seltzer & Krauss, 2001; Turnbull, Brown, & Turnbull, 2004). Family Quality of Life (FQOL) developed from the work of individual QOL (Schalock, 2004b), but focused on quality within the family unit as a whole, including the impact of disability services on outcomes for the family (Isaacs et al., 2007). The importance of a multi-element QOL framework encompassing the desired states of emotional, material, and physical well-being; interpersonal relations or interactions; personal development; self-determination; social inclusion; and rights, has become widely accepted (I. Brown, Brown, et al., 2000; Hoffman, Marquis, Poston, Summers, & Turnbull, 2006). Understanding the potential of the QOL model and its application has also become important to social policy, support services, and programs (e.g., education, health, and social) and their evaluation (I. Brown, Brown, et al., 2000; Schalock,

F. Rillotta (✉)
School of Psychology, The University of Adelaide, Adelaide, SA, Australia
e-mail: fiona.rillotta@adelaide.edu.au

R. Kober (ed.), *Enhancing the Quality of Life of People with Intellectual Disabilities*, Social Indicators Research Series 41, DOI 10.1007/978-90-481-9650-0_17,

2004a). Moreover, the value of researching FQOL is recognized insofar as the family constitutes a structure that is important to society's functioning and stability, and because well-functioning families and good FQOL are viewed as a positive social resource (Isaacs et al., 2007). The ultimate purpose of FQOL research is to focus on, and understand, global, positive, and universal aspects of family life (Isaacs et al., 2007; Poston, 2006); and to use the QOL framework to influence service outcomes aiming to improve the general well-being of people with intellectual disabilities and their families.

"Family"

In today's society the definition of a "family" has become complicated partly due to the changing nature of family structures. In Western societies "family" has traditionally been based on the nuclear model of biological parents and offspring. However, it now may include: step, foster, adoptive, or single-parent families; a non-related group of people; blended families; extended families residing together; etc. For example, the Australian Bureau of Statistics (ABS, 2001, 2006) census results showed that between 1996 and 2006, there was a 4.7% drop in couple families with children; a 3.2% rise in couple families without children; a 1.9% rise in single-parent families; and a 0.1% drop in "other" families. Currently, in the United States, only about a quarter of all households consist of nuclear families (24.1% in 2005 compared to 40.3% in 1970), due to a rise in other family arrangements such as blended families, binuclear (step) families, and single-parent families (Williams, Sawyer, & Wahlstrom, 2005). The definition for "family" used in this chapter is based on a combination of those presented in the two FQOL surveys considered in this chapter (Beach Center on Disability, 2003; I. Brown et al., 2006): "People who are closely involved in the day-to-day affairs of your household and support each other on a regular basis; whether related by blood, marriage or by close personal relationship."

Why Compare Two FQOL Measures?

This chapter does not summarize all findings associated with family-centered research within the field of disability because it focuses primarily on the use of two measures of FQOL (Beach Center on Disability, 2003; I. Brown et al., 2006). However, a brief overview of such findings is presented, including specific reference to Australian research. At the 2006 E-IASSID conference, Quality of Life Special Interest Research Group presenters (N. Baum, I. Brown, D. Poston) explained that the International FQOL Survey was being used in several countries (including in Australia by the authors of this chapter) and with families that had members with various intellectual disability types and ages, whereas the Beach Center Survey was only being used in the United States, mostly for families with children younger than 12 years of age, and was not disability specific (i.e., not only intellectual disability). Since the two surveys had essentially the same purpose, it was considered useful to explore convergent validity by comparing the information collected using both measures with the *same* families, as suggested by Isaacs et al. (2007). The study described in this chapter aimed to do this, using both surveys with a sample of families in Australia.

Given that FQOL is a relatively new area that is considered critical to policy, service, and research for enhancing the QOL of people with a disability and their families, the aims and benefits of comparing the two surveys are to identify the best features of each and contribute to the future developments of improved FQOL measures. The research discussed in this chapter also investigated FQOL more generally in order to identify important features that may not currently be included in either of the existing measures, and which may also contribute to an increased understanding of FQOL. Further development of FQOL measures will assist in applying the FQOL concepts to program planning, service delivery and evaluation. It will also facilitate further research into FQOL, moving from conceptualizing a QOL "model" (inputs, activities, outputs, outcomes) to a "framework" (factors, domains, indicators) applying the principles of QOL (Schalock, 2007).

The practical benefit of this study was to provide main disability service providers with relevant service information on FQOL issues. Previous family-centered research in Australia (e.g., See Brown et al., 2004; Eacott, 2002; Kristine Peters Project Management Pty Ltd, 1998; Shearer, 2000; and refer to section of this chapter "FQOL Research in Australia") did not use such comprehensive FQOL measures. Management and staff of the disability service provider that facilitated recruitment of participants were interested in applying research findings to their services for families with a member with an intellectual disability. The longer term benefit of this study was to have an FQOL measure that could be used to identify service needs of families and evaluate their effectiveness.

Overview of Previous Research

Recent Australian and international literature has supported the idea that FQOL is a useful construct in the field of disability (Aznar & Castanon, 2005; I. Brown & Brown, 2004; R. I. Brown & Brown, 2006; Davis & Gavidia-Payne, 2009; Hoffman et al., 2006; Isaacs et al., 2007; Neikrug, Judes, Roth, & Krauss, 2004; Poston, 2006; J. A. Summers et al., 2007). Research has shown that the member with a disability becomes the focal point of the whole family. For example, a study concerned with family spontaneity in recreation activities found that the member with a disability often played a decisive role in determining the activities that the family could and could not undertake, because of skill limitations, challenging behaviors, difficulties in coordinating busy schedules, and limits in availability of service information (Mactavish & Schleien, 2004). There also appears to be a lack of congruence in everyday family life between meeting the needs of the child with a disability and those of other family members; such that the child with a disability is often not integrated into everyday family life or into the wider community (Llewellyn, Dunn, Fante, Turnbull, & Grace, 1999; Owen, Gordon, Frederico, & Cooper, 2002).

Variables such as the age of the member with a disability and/or the age of parent carers and the type of disability (or "diagnosis") have also been found to influence stress levels in the family as well as the family's coping mechanisms for dealing with the challenges that come with having a child with a disability (Blacher, 2001; Eisenhower, Baker, & Blacher, 2005; Jokinen & Brown, 2005; Schneider, Wedgewood, Llewellyn, & McConnell, 2006). It has also been found that parents' own health and well-being becomes second to their child with a disability's needs; and parental carer well-being falls significantly below the population norms for Australian families (Mackey & Goddard, 2006, 2007; McVilly, 2007a, b). Parents caring for children with an intellectual disability also display poorer states of mental health and vitality than Australian norms (Llewellyn, Thompson, et al, 2003; McVilly, 2007b). These findings are consistent with the theory that poor personal well-being is an indicator of a breakdown in homeostasis regarding life satisfaction and subjective well-being, and also indicates the emergence of psychopathology (Cummins, 2003, 2005; Cummins, Eckersley, Pallant, Van Vugt, & Miasjon, 2003).

FQOL Research in Australia

A number of studies in Australia associated with families that have a member with a disability have focused on particular aspects of FQOL, such as parents' health and stress levels, caregiver burden, parent–professional relationships, or sibling issues (R. I. Brown, Davey, et al., 2004; Cummins, 2007; Eacott, 2002; Llewellyn, 2004; Mackey & Goddard, 2006; McVilly, 2007b; Owen et al., 2002). In a very recent Australian study, Davis and Gavidia-Payne (2009) found that parental experiences and perceptions of family-centered professional support was a strong predictor of FQOL; and support from extended family, the child's behavior problems, and family income also had an impact on FQOL. These findings highlighted the need for professional supports to respectfully consider family-centered outcomes to service provision. The current study is the only Australian study using two established measures of FQOL and their associated FQOL domains (Beach Center on Disability, 2003; I. Brown et al., 2006). As indicated by Llewellyn, Thompson, et al. (2003), policymakers and service providers in Australia are interested in finding effective and efficient processes that will encourage families to continue caring for their children with disabilities at home.

There have been a few studies exploring FQOL issues and intellectual disability in the state of South Australia (R. I. Brown, Davey, et al., 2004; Eacott, 2002; Kristine Peters Project Management Pty Ltd, 1998; Shearer, 2000). Roy Brown and his colleagues began research in FQOL in South Australia in 1997, using a similar tool to the current International Survey (I. Brown et al., 2006. See Section on "Measurement of FQOL" in this chapter). They found similar results to other studies from Australia and to those of international FQOL studies. In particular, having a member with an intellectual disability significantly influenced FQOL, and each family member was found to be affected in different ways. Examples included; stress and poor health of carers whose child's needs were paramount in the family and who were physically, mentally, and emotionally demanding; restricted employment options for carers to accommodate the needs and schedule of the member with a disability, which often resulted in financial constraints for the family, and was especially difficult due to the additional and sometimes excessive expenses involved for some people with disabilities; and family social isolation with an associated lack of community involvement (R. I. Brown, Davey, et al., 2004; Eacott, 2002; Kristine Peters Project Management Pty Ltd, 1998; Shearer, 2000). With respect to sibling development and individual attention to all family members, some families reported the positive impact of respite services or recreational services that take the person with a disability away from the family every so often, to give siblings a break from the demands that accompany caring for a person with a disability (R. I. Brown, Davey, et al., 2004; Kristine Peters Project Management Pty Ltd, 1998). Dissatisfaction with the supports and services available for the family and for the individual with a disability, including insufficient amounts of respite, childcare and funding, was also expressed in these studies. Results from the current Australian study, using a similar measure for FQOL, have revealed similar service issues as those identified by R.I. Brown, Davey, et al. (2004) and Eacott (2002). However, current results also contribute additional information about implications for the measurement of FQOL.

Measurement of FQOL

There is a consensus in the QOL literature that it is necessary to obtain both qualitative and quantitative data when conducting QOL research (I. Brown, Brown, et al., 2000). Qualitative measures are useful to assess family outcomes involving personal experiences that can only be explained by considering the perceptions of the family members themselves, because ultimately it is these subjective perceptions that determine the individual's approach to life and how satisfied they are with life (Bailey et al., 1998; I. Brown & Brown, 2004). There are many measurement tools that have been used for research involving families, but most tend to measure aspects of family life as separate issues; such as financial well-being, caregiver/parental health, and burden or stress. They do not draw together these various components or encompass the holistic notion implied in the concept of FQOL and its frameworks (Isaacs et al., 2007). The FQOL framework attempts to bring together a wide range of objective and subjective aspects of family life, including family income and the amount spent on disability-related needs; the number of hours friends/relatives spend supporting the family; employment; and clubs/organizations to which family members belong (Isaacs et al., 2007). The two surveys described next aimed to integrate these and other aspects of FQOL within concepts commonly accepted for individual QOL research, such as levels of satisfaction.

International Survey

The Family Quality of Life Survey (I. Brown, Neikrug, & Brown, 2000) was originally developed by experts in the field of QOL and stakeholders (Isaacs et al.,

2007). Nine domains of FQOL were identified, forming the basis of the survey: "Health," "Financial Well-Being," "Family Relationships," "Support from Other People," "Support from Disability-Related Services," "Spiritual and Cultural Beliefs," "Careers and Preparing for Careers," "Leisure and Enjoyment of Life," and "Community and Civic Involvement." These domains were formed by reviewing FQOL research; input from researchers from nine institutes and universities; feedback from family members (with and without a family with an intellectual disability); and feedback from prospective users of the tool, professionals, and academics (Isaacs et al., 2007).

The original version of the survey (I. Brown, Neikrug, et al., 2000) was also later field tested. It was piloted internationally over the course of 4 years with over 300 family members (mostly mothers and fathers of relatives with various intellectual disability types including Down Syndrome and Autism). It was used as a measure of FQOL in Australia (R. I. Brown, Davey, et al., 2004; Shearer, 2000), Canada (I. Brown et al., 2003; I. Brown, Isaacs, McCormack, Baum, & Renwick, 2004), Israel (Neikrug et al., 2004), South Korea, and Taiwan. The survey resulted in similar findings across these different cultures in terms of main caregiver's concerns for their family and the life of the member with an intellectual disability. For example, it was consistently found that the main burden of care was placed on the mother of the family, and that the main concern for the relative with a disability was social isolation. As described by Isaacs et al. (2007), analysis of the international data also indicated high reliability and validity of the first version of this scale, and the nine domains were deemed feasible subscales for measuring different aspects of FQOL. However, due to the small sample size, confirmatory factor analysis was not conducted. Some wording changes and clarification of the Likert scales were found to be necessary. Respondents also indicated their desire to provide supplementary qualitative information, to explain their quantitative ratings. Subsequent work on the FQOL domains was conducted accordingly and participants' interpretations of the concepts were analyzed. For example, "civil involvement" was considered to be irrelevant to some families because they interpreted it to mean involvement in official civic duties. Also, there was a need to elaborate on what was meant by "stability" in terms of the anticipated future for disability supports, which may have been viewed as either a positive or negative element of family life (See Isaacs et al., 2007 for further detail). The older version of the survey was also deemed to be quite long (1.5–2 h) and while that was appropriate for research purposes, it was less appropriate for other purposes such as outcome evaluation or administering large numbers of surveys in order to statistically compare groups (Isaacs et al., 2007).

An updated version of the survey was published in 2006 (I. Brown et al., 2006) with revised FQOL domains; "Health," "Financial Well-Being," "Family Relationships," "Support from Other People," "Support from Disability-Related Services," "Influence of Values," "Careers and Preparing for Careers," "Leisure and Recreation," "Community Interaction," as well as two extra sections of the survey – "Family Background" and "Overall Family Quality of Life" (See Isaacs et al., 2007). The assessment concepts associated with the questions in each of these domains include: *Importance* (the degree of value the family places on that particular element), *Opportunities* (the options that are available to families), *Attainment* (the degree to which the family is able to accomplish or obtain what they need), *Initiative* (the degree to which families take advantage of available opportunities), *Stability* (the degree to which circumstances are likely to improve, decline, or stay the same), and *Satisfaction* (overall perception about important aspects of family life) (see Isaacs et al., 2007). In the current study, the International Survey took between 1 and 3.5 h to administer by interview. It is currently being used in 19 countries and has been translated into 12 different languages.

Beach Center Survey

The Beach Center Family Quality of Life Scale (Beach Center on Disability, 2003)[1] was developed at the Beach Center, The University of Kansas. It was trialed in three States of America (Kansas, Louisiana, and North Carolina) and was developed in three phases in order to be used for both research and program or policy evaluation. The first phase sought to understand people's perceptions of the meaning of FQOL with or without having a member with a disability. Qualitative interviews were conducted with over 100 people including family members of children and youth with and without disabilities, service providers, and administrators (Poston et al., 2003). The second phase was undertaken to develop 10 specific domains of FQOL. During this phase focus groups and interviews were conducted with family members, including those with disabilities, and service providers. The domains were: "Family Interaction," "Parenting," "Daily Life," "Financial Well-Being," "Emotional Well-Being," "Social Well-Being," "Health," "Physical Environment," "Advocacy," and "Productivity" (J. A. Summers et al., 2005). The third phase was dedicated to developing a statistical model based on the qualitative data and field tests, using exploratory factor analysis to form subscales from a 5-factor solution; Family Interaction, Parenting, General Resources, Health and Safety, and Support for Persons with Disabilities (see Hoffman et al., 2006; Park et al., 2003 for more detail). Items that were rated low on importance were removed; however, the literature does not report what these items were, or any possible reasons why they were not rated as being as important as other items. The end result of these statistical analyses and rewording of items was a 25-item survey (plus a section on General and Individual Family Information), including five FQOL domains: "Family Interaction," "Parenting," "Emotional Well-Being," "Physical/Material Well-Being," and "Disability-Related Support." Questions in the survey were designed to also assess these domains in terms of the concepts of Importance and Satisfaction.

---

[1]For some of the data collected in the present study, The Beach Center Partnership and Family Quality of Life Survey was used, which included a preliminary section on Support and Services (disability-related or otherwise). For the purpose of this chapter, only FQOL data are presented. Results from Partnership and Support Services sections of the survey are relevant for other analyses.

Poston et al. (2003) outlined preliminary limitations in the initial study used to develop The Beach Center FQOL Scale, including the fact that confirmatory analysis of the data examination procedures by a professional peer was not conducted. Also, given that it was based on a qualitative analysis with selected people, results may not necessarily be generalized to all families. However, in a later study with 280 family members (mostly mothers) of children with mostly "moderate" levels of disabilities (including but not limited to Autism, Developmental Delay, learning difficulties, emotional disorders, and physical health conditions) Hoffman et al. (2006) confirmed (from psychometric evaluation) the 5-factor solution for the FQOL domains. They concluded that the scale is an effective tool for researching FQOL, as well as for applied research to examine the outcomes of family services and policies.

The Beach Center Survey has so far been used with over 1,000 participants in American populations, including a translated Spanish version used in Colombia (Verdugo, Córdoba, & Gómez, 2005; Wang et al., 2004; 2006), and it has been used in a multi-survey study self-administered by 64 families in Australia assessing the impact of child, family, and professional support characteristics on FQOL for families with young children aged 3–5 years (Davis & Gavidia-Payne, 2009). No other uses of the Beach Center Survey are known to the authors. Studies describing the data obtained from using this measure (e.g., Hoffman et al., 2006) did not specify how long participants took to self-administer the survey. However, the Spanish version (Verdugo et al., 2005), administered by interview, was reported to have taken 45 min. Similarly, in the current study interviews took between 30 min and 1 h.

Methodology of the Current Study

The data discussed in this chapter ($n = 15$) came from a larger sample of 53 main caregivers of people with a disability who participated in the Australian Family Quality of Life study. Main caregivers were interviewed in their homes in a semi-structured manner using one or the other, or both of the surveys. Not all families completed both surveys; depending on how much time they had available. Most completed the International Survey only ($n = 29$) and the remainder completed the Beach Center survey only ($n = 9$). The data from the 15 families who had time to complete both surveys were considered a useful indication of the similarities and differences between the two measures. Further observations on each measure could also be made from the results of the 38 participants who only completed one of the measures, as well as from responses to any additional questions asked during the time spent with these families.

Participant Demographics

Table 17.1 shows demographic details of the 15 main caregivers who completed both surveys. Main caregivers were all biological mothers and they varied in

Table 17.1 Demographical details of participants who completed both measures

	Age	Gender	Marital status
Participant (main caregiver)	Range: 25–76 Mean: 45 years *SD*: 12.64	$F = 15$ $M = 0$	Married = 8 Divorced = 2 Separated = 2 Not married = 2 Widowed = 1
Member with intellectual disability[a]	Range: 2–39 Mean: 16 years *SD*: 12.20	$F = 6$ $M = 9$	N/A

[a]Six families had more than one member with a disability. Since the Beach Center Survey did not ask about each family member with a disability separately (the International Survey did) the family member with the most impact on the family has been discussed for comparison purposes (see section of this chapter on "Findings from Australian Data Comparing Two Measures – more than one family member with a disability").

age from 25 to 76 years. Nine families were two-parent families and six were single-parent. The Beach Center Survey question about financial income, asking participants to select from 10 options (from $15,000 to above $75,000), was found to be too personal or challenging for some to answer; therefore it was not usually asked. One mother responded, "Nope, I'd rather not answer that ... I don't like them asking that question ... I don't even know how much my husband earns." Pilot study participants indicated that they preferred the equivalent question from the International Survey, which requested that participants select from five options ("well below average" to "well above average") based on the average income of their country. The vast majority (87%) of participants selected an "average" income level; one participant selected above average, and another selected below average). This suggests that asking about level of income may not be a useful question. However, this needs to be explored in larger samples, along with qualitative data about financial well-being. In addition, the vast majority of families had an Australian cultural background, with a few who were English, German, or Croatian descendants.

Table 17.1 also shows that members with an intellectual disability varied in age, and that there were slightly more males than females. The "diagnoses" for the 15 family members with a disability varied; Autism Spectrum Disorder ($n = 4$); Intellectual disability ($n = 3$); Developmental Delay or Early Childhood Disability ($n = 3$); Down Syndrome ($n = 3$); Cerebral Palsy ($n = 1$); and Chromosomal Disorder III ($n = 1$). Almost all had one or more secondary conditions including behavioral problems, mood, or expression challenges, physical impairments, or speech/language/communication difficulties. The Beach Center Survey asked about level of disability (mild, moderate, severe, unknown) whereas the International Survey did not. Based on responses of the participants, asking for this information did not prove to be useful, because most participants found level of disability difficult to describe. This was not surprising since Australian disability services describe a person in relation to their service needs rather than their level of disability and they no longer classify level of disability. The equivalent International

Survey background question asking about level of disability support required was more suited to the Australian participants. The mean score from the participants in the current study was 2.15 (equivalent to "requires disability-related support for most, but not all, aspects of life"); no participants selected "does not require disability-related support"; two participants selected "only a few aspects of life"; three selected "some aspects of life"; three selected "most, but not all, aspects of life"; and five selected "almost all aspects of life" (two respondents did not indicate a level of disability-related support). Therefore, this question was useful in discriminating between participants in terms of differing levels of support needs.

Pilot Study: Modifications to Surveys and Cultural Considerations

A pilot study was conducted with four families selected by a regional manager of the disability service provider. The pilot study resulted in adding supplementary questions about relevant *past* family circumstances to each section/domain of the International Survey (See section on "Past and Distant Future" of this chapter). It was also considered necessary to distinguish between the provision of practical (or material) support and emotional support in the "Support from Other People" domain of the International Survey because pilot study participants identified these as two separate constructs. For example, practical support referred to monetary support or assistance with babysitting or housework, etc., whereas emotional support included listening when needed or being "a shoulder to cry on" at times of grief or distress. The Beach Center Survey questions about support from others were broader in that they did not specify "practical" or "emotional" support. However, questions were worded so that it was left up to the individual's interpretation. For example, the Beach Center Survey asked about the importance of, and satisfaction with, "the support we need to relieve stress," "friends or others who provide support" and "outside help . . . to take care of special needs of all family members." Generally, participants in the current study responded to these Beach Center Survey questions about support from others without asking for clarification of the *kind* of support. Results of the pilot study suggested that modifications to the Beach Center Survey (with the permission of the survey's authors) were only required in terms of culture specific demographic questions to fit with Australian terminology (e.g., educational qualifications and race/cultural background). These changes were necessary because the Beach Center Survey had only been used in the United States, and it was not originally designed for international use.

With further respect to cultural context, Aznar and Castanon (2005) suggested that Latin American families may have different values, understandings, and priorities than those encompassed in commonly reported FQOL "domains" developed in Anglo-American cultures, such as the International Survey. Aznar and Castanon (2005) therefore developed an FQOL measure, including domains worded appropriately for their culture; "Emotional Well-Being," "Personal Strength and Development," "Rules of Cohabitation," "Physical/Material Well-Being," "Family Life," and "Interpersonal and Community Relations" (See Aznar & Castanon, 2005, for further information). Also, S. Devi from India (Devi, 2006), who had hoped to use the International FQOL survey in her country, indicated that an additional domain associated with superstitions and religion would be necessary because these elements help guide the people of India through their everyday lives and hence their family life (Devi, 2006). Therefore, if research is to effectively inform policies associated with disability in different cultures, there is a need for FQOL measures to be sensitive to cultural differences.

To the best of the authors' knowledge, no further culture specific (or other) changes have been made to the published surveys, and there is no evidence from previous studies or from the current pilot study suggesting any other necessary rewording for either of the surveys.

Findings from Australian Data Comparing Two Measures

While both surveys attempt to measure the same construct (i.e., FQOL), and they seek similar information from families about their FQOL in slightly different ways, they also differ considerably in various elements including: length; user-friendliness; time taken to administer; methodology (i.e., self-administered versus face-to-face; and qualitative versus quantitative); and the expertise or personal traits required to administer the surveys. Comparisons between the two measures were also considered in terms of the FQOL aspects that were included in one survey but not the other, such as: provision to report information about more than one family member with a disability (in the International Survey). As noted by Poston et al. (2003), the Beach Center Survey "domains" were broader; and while the Beach Center Survey included the domain of "Parenting," the International Survey included the domain of "Influence of Values"; The overarching measurement "concepts" that the Beach Center Survey used within each domain were the same as the major measurement concepts used in the International Survey (i.e., Importance and Satisfaction), but the International Survey also assesses Opportunities, Initiative, Attainment, and Stability. Table 17.2 summarizes the main differences between the two surveys, and these differences are then discussed in light of the Australian data.

From Table 17.2 it can be seen that there are considerable similarities between the five Beach Center Survey domains and the nine International Survey domains (domain comparisons were adopted with permission from Zuna, Beach Center on Disability, & Hu, 2007). For example, certain items from the "Emotional Well-Being" domain of the Beach Center Survey align with three of the International Survey domains; "Support from Other People," "Leisure and Recreation," and "Community Interaction" (See Table 17.2). The International Survey has separate domains (and more detailed survey sections) for "Influence of Values," "Community Interaction," "Leisure and Recreation," and "Careers," but the Beach Center Survey only had one survey item which could be linked to these domains respectively; "teach the children to make good decisions," "safety at home, work, school and

Table 17.2 Summary of face-value comparisons

Comparison area	International survey	Beach Center Survey
Development	Researchers (9 institutes/universities)	Qualitative inquiry
	Field tested 300+ International sample from 3 countries (Canada, Australia, Israel)	Field tested 150+ sample from 3 States of USA (Kansas, Louisiana, North Carolina)
Number of pages	39	15
Time to administer interview	45 min–3.5 h	20 min–1 h
Number of items per survey section	**121**	**69**
	About your family (13)	Support and services (28)
	Health of family (10)	FQOL (25)
	Financial well-being (13)	Physical/material well-being (5)
	Family relationships (10)	Emotional well-being (4)
	Support from other people (12)	Family interaction (6)
	Support from disability-related services (10)	Disability-related support (4)
	Influence of values (12)	Parenting (6)
	Careers and preparing for careers (13)	General individual and family information (16)
	Leisure and recreation (10)	
	Community interaction (11)	
	Overall FQOL (7)	
Comparison of FQOL Domains in the two surveys (Adopted with permission from Zuna, Beach Center on Disability, and Hu (2007))	Health of family	Physical/material well-being (2 items; medical care, dental care)
	Financial well-being	Physical/material well-being (1 item; take care of expenses)
	Family relationships	Family interaction (whole domain; 6 items)
	Support from other people	Emotional well-being (3 items; support to relieve stress, friends or others who provide support, outside help available)
	Support from disability-related services	Disability-related support (whole domain; 4 items)
	Influence of values	Parenting *Questionable*[a] (1 item; teach children to make good decisions)
	Careers and preparing for careers	Emotional Well-Being *Questionable*[a] (1 item; pursue own interests)
	Leisure and recreation	Family interaction (1 item; enjoy spending time together)
		Emotional well-being (1 item; pursue own interests)
	Community interaction	Physical/material well-being (1 item; feel safe at home, work, school, neighborhood)
		Emotional well-being (2 items; friends or *others* who provide support, outside help available)

Table 17.2 (continued)

Comparison area	International survey	Beach Center Survey
Provisions For. . ..	More than one family member with an intellectual disability (up to 3)	The member with a disability who has the *most* impact on family life (despite how many family members there are with a disability)
	State siblings and any other people considered to be immediate family (i.e., not just parents of the relative with intellectual disability)	Only asks about the participant in the study (i.e., main caregiver/usually the mother)
Measurement	Quantitative with some provision for qualitative explanations	Quantitative only; no opportunity for Qualitative explanations (other than in the General Information/demographics section)
Measurement concepts	Importance Opportunities Initiative Attainment Stability Satisfaction	Importance Satisfaction
Five-point Likert scale (importance)	Very important Quite important Somewhat important A little important Hardly important at all	Critically important (blank) Important (blank) A little important
Five-Point Likert Scale (satisfaction)	Very satisfied Satisfied Neither satisfied or dissatisfied Dissatisfied Very dissatisfied	Very satisfied (blank) Neither (blank) Very dissatisfied

[a] *Questionable* means that it is debatable as to whether cr not these items from the Beach Center Survey fit into the equivalent International Survey domain.

in the neighborhood," and "time to pursue own interests" (which could be interpreted to represent either International Survey domains of "Leisure and Recreation" or "Careers" or both). This implies that the Beach Center Survey questions are not as extensive in their coverage of these issues as those in the specific sections of the International Survey, which means that participants cannot expand on issues associated with quality and quantity of education, leisure, involvement in groups or clubs, and careers as they can in the International Survey.

Survey Completion Time

Interviews with the International Survey took between 45 min to 3.5 h (average 1 h and 55 min, *SD* = 50.86), which is similar to the results reported by Isaacs et al., 2007 with the first version of the survey (i.e., 1.5–2 h to administer). The Beach Center Survey interviews took between 20 min to 1 h (average 55 min, *SD* = 13.78). Previous literature reporting use of the Beach Center Survey has not specified the time taken, so comparison was not possible. Surveys that were self-administered by the main caregiver were estimated (by means of the researcher filling out the survey based on their own family life, prior to distributing it to participants) to take less time than the face-to-face interview format (i.e., approximately 40 min for the International Survey and 20 min for the Beach Center Survey). However, of the total 15 participants in this study, only three chose to complete the surveys on their own and they were not asked to record how long they took to complete the survey. The International Survey took longer to complete because it contained more items, and due to the open nature of some of the questions, participants were more stimulated to add comments and explanations than they were with the Beach Center Survey.

Methodology and Survey Designs (Qualitative versus Quantitative; Interview versus Self-administered)

The Beach Center Survey is predominantly quantitative, requesting that participants *only* mark a circle for their responses without providing comments on the form (other than in the General Information section). The International Survey has some open questions and allows for participants to elaborate on the information in each domain. However, when participants self-administered the surveys ($n = 3$), they provided relatively little qualitative information in the International Survey, even though they were given the opportunity to do so. For example, in response to the question about disability-related services needed that they were not currently getting, a self-administered response was: "Social Skills training. Friendship Groups"; and the response from another participant who was interviewed face-to-face was more detailed: "more support from talking to people ... groups and things like that ... some more friends ... and some friends for [member with intellectual disability] ... Someone like him, some other kids that he can have to play with, he's got no one ... go somewhere and meet other kids with special needs and be able to play with them and communicate with them."

When both surveys were conducted in an interview format, far more qualitative information was obtained. During the interview with the Beach Center Survey, the same participant as in the above example provided the following explanation; "I haven't got many friends ... could do with a bit more ... he [member with intellectual disability] needs a lot more support [to make friends] ... I don't know how to work with him ... I think he needs more friends." Although the response to the Beach Center Survey question was not as detailed as the explanation given in response to the International Survey question, it was more than what was provided from self-administered surveys. Another critical point was the wording of the survey questions which led to these explanations by the participant. The first example given above was in response to the International Survey item, "disability-related services you need that you are not currently getting," and hence the participant may have felt motivated to explain more in the hope that the information might be fed back to the services and something would be done about it, whereas the Beach Center Survey did not specifically ask about services needed. The comparative Beach Center Survey questions only asked about the importance of, and satisfaction with, "friends or others who provide support" and "family member with a disability has support to make friends." Thus, participants were asked to provide a more general explanation of their situation and not refer specifically to disability services.

Therefore, both surveys, as currently worded, elicited detailed qualitative information and feedback for services when administered in a face-to-face interview format, but only minimal or no qualitative data when self-administered. There were benefits to both qualitative and quantitative data collection approaches. For self-administration, quantitative methods were appropriate and convenient for the participant (with respect to time to complete and ease of completion). However, if time and resources permit, the face-to-face interview format has been preferred by the developers of the surveys (e.g., see Park et al., 2003) and by those using the surveys, because it can provide supplementary qualitative information concerning the unique needs of family members, including clarification of certain questions, to prevent misinterpretation. This method also assists family members who may not be able to read the surveys – a group who could have been excluded if self-administration was the only option (Park et al., 2003). An advantage of the quantitative method of the Beach Center Survey is its scanning technology, which can be used for convenient and easy entry of the quantitative data points. Both surveys provide quantitative data that can be used for statistical analyses as part of FQOL assessment, but the International Survey also requires expertise in qualitative analysis.

Surveys' Structures and Participants' Experiences of the Interviews

The Beach Center Survey was not split into sections according to FQOL domains, and questions were in random order; therefore, participants were not as aware of the question that was to come next; whereas in the International Survey all questions regarding the same domain were grouped together, meaning that participants felt comfortable once the domain was mentioned to adjust their responses accordingly and provide information about their family situation concerning whatever issue was being asked about. This may have been partly why the International Survey took longer and stimulated more comments. Some participants were uncertain about the exact content of the survey at times. For example, one participant said, "do you want me to talk about that now, or will it be asked about later?". Another participant specified (in the "Health" domain of the International Survey) that there were *no* major physical and/or mental health concerns for other family members; however, at the end of that section she stated, "I was just going to say, with health ... would that [include] depression and stuff like that, because I've been on antidepressants for a while – I just thought of that as well."

Although some participants seemed initially to be apprehensive about providing information (evident by their short answers at the beginning of interviews), once rapport had been established with the interviewer, they seemed to enjoy the opportunity to express their feelings about family life in the context of having a member with a disability. For example, participants made comments after completing the International Survey such as; "it was good to let everything out." Although responses from the Beach Center Survey were generally not as detailed, one mother who only had limited time for the interview with the Beach Center Survey nevertheless commented at the end, "there we go, we got it done in time after all and I got to tell you all about the family," indicating that she felt the survey had adequately considered her FQOL.

Empathy and listening skills of the interviewer were important in order to create a more pleasant experience for the participant. A number of participants had moments of tears and/or deep reflection during the interviews with the International Survey. First, this seemed to be due to the personal and emotional nature of the topics such as, "Support from Other People," which may or may not have been forthcoming. The questions added to the International Survey by the current authors about the past also triggered emotional reactions as family members often reflected on life before the child with a disability, or what family life might be like without the member with a disability. Second, the time spent elaborating on the quantitative questions of the International Survey with qualitative responses enabled participants to reflect on the support (or lack of) that they received, as well as to consider their satisfaction with each FQOL domain. For example, in one case, the interviewer decided not to ask questions associated with "Support from Other People" but instead moved straight on to the next section of the survey, because this participant began to cry as soon as the topic was mentioned. She explained that she did not wish to talk about that aspect of family life because all her relatives were overseas and she did not have anyone else. There were less emotional reactions of this kind to the Beach Center Survey because questions were all quantitative in nature and did not ask about one topic with additional qualitative questions before moving on to another topic. For the same participant as described immediately above, quantitative questions in the Beach Center Survey concerning, "have friends or others who provide support" or "outside help available to take care of special needs of all family members" did not elicit the same emotional reaction. Perhaps this was because the participant did not associate either of these Beach Center Survey questions with her overseas relatives or perhaps these questions led her to think more in terms of formal service provisions. Neither question specifies who "others" or "outside help" may include. Also, since the next item in the Beach Center Survey that follows these questions was not related to the same topic, the participant was not given much opportunity to reflect on the issue that saddened her when she was answering the equivalent International Survey questions.

Empathy and interviewing expertise was also needed for the Beach Center Survey since one person did cry during the interview with it. However, in this case, the tears were due to the participant raising a topic that was not part of the survey; in particular, she expressed feelings of resentment related to having a child with a disability, and how different life could otherwise be. The survey question that was asked prior to this reaction concerned the importance and satisfaction related to "family members talk openly with each other." After giving her quantitative response, the mother went on to explain that it was important for her to have talked with her other children when she was at a very low point in life and that is when she began to cry; "and I told them my concerns of . . . leaving her . . . they have seen me at my worst." She also explained that "when we moved into this house . . . I remember thinking; now, should I put [sibling without disability] in that room or should we put [member with disability] in that room, because what if a car went through . . .?" Here the mother was referring to the fact that she would have preferred her daughter with a disability to have endured the consequences of an accident, over her other children without disabilities. Therefore, interviewing and basic counseling skills were required to deal with the extent to which FQOL questions, whether quantitative or qualitative, elicited emotional reactions of this kind. If controlled and dealt with appropriately, these emotional reactions can make service providers aware of the severity or sensitivity of some FQOL issues. This information might be extremely useful for evaluative purposes in prioritizing different kinds of services for certain families. A suggested addition to the analysis of data from the two surveys would be to record the degree of emotion that arose about particular FQOL issues.

In summary, interviews conducted with both surveys indicated that their structure in terms of FQOL topics was logical and appropriate. However, the International Survey was slightly better in this regard since all items associated with a particular FQOL domain were grouped together, enabling participants to elaborate more easily on that particular aspect. During the development process of both surveys, only those domains considered important to families involved in the pilot studies were included. The current study also confirmed the relevance and importance of the domains insofar as most participants had something to say about each of the FQOL issues. Interpersonal and professional interview skills were also important with respect to ethical considerations in the delivery of both surveys. It is recommended that interviewers receive specific training, and that information be provided to participants about who they could contact to obtain appropriate advice and assistance (e.g., the government's main disability service provider). These ethical considerations were put in place for the current study and proved to be effective, although no one asked for, or was considered in need of, additional counseling. It should be noted that even though participants became emotional when reflecting on their family life during interviews with the International Survey, there was no evidence to suggest that they felt particularly uncomfortable in the interview situation, because no one chose to withdraw from the study, despite being free to do so.

More than One Family Member with a Disability

Six of the 15 (40%) families who completed both surveys had more than one member with a disability. A major advantage of the International Survey is that it has provision for this family demographic by asking participants to talk about each family member with an intellectual or developmental disability separately. The Beach Center Survey does not provide an option for participants to discuss how FQOL is affected by more than one family member with a disability. Instead, it specifies that participants should "consider the one who has the most impact on your family life." Of the six families that had more than one member with a disability, it was notable that all members of the family with a disability had an impact on the family and in different ways. For example, it was revealed in responses to the International Survey, that one family had an 18-year-old child with a developmental disability and behavioral problems including physical aggression toward his mother, while his 10-year-old brother who also had developmental disability did not have any behavioral issues, but was in and out of hospital due to his physical health conditions. This participant also explained that: "[10 year old] has always been jealous of [18 year old brother]." These facts and explanations were not evident in the same participant's responses to the Beach Center Survey. Also, another participant who had two children with a disability was not able to choose one satisfaction rating for the question about "family member with a disability having support to make friends" from the Beach Center survey, because, "[daughter with disability] does alright . . . but [son with disability] needs a lot more . . . [Daughter with disability] is slowly making friends, but [son with disability], needs a lot more support." Even though the Beach Center Survey asked about the family as a whole, there was no opportunity to comment on both family members with a disability and the separate impact of their disabilities on the family. These results indicate that when assessing FQOL, it is necessary to ask about all members with a disability and their individual affects on the family.

"Parenting" Domain – Beach Center Survey

The Beach Center Survey included the FQOL domain "Parenting" while the International Survey did not. The six Beach Center Survey items associated with "Parenting" were: "help children learn to be independent"; "help children with schoolwork and activities"; "teach children how to get along with others"; "teach

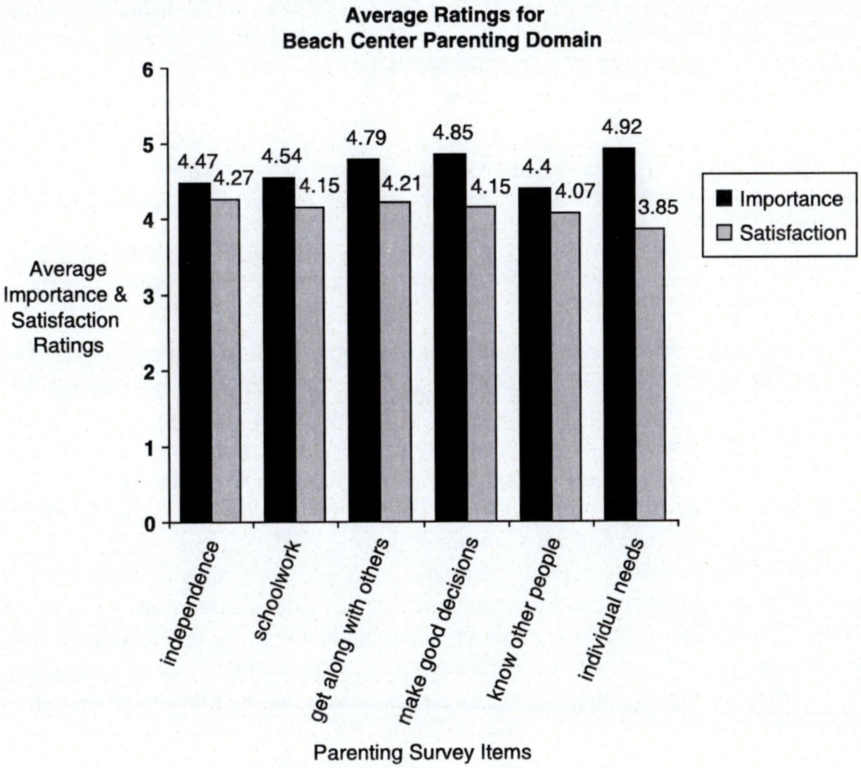

Fig. 17.1 Average ratings for beach centre domain – "parenting"

children to make good decisions"; "adults in my family know other people in the children's lives (friends, teachers, etc.)"; "adults in my family have time to take care of the individual needs of every child." As can be seen in Fig. 17.1, on the Importance scale of 1–5 (from 1 = a little important to 5 = critically important), all participants from the current study rated 3 and above for all of these items except for, "knowing other people in the children's lives," for which one participant specified "a little important." Figure 17.1 also shows that in terms of Satisfaction, the majority were "very satisfied" with "helping children learn to be independent," "helping children with schoolwork," and "teaching children to get along with others." There was more variation in the responses for "teaching good decisions" and "knowing others in the children's lives," but with both still having an average rating of 4 (equivalent to "satisfied").

While all other items associated with "Parenting" were important to participants, the item associated with having "time to take care of the individual needs of every child" in the family was rated the highest in importance yet lowest in satisfaction, suggesting that it is an area of concern in some families, which should be asked about in FQOL measures. In general, participants provided slightly lower satisfaction ratings (Mean = 3.85) to this item, despite the fact that all participants rated it as "critically important" (except one who rated it just below "critically important"). The impact of this issue on FQOL was also evident in the qualitative comments that accompanied these ratings to the Beach Center Survey; for example:

> It is absolutely vital [to take care of the individual needs of every child] . . . but it's not practical . . . it is extremely hard to make sure that all 3 are totally satisfied, especially when you've got a high needs child.
>
> [For] so many months we look[ed] after [member with intellectual disability] but we have another son, we love him too . . . [Member with intellectual disability] needs more care but he [older son] needs love too.

Throughout interviews using both measures almost all participants referred to their other children (i.e., siblings of member with a disability), even though the International Survey did not include any direct questions about this issue. These results suggest that it is very important to explore the impact of having a family member with a disability on siblings – an area of research which has received separate attention in the literature (for example, Hodapp, Glidden, & Kaiser, 2005; M. M. Seltzer, Greenberg, Krauss, Gordon, & Judge, 1997; Strohm, 2002). In many cases, examples were provided by participants in the current study of drastic effects on siblings, which in turn had impacted on FQOL. For example, in response to the Beach Center Survey question a mother explained that it was a very emotional time for her whole family when she started working again and the second sibling had some concerns that she had spoken to a person who ran a siblings support group about; "[sibling 1] had her baby and moved on; [father] was at work; I [mother] was sort of finding my pathway; and all of a sudden she [sibling 2] found out that she was home and [member with disability] was all she had left really, so she was a bit lost, it was the first time that she had seen her sister [member with disability] for who she was and there was no one to talk to . . . it was emotional for us *all*."

Participants also expressed their concerns for siblings when responding to the International Survey, mostly in response to the demographics question that asked participants to state who their other children were. For one mother, the biggest cause for concern for her FQOL was the sibling of the member with an intellectual disability. For example, "they say when somebody in your family has got cancer everybody has got cancer, it's the same . . . he [sibling] gives me a hard time . . . he's [sibling] doing some bad things . . . it's affecting him [sibling] too. . . ." She went on to explain in the section about "Family Relationships" that "I don't receive enough help for [member with intellectual disability] . . . I think sometimes if I receive enough support for [member with intellectual disability's] health, then I'll spend more time with my other son [sibling] when he plays sport . . . maybe I should be there more often . . . things might be different . . . but I can't go . . . can't bring [member with intellectual disability] because he's in a nappy . . ." and "he's [sibling] full of anger." This participant continued to raise this issue throughout the interview with the International Survey. While there was no comparable data from the same participant using the Beach Center Survey, it was clear when comparing these comments to those previously described in response to the Beach Center Survey question, "time to take care of the individual needs of every child," that responses to the Beach Center Survey were a lot shorter and less detailed, but presented the same kinds of issues.

Ratings and averages for groups need to be interpreted with caution, because in this study there were only 15 participants, but for larger samples there may be more variation around the mean. Therefore, it is important to consider not only mean scores, but also any outliers or cases that particularly deviate from the norm. For example, in Fig. 17.2, which shows the individual scores of participants for importance and satisfaction in the Beach Center parenting domain, it is clear that participant 3, who had a learning disability herself, stands out from the other participants. She had indicated that *all* parenting domain items were "critically important," but she was "dissatisfied," implying that she would require further support, as displayed in her response to the question about adults in the family teaching children to make good decisions; "I try but probably it's not perfect enough, but I do try ... I suppose that's probably why I'm seeing a doctor too, because I don't get enough credit for myself for anything .... "

In summary, results show that the Beach Center Parenting domain is an important element of FQOL. However, the most interesting results were in terms of "taking care of the individual needs of every child" and exploring the cases who presented as outliers. FQOL measures should question those elements of Parenting that are important to families. This can be done in a briefer manner than the six questions of the Beach Center survey of presenting. It is suggested that FQOL measures include an open question asking participants to explain any impact of parenting on their

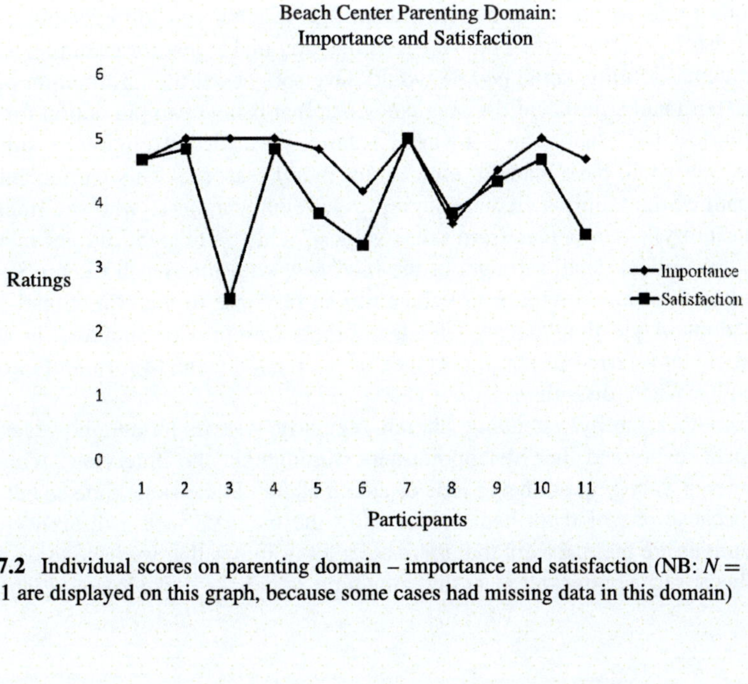

Fig. 17.2 Individual scores on parenting domain – importance and satisfaction (NB: $N = 15$, but only 11 are displayed on this graph, because some cases had missing data in this domain)

FQOL; for example, "are there any elements of raising/bringing up the children that are particularly important to your FQOL, such as taking care of the individual needs of every child; if there are, please explain."

"Influence of Values" Domain – International Survey

The International Survey included the domain "Influence of Values," while the Beach Center Survey did not contain any questions associated with this aspect of FQOL. Every participant who completed the International Survey and responded to the "Influence of Values" section indicated that they held personal values, including personal morals such as; knowing right from wrong ($n = 11$, 73%), but less participants specified that the family had religious ($n = 6$, 40%), spiritual ($n = 4$, 27%) or cultural ($n = 4$, 27%) values. These values were, on average, using a scale of 1–5, rated as "very important" to FQOL ($M = 4.40$, $SD = 1.27$); and most participants were "satisfied" with the degree to which values contributed to FQOL ($M = 4.00$, $SD = .67$). There were no apparent outliers for satisfaction with Values from the 15 participants – all participants had selected from the middle satisfaction option and above. For importance, one participant differed to most of the others in that they selected "hardly important at all" and then went on to select "neither satisfied or dissatisfied," whereas most others had selected "quite" to "very" important. With larger samples, participants who differ substantially from the mean would need to be considered further. Two participants stated that their family held all four areas of values (i.e., personal, religious, spiritual, and cultural), and they provided detailed explanations placing more emphasis on the importance of the "Influence of Values," to their FQOL. For example, one participant explained that "[religious values] has very little to do with ... our beliefs except that it helps you to understand ... It [values] has a profound effect on decisions that you make; just for example, having a child with disability, some people would have sought out the information before she was born and terminated the pregnancy, but that is not even [an option for consideration] for us ... and even if it wasn't a choice we made for religious or spiritual reasons, we would have made it anyway, for moral reasons." This participant further qualified the family's view by saying, "Our appreciation of who she [member with disability] is ... comes from those values." This participant did not mention any of this critical detail throughout the interview with the Beach Center Survey. The only hint of any reference to values was in response to the "Emotional Well-Being" domain question "having friends or others who provide support," in which the participant referred to the importance of having someone to *love and care* for the member with a disability.

For another family, attending church regularly was important; however, the participant expressed her disappointment throughout the interview with the International Survey at not being able to attend church at the same time as her husband, because one of them had to look after the member with a disability; "the opportunities are there, except that there are a lot of things that we have to do alternately because we both can't go at the same time, which we'd like to do ... when he [member with disability] goes to [respite] we go together." In this case the presence of a member with a disability in the family led to restrictions on the family being able to do what they would like to do to maintain their values. This same participant did not refer to their family's values to the same extent during the interview with the Beach Center Survey, despite their obvious importance to the family. The only reference throughout the Beach Center Survey that was associated with religious values was in response to the "Emotional Well-Being" domain of "family members being able to pursue their own interests," in which the participant stated that they belonged to a church choir and a church group, but there was no further detail provided, other than that these groups were "critically important" to them and that they were "very satisfied" with having time to pursue their own interests. Thus, there was an apparent discrepancy between the International Survey qualitative response and the Beach Center Survey Satisfaction rating, insofar as the participant had explained in the International Survey domain on "Influence of Values" that she was disappointed that she could not go to church together with her husband, yet still reported being "very satisfied" with "having time to pursue own interest" in the Beach Center Survey. This suggests that the differences in wording between the two surveys allows for differences in interpretation. Questions therefore need to be as specific as possible, so that participants are prompted to provide specific informative details in their responses.

These results suggest that even though the Beach Center Survey did not have a specific question related to "Influence of Values," participants still had the opportunity to raise issues associated with the "Influence of Values" domain in response to certain questions (for example, in the "Emotional Well-Being" domain) but not to the same extent as was provided by the direct questions on values in the International Survey. There also seemed to be some implied emphasis on values in the Beach Center Survey "Parenting" domain item: "adults in my family teach the children to make good decisions," because at least two participants responded to this question in relation to teaching personal *values*, such as right from wrong; and choices, such as experimenting with illicit substances; for example, "I've done my best ... I've always taught them good values ... I trust my kids ... none of them are [alcohol] drinkers or on drugs or nothing." This information was provided from extra qualitative questions asked by the interviewer, which emphasizes the importance of the interviewer seeking clarification, and it also suggests that all domains of FQOL can be interlinked, depending on the wording of survey items. The difference with placing this item in the "Parenting" domain is in the words "adults in my family *teach* children ..."; if the question purely asked for the importance and satisfaction of "making good decisions" then it would be more appropriately placed in a "Values" domain. The words "adults in my family" also indicate that this is referring to perceived competency of the *adults*, whereas in the International Survey, items related to personal values (which may include personal values of making good decisions), referred to the *family* as a whole.

Given that only 13% (2 out of 15) discussed the "Influence of Values" comprehensively in their responses to the International Survey, it is not necessarily the case that a whole domain or section of the survey should be dedicated to values. However, since participants did mention church groups, religious morals, or personal values such as knowing right from wrong, throughout the International Survey, it is necessary to at least provide the participants with some explicit opportunity to comment directly on how these may or may not influence the ways in which the family deals with disability or copes with stress, etc. For example, participants could be asked: "does your family hold personal, spiritual, cultural, and/or religious values that are important to your FQOL (yes or no)?" and then "if yes, please comment or discuss how they affect FQOL." If the answer is "no," then there need not be a whole domain of questions dedicated to family values.

Transportation

The topic of "transportation" was incorporated into both surveys, but it was not considered in as much detail throughout the International Survey as it was in the Beach Center Survey. During the Beach Center Survey participants were asked "does your child currently need transportation and/or mobility services" (item 9) and "does your family currently need transportation" (item 19). Both were followed by "if yes, how much service does your family get?" In the FQOL section of the Beach Center Survey under the domain of "Practical/Material Well-Being," the questions "how important is it that my family members have transportation to get to the places they need to be," followed by "how satisfied am I that my family members have transportation to get to the places they need to be" (item 6) elicited much discussion by family members. The International Survey did not specifically ask about transportation, but it was a response option included in the "Health" domain as a possible barrier to the family accessing health care; and then in the "Support from Services" domain as an option for why the family was not receiving the disability-related services they need.

Four (27%) participants mentioned transportation as an issue affecting FQOL during the interview with the International Survey. Of these four, only one also mentioned the same specific transportation issue in the interview with the Beach Center Survey and the other three cases (see examples below) did not present any concerns with transportation throughout the Beach Center Survey.

1. "Support from Services" domain: In response to the question: "Are there disability-related services you need that you are not currently getting?", the participant explained a need for transportation training; "Bus training . . . anytime that she had to go anywhere by bus . . . ." This mother explained that she had to train her daughter herself to be able to independently catch public transport, but she would have liked some formal assistance from the services with incorporating this critical skill into her child's life. This was not discussed in any part of the interview with the Beach Center Survey, but instead lack of funding and the need for more mobility allowance was mentioned with respect to transportation.
2. "Support from Services" domain: In response to the question "Why are you not receiving the disability-related services you need?" the participant had at first

said that transportation was not a problem, but later recalled; "Come to think of it, transport can be a problem; one of the reasons is because they need 10 days notice to change anything for the transport to and from school if we use it ... and the other thing is that you never quite know when they're going to arrive ... the kids have to go to two separate schools ... the issue I have is ... how do I coordinate?" [PCM0032]. There was no mention of transportation issues in any part of the interview with the Beach Center Survey for this participant.

3. "Financial Well-Being" and "Leisure and Recreation" domains: "The car I had, I had problems with it, then I brought this one, now I've got problems with it ... as it is now, I've got to borrow the money so I can go get the starter motor and things fixed ..." and then later on the participant was talking about the activities that the family takes part in, such as going to the Christmas pageant; "At the moment ... I can't live without a car ... when you do have transport, life's a lot easier." Once again, these issues were absent from comments and explanations in the Beach Center Survey.

Results from the Beach Center Survey showed that 12 (80%) family members considered transport as "critically important"; two (13%) rated it just below "critically important," and one (7%) indicated that it was "important." There were more varied responses for participants' satisfaction with transport; just over half (eight participants, 53%) were "very satisfied," three (20%) were "satisfied," three (20%) were "neither satisfied nor dissatisfied," and one (7%) was "very dissatisfied." Of the six (40%) participants who presented problems or negative concerns associated with transportation, only one of these same issues had also been mentioned in the interview using the International Survey. This means that these problems with transportation would not have otherwise been presented by participants with just the International Survey, suggesting that even though "transportation" was incorporated into other domains of the International Survey, the wording of such questions elicited different interpretations and hence different responses from participants.

Fifty-three percent of participants commented on the importance of having a family car to get around and that it was critical for at least one of the parents to have a driver's license; "I couldn't imagine catching buses ... if I had to catch a bus I just wouldn't go anywhere." All of these families, except one who selected "neither" satisfied or dissatisfied, indicated that they were "satisfied" or "very satisfied" with respect to transportation at the moment. For example, two participants discussed how it may become more difficult once the father of the member with a disability becomes too old to be able to drive a car; "Having a car to get around is important and as long as [father of member with disability] can still drive then it's okay" and, "One day when [father] loses his license ... at the moment we don't need [help] ... in future, yes [we will need help with transport]." These comments suggest that there is a need to ask about any future concerns with respect to family issues although neither survey specifically asked about this. Even though many (40%) commented on the availability of public transport (i.e., trains and buses), some (33% of participants who commented on public transport) expressed dissatisfaction with certain elements of it, such as running late or not being able to read timetables easily; for example, "There could be more transport at a lot of different places ... places where I can't go, which I'm too frightened to go because I don't think there's any bus routes there ... so if there's not bus routes and you don't know how to get there well you can't go." Furthermore, a few participants (33%) discussed the use of Taxi services, particularly to and from school, which was usually a service that families considered critical and was free to families having a child with a disability. Some children's access to school is provided for by the public education system but not all, and adults do not receive such assistance with transport to work or day activities. Another cause for dissatisfaction with respect to transportation was that there was no extra funding to help pay for transportation. A few participants (20%) talked about "mobility allowance" and the little amount of government support they received to help cover the cost associated with transporting the family member with a disability; "we have got two cars, it's more just the cost associated with them that is a problem." For another participant, the school bus, which used to be a free service, was no longer being provided to her daughter due to her behavior and her refusing to wear a seat belt correctly, so now she was expected to pay for transportation herself; " ...she [member with disability] played up last week and the bus driver said 'nup [nope] she's not coming back at all' ... they won't have her back on the bus ... she got booted off [the school bus] ... it's costing me 80 dollars a week in petrol at the moment." These results suggest that there should be some questions concerning the costs of family transport in the financial section of FQOL surveys, as well as an opportunity for participants to discuss transportation openly as an issue impacting FQOL. In conclusion, judging from responses to the Beach Center Survey items associated with transport and the few comments received in response to the International Survey, transportation and its associated costs are important elements of FQOL that should be directly incorporated in to FQOL surveys, either in a separate domain or in the domains "Support from Services" or "Financial Well-Being."

Differences in the Measurement Concepts of Both Surveys

The measurement concepts of Importance and Satisfaction were used in both surveys; however, measures for Opportunities, Attainment, Initiative, and Stability were only used in the International Survey. Results from the current study are discussed mainly in terms of comparisons in the use of the Importance and Satisfaction ratings, but comments are also provided on the Opportunities, Attainment, Initiative, and Stability concepts.

Importance and Satisfaction

Table 17.3 shows that for the 15 participants in the current study there were some consistencies and inconsistencies between the responses from the two measures in terms of what was considered to be most and least important, and elements

Table 17.3 Most and Least Important and Satisfied Domains from Both Surveys ($N = 15$)

	Importance		Satisfaction	
	Most	Least	Most	Least
International survey	1. Health $M = 5.00$ $SD = 0.000$	1. Practical support from other people $M = 3.60$ $SD = 1.647$	1. Family relationships $M = 4.77$ $SD = 0.439$	1. Financial well-being $M = 3.15$ $SD = 0.899$
	2. Family relationships $M = 5.00$ $SD = 0.000$	2. Emotional support from other people $M = 4.09$ $SD = 1.221$	2. Practical and emotional support from other people $M = 4.09$ $SD = 0.831$	2.Community interaction $M = 3.89$ $SD = 1.054$
	3. Financial well-being $M = 4.58$ $SD = 0.515$	3. Support from services $M = 4.38$ $SD = 1.121$	3. Leisure and recreation $M = 4.08$ $SD = 0.669$	3. Support from services $M = 3.92$ $SD = 0.760$
Beach center survey	1. Family interaction: Love $M = 4.93$ $SD = .258$	1. Emotional Well-being: Outside help available to help the family $M = 4.00$ $SD = 1.363$	1. Disability-related support: to accomplish goals at home $M = 4.46$ $SD = 0.519$	1. Emotional well-being: outside help available to help the family $M = 3.25$ $SD = 1.288$
	2. Physical/ material well-being: Medical $M = 4.93$ $SD = 0.258$	2. Disability-related support: relationships with the service providers $M = 4.40$ $SD = 0.910$	2. Physical/ material well-being: Medical $M = 4.27$ $SD = 1.100$	2. Emotional well-being: Time to pursue own interests $M = 3.46$ $SD = 1.56$
	3. Physical/ material well-being: Safety $M = 4.93$ $SD = 0.258$	3. Parenting: Learn independence $M = 4.47$ $SD = 0.743$	3. Parenting: Learn independence $M = 4.27$ $SD = 1.100$	3. Physical/ material well-being: Having a way to take care of expenses $M = 3.47$ $SD = 1.302$

of FQOL that families were most and least satisfied with. Consistencies included high importance placed on: "Family Interaction" ("Family Relationships") and "Physical/Material Well-Being" ("Health"; "Financial Well-Being"). Participants also consistently reported that "Support from Other People" (including service providers) was slightly less important, although it was still well above an average rating. The results were less consistent with respect to satisfaction insofar as the International Survey showed highest satisfaction with "Family Relationships," while the Beach Center Survey showed highest satisfaction with "Disability-Related Support: To accomplish goals at home." Similarly, the lowest satisfaction scores were in the domain of "Financial Well-Being" for the International Survey, and "Emotional Well-Being: Outside help available to help the family" for the Beach Center Survey. However, as with importance, all satisfaction scores were above an average rating. Some of the varied responses between the two surveys for satisfaction and importance ratings of FQOL can be attributed to the different wording used in each survey. For example, participants reported that they were "satisfied" with "Leisure and Recreation" in the International Survey, but this was not a domain included in the Beach Center Survey. Similarly, for the Beach Center Survey participants reported that teaching their children to learn to be independent was important, but this was not a question in the International Survey. Importantly, even though these variations between the two surveys exist, participants generally reported that all FQOL domains were important. Even though participants were "dissatisfied" in some areas, the mean satisfaction ratings were still reasonably high for most of the domains in both surveys. However, these data are based on only 15 participants from Australia. More data need to be collected and further comparisons need to be made in order to generalize results about the concepts of Importance and Satisfaction. When interpreting quantitative results, however, it is important to consider not only mean scores and standard deviations, but also individual differences and any outliers. In practical terms, there may be "outlier" families who might be in desperate need of urgent assistance. For service providers, just looking at high mean satisfaction scores for a group might suggest there is no need for any urgent interventions or any change in services; whereas investigating cases who stand out from the rest (e.g., those who score low satisfaction in domains that other participants are satisfied with) can enable further support and assistance to be provided and/or facilitate changes in service provision. A particular strength of both surveys' measurement concepts is that they allow participants to express dissatisfaction in elements of FQOL that they have indicated as being important to their families.

In spite of some inconsistencies in relative ratings, the generally high mean Importance and Satisfaction ratings in both surveys support their concurrent validity. In order to assess their concurrent validity further, correlations were run on the survey items that were directly related. Table 17.4 shows three areas of FQOL that were included in both surveys and it can be seen that they correlated highly, with Pearson's Correlation Coefficients between .5 and .9. While definite conclusions cannot be drawn on the basis of only 15 participants, the results do suggest that the surveys measure similar constructs within the FQOL domains.

Opportunities, Initiative, Attainment, Stability

A few participants did not seem to know how to respond to, or they did not understand what was meant by, the International Survey's concepts; Opportunities, Initiative, Attainment, and Stability. Certain questions such as: "are there opportunities for members of your family to . . . ?" (Opportunities) or "to what degree do

Table 17.4 Correlations between specific survey items (Importance and Satisfaction)

	Beach Center Survey items				
International survey domains	Medical (satisfaction)	Take care of expenses (importance)	Take care of expenses (satisfaction)	Time to pursue own interests (importance)	Time to pursue own interests (satisfaction)
Health (satisfaction)	$r = 0.744$ $p = 0.004$*	–	–	–	–
Financial well-being (importance)	–	$r = 0.683$ $p = 0.014$**	–	–	–
Financial well-being (satisfaction)	–	–	$r = 0.597$ $p = 0.031$**	–	–
Leisure and recreation (importance)	–	–	–	$r = 0.553$ $p = 0.077$	–
Leisure and recreation (satisfaction)	–	–	–	–	$r = 0.842$ $p = 0.002$*

NB: Health/medical (importance) has not been included here because for the international survey all participants selected "very important," meaning that the variable was constant.
Significant at the *$p<0.01$ level; **$p < 0.05$ level.

members of your family enjoy good health?" (Attainment) resulted in participants asking "what does that mean?". These International Survey questions sometimes required further explanations by means of the interviewer elaborating on exactly what was being asked and rewording the question. For example, "are there opportunities for your family to . . . ?" was changed to "is it possible for your family to . . .?" or "are there restrictions on . . . ?" and only then was the participant able to select from the quantitative options. This lack of understanding the question at first could be due to vagueness of the words "opportunities" or "enjoy." While these difficulties in interpreting the concepts only occurred to a limited extent in the current study, with larger samples it could be problematic, particularly if the survey is being self-administered because there is no opportunity available for an interviewer to explain the concepts.

Furthermore, three of the 15 (20%) main caregiver participants from the current study stated that they had learning disabilities themselves, and these participants needed to be carefully considered and accommodated accordingly. For example, the items associated with the measurement concepts in the International Survey needed to be reworded, but this was not the case for any of the Beach Center Survey questions. For people self-administering the surveys who may have difficulties reading and/or understanding the questions due to their own disability, it is important to provide easily understood questions and ratings. For example, one participant stated at the very beginning of the interview using the International Survey that "we [participant and her 9 year old daughter] have problems understanding what people say ... so you have to explain it over and over again so we understand what you mean ... ." In order to ensure ease of understanding, it is important for individual questions to only address a single issue. Future research needs to explore this issue further to ensure that questions are worded so that participants are capable of providing accurate FQOL information and that missing data and/or very low scores indicate a real need for support, and not just a misunderstanding of questions.

Repetitiveness of Measurement Concepts and Limitations to Likert Scale

During interviews using the International Survey, when responding to questions from Section B of each domain (i.e., the six measurement concepts), many participants found the concepts and their associated quantitative options repetitive. For example, by the time the survey reached Section 6 ("Values" domain) and after 2 h of being interviewed, one main caregiver said "this is getting a bit repetitive isn't it?". Problems with the repetitive nature of parts of the International Survey were also illustrated by one mother, who when phoned and invited to participate in the Beach Center Survey, after having completed the International Survey previously, stated that she was happy to participate again, "as long as it is not as repetitive as the last one." When questioned about this comment, the participant indicated that she was referring to Section B (the six measurement concepts) of each part of the International Survey. This participant did not make similar comments about the Beach Center Survey, but instead commented at the end of the interview: "that was OK." However, participants did express some concerns about the repetitiveness of the quantitative questions for *both* surveys. To avoid the Beach Center Survey also becoming tedious due to its predominantly quantitative nature involving ratings, the interviewer found it necessary, in order to maintain rapport and to supplement the quantitative information, to ask extra questions, such as "what do you mean by that?" or "can you please explain that?" For example, the interviewer added to the Beach Center FQOL question about support to relieve stress, "what sorts of avenues do you go to for that kind of support, when you need to relieve stress?" and the participant responded, "I just talk to family that's all ... my mum ... and friends." It is recommended that such questions be added to the surveys, not only to avoid repetitiveness, but also in order to check that participants have understood and interpreted the questions correctly, as well as to better understand the details associated with satisfaction or dissatisfaction. In the above example, it was unclear until the additional open question was asked, as to who or which service the participant was referring to when she stated that it was "critically important" and that she was "very satisfied" with having support to relieve stress.

Many participants found the 5-point Likert scale options in both surveys to be limiting, and most chose to explain their situation further whether or not there was a direct qualitative question being asked of them. "Missing data" from the current study was not necessarily the result of participants misunderstanding the questions, or from accidentally missing questions when completing the surveys themselves, but may have also been because participants found it difficult to select a rating. For example, for the Beach Center Survey FQOL question asking about the degree of satisfaction with the family enjoying spending time together, one participant chose not to select a satisfaction rating, but instead differentiated by saying that when the family does get the chance to spend time together it is good; "Are you talking about the quality or quantity? . . . I am happy with the quality, not happy with the quantity." This same participant also broke down his satisfaction ratings for the Beach Center Survey FQOL question about outside help to take care of the family; "Are we talking about [disability service provider/Autism service provider] or are we talking about family wise . . .? The services we are very happy . . . [but with relatives, friends and neighbors we are] neither [satisfied or dissatisfied] . . . they are too busy." In some instances participants decided not to select a general satisfaction rating for the whole family, because it was very different for different family members. For example, in the interview with the Beach Center Survey, one mother explained that she was "very dissatisfied" with having time to pursue her own interests, because she needed sleep and was doing housework whenever she had a free moment; but she was "neither" satisfied or dissatisfied with the kids having time to pursue their own interests, because they were all able to do what they wanted to. Similarly, in response to the Careers – Opportunities question from the International Survey, one participant felt that she could not select a rating, because it was different for her and her husband; "very limited for me . . . with my husband yes [there are opportunities] and that's our choice that it would be him that would pursue it rather than me . . . the reality is that there aren't too many three day a week jobs where we can each have a three day a week job . . . and he can probably earn more in his one job pursuing his career than we could doing that anyway." These results once again emphasize the need for questions in both surveys to be revised and worded carefully to avoid perceived ambiguity as much as possible. These issues also support the use of the interview format whenever possible, which enables additional questions to be asked to clarify the participant's interpretation, and to understand participant's family experiences more clearly.

High Importance, Consistencies, and Contradictions of Ratings

Consistent with the literature and previous results using both surveys, participants in this study often selected at the high importance end of the scale (i.e., "very important" or "critically important") for almost all elements of FQOL in both measures. As explained by Hoffman et al. (2006) the little variation in responses to importance was expected, given that the surveys were designed to efficiently represent factors that were of high relevance to FQOL. The same result is evident in the sample Standard Deviations in Table 17.3 where it can be seen that all FQOL items were relevant to all families, because there was very little dispersion around the mean and the mean was usually closest to the highest importance rating. As a result, responses tended to become quite repetitive. Arguably, since we already know (from the background development of both surveys and the current results) that the FQOL indicators presented to participants are important to FQOL, the value of continuing to ask participants about importance is questionable. However, the case for continuing to ask about importance is that it is useful to explore outliers, in which particular caregivers stand out from the rest, because they have specified that certain elements were not important to their family. In these instances it is critical to obtain explanations of why certain elements are not so important to FQOL. For example, for one participant, Support from Services was "not very [important] but it's nice to know it's there ... For me ... individually it's nice to know that it's there but for others it'd be very important. ... ." This participant was viewing her family's situation in light of what it could be like or in comparison to other families, and this critical explanation may not have been obtained if the survey was self-administered.

An advantage of the International Survey was that participants had the chance to explain their family story or circumstances first in each of the domains, and then they were able to reflect on how important various elements were and how satisfied they were with them. In addition, the second to last question of the International Survey asked participants to rate how satisfied they are with their FQOL overall (from 1 = "very dissatisfied" to 5 = "very satisfied"). Overall satisfaction ratings were found to be consistent with the satisfaction ratings that participants chose for the individual domains. The Beach Center Survey did not allow for participants to explain their situation first, nor did it ask for an overall FQOL rating. This resulted in some notable inconsistencies between quantitative ratings and qualitative explanations. For example, one mother selected "very satisfied" to the Beach Center Survey FQOL item "family enjoys spending time together," but then went on to explain that, "[sibling 1] is jealous of [sibling 2] and they don't get on too well. This disappoints [their father]," and even though the participant had responded with the quantitative option just before "very satisfied" about family members supporting each other to accomplish goals, the participant then went on to state: "sadly I don't think it happens." These comments would be more consistent with a rating at the "dissatisfied" end of the scale. There were some contradictions between quantitative and qualitative responses to the International Survey too. For example, one respondent did not select an Importance rating for the domain of "Leisure and Recreation," because "I don't know how important it is because I don't have it," but then went on to indicate "satisfied" for the satisfaction rating of the same domain. The extent of such inconsistencies needs to be explored with larger sample groups since they only occurred for a few individuals in the present study. These examples once again indicate the need, whenever possible, to obtain qualitative explanations to accompany the quantitative ratings in both surveys, in order to check the accuracy of ratings and to better understand FQOL.

Summary and Conclusions Associated with Measurement Concepts

Questions concerning Opportunities, Initiative and Attainment (in the International Survey) were designed to determine whether participants made efforts or were actually able to acquire particular elements of FQOL, such as socializing outside the family and receiving practical and emotional support. However, some participants had problems understanding some of these concepts and their ratings. The usefulness of asking about Opportunities, Initiative, and Attainment *separately* was also found to be questionable, because most participants indicated that the opportunities do exist but restrictions placed on the family by having a child with a disability mean that the opportunities cannot be taken up. For example, one mother explained that when it comes to socializing outside of the family, "often you decline invitations because ... then you think about will [member with disability] be home alone ... tend to not bother, it's too hard." Accordingly, quantitative results need to be interpreted with caution; and interviews are recommended whenever possible in order to clarify the participants' understanding of the measurement concepts; and to obtain further explanations of why participants chose certain options for each of the additional measurement concepts.

The Initiative concept was designed partly to determine whether the reason for not obtaining certain elements of FQOL was due to lack of effort by the family to acquire them. For example, one mother became very emotional when responding to the Support from Other People section as she indicated that the family makes "a little" bit of effort ("Initiative") to get practical and emotional support; and followed again by explaining in response to the "Attainment" question that the family does not receive as much support from others as they would like, "...but then that's probably our fault as well, because you don't tend to ... you don't ask for it." This was a common theme for many participants, particularly those who indicated that they were more likely to put in the effort to make themselves heard, resulting in obtaining what they required. These participants commented that they believed that they can attain particular elements of FQOL if they make the effort. For example, when talking about Support Services one mother said, "...I've done it all ... if I wasn't the sort of person that I was, [my son with a disability] would have fallen through the cracks, because there isn't enough out there ... I worry so much for the ones that just don't give a damn about their kids ... there must be a lot of children falling through the cracks, which is a damn shame." This discussion about the amount of effort or initiative needed in order to obtain required services was also present in the qualitative responses to the Beach Center Survey, even though it was not directly asked about. Generally, when participants were provided with the opportunity to discuss obtaining their service needs they would mention that they personally had to put in a lot of effort. For example, with respect to physical/occupational therapy, one participant explained that "they [special school] do [provide it], but only if you ring up and say you want something ... ." These results suggest that the measurement concepts of Opportunities, Initiative, and Attainment the International Survey are interrelated and should continue to be asked about and assessed in FQOL measures. However, they may be more accurately assessed by not asking them as separate constructs and not as quantitative ratings. Such a question could be reworded as, "Discuss what is *possible* and what is *difficult* to obtain with the *effort* your family makes to *obtain* the *desired* outcome for [each FQOL domain]?" With the key words (in italics in the above statement) in place, FQOL surveys could add qualitative questions such as "please comment" or "please provide examples."

The Stability concept served the purpose of finding out about the families' perceptions of their future, with respect to whether they think certain areas of FQOL will improve, stay the same or decline. While all participants understood this question, a common response was "I don't know." The majority also indicated that while they would *like* and *hope* for it to improve, they were uncertain as to whether or not that would be the case. Uncertainty about the future was found to impact on present FQOL, particularly with respect to "fear of the unknown." This supports the inclusion of questions about Stability to fully understand present FQOL (see section on "Past and Distant Future" of this chapter for further details and evidence).

Overall, questions on Opportunities, Initiative, Attainment, and Stability enabled the International Survey to cover FQOL far more comprehensively than the Beach Center Survey, which needs to incorporate similar types of questions. However, while the current results support the validity of the Importance and Satisfaction measurement constructs, it also confirmed that all FQOL domains were generally important to most families. Accordingly, it is questionable whether it is worth the additional time required to repeat this question for all domains. It might be worth considering a more general question as to whether there are any of the domains, or aspects of them, that are particularly important to the participant and if so, why? It could then be asked if there are any domains, or aspects of them, that are of little importance to them, and if so, why not? For domains indicated as being of little importance there may be no need to continue to ask about them, once it has been explained as to why/why not that area is/is not important to the family.

Past and Distant Future

> As [member with intellectual disability] gets older it's harder to get respite from the responsibilities of caring for her, it's harder to get people to be willing to take caring for her on. And that in turn affects all of us ... when she was younger she was just a baby like any other baby to care for ....

Previous research has not explored the effects on present FQOL of significant events in the past, or those anticipated in the more distant future. Family well-being is subject to change (for better or worse) depending on events or transitions that may enhance, disrupt, or unsettle everyday family routines (R. I. Brown, Davey, et al., 2004; Llewellyn, Thompson, et al., 2003; Owen et al., 2002; Rapanaro, Bartu, & Lee, 2008). Esbensen and Benson (2006), who conducted their research on individuals with disabilities and not their families, found that people with intellectual disabilities who experienced more life events, such as changes associated with family, work, and social activities, reported more depressive symptoms and more behavior problems. These results highlight the importance of gaining information about life events or issues in the past and anticipated for the distant future. Research to date has not explored these issues in relation to FQOL; and neither the International Survey nor the Beach Center Survey questioned how elements of the family may have changed over time, particularly with respect to the significance of past events.

Based on comments made by family members in the present pilot study, asking about past circumstances or events was important, and in some cases essential, to understand how FQOL had changed over time and how present FQOL continued to be affected by past events. Accordingly, the following questions concerning the past were added to the interviews:

1. Has your immediate family changed over the past few years and, if so, in what ways?
2. In the past, has your family's [Health/Financial Situation/Relationships/Support from Others/Support from Services/Values/Careers/Leisure and Recreation/Community Interaction – i.e., for each domain/section of the International Survey] been any different to what it is now? If yes, please explain when and why (including before children were born)?
3. In the past, has your *overall* family quality of life been any different to what it is now (including before the child with a disability was born, or at relevant transitional periods)?

In the current study all except one of the 15 participants (93%) presented issues about significant past family event/s that impacted negatively on their present FQOL including, a major health concern for any family member; a change in career, such as main caregiver giving up their job in order to care for the member with a disability; or illness/death of close relative who had provided support in the past, leading to a decrease in FQOL. Seven participants (47%) described a change for the better including, a new partner to the main caregiver, resulting in extra support for the whole family; or more support services now, such as extra respite. These concerns were raised in response to the additional questions added by the current researchers, and not in response to direct questions as part of the existing surveys. Of the 15 participants, only about 4 (27%) raised these issues incidentally, during informal discussions throughout interviews. This indicates that participants are not likely to mention such points, unless the additional direct questions about the past are asked. Nevertheless, issues of the past can impact on present FQOL. For example, a father explained that "if you came to me, say 5, 6 years ago this [answers to the survey] would have been totally different." This participant explained that he was very stressed out in the past, due to being home constantly with his son who has an intellectual disability and significant behavioral issues. Under the doctor's advice, this participant stated that *now* FQOL is far better, because he has returned to work and the member with an intellectual disability participates in day activities. Therefore a significant change made in the past resulted in better present FQOL.

With respect to the possible effect of concerns about the future on present FQOL, the International Survey did ask participants about their perceptions of the Stability of FQOL domains in the *near* future (e.g., over the upcoming couple of years), in terms of whether they anticipated improvement or decline, but neither survey directly asked about how participants anticipated the *distant* future (e.g., over the next 10–20 years). In the current pilot study, none of the participants mentioned issues about the distant future and so no questions of this kind were added to the two surveys. However, such issues about the distant future did emerge, suggesting that questions about concerns related to the distant future need to be added to FQOL surveys. In response to questions about the future in the International Survey and/or as part of general comments throughout interviews, most participants in the current study mentioned that in their experience, medical, vocational, and accommodation services, which are more important in adulthood and which can be expensive, must be sought out by parent-caregivers and paid for by the family. For example,

> We [parents] can get a bit down from time to time because we have anxieties for the future of the children. Will they get jobs or the careers they want? Where will they be? . . . People have told them just to take their pension and be happy with that . . . that crushes any hopes of being able to work "normal" jobs . . . they can work with normal people and not just earn a measly $10 per week . . . people give the impression that because they have a disability then they cannot work in the mainstream.

Present FQOL was also found to be negatively affected by the belief that fewer resources would be available when the member with a disability is older, than were available when the child with a disability was younger. These concerns were only raised incidentally throughout interviews. The following examples from interviews illustrate how concerns for the near and distant future, including transition from school to adulthood (a separate area of research, e.g., Blacher, 2001; Glidden & Jobe, 2007; Jokinen & Brown, 2005; Nuehring & Sitlington, 2003); accommodation; and what will happen to the child when the parents die, can impact on current family life:

> [When member with disability leaves school] I've pretty well been told that she won't get anything – none of the workshops, because of her behavior . . . Options [disability service] won't do anything until she's actually ready to leave school.
>
> They [disability-related support services] will be somewhat important later I think . . . when he's out on his own . . . because that's a bit of a problem . . . we [main caregivers] can't live forever and whether it's more important to get [member with disability] settled before we "move on" [die] . . . I don't know . . . we've already got his name down for housing trust and accommodation . . .
>
> I want *** [member with disability] to go [die] before me coz [because] then I won't have to worry about her . . . Do I take her with me [when I die]? . . . how do I take her with me? . . . who can look after her? . . . who's gonna [going to] put up with her? . . . They [sisters] know that they won't be left with caring for ***.

These examples show that parents were worried at the present time about these anticipated future issues, and a considerable amount of time was being spent looking for viable options for the future. Supports from services for these areas of future need (e.g., careers and accommodation) were often not forthcoming. Despite their apparent influence on current FQOL, especially evident by the fact that family members felt the need to talk about these issues during the interviews, neither survey addressed such issues concerning the distant future and their possible affects on present FQOL. Instead, these issues were raised incidentally in response to other questions. For example, in response to the Beach Center Survey question about making friends, which did not specify anything about the past or the future, one participant said, "when he gets to a group home it'll be important." This indicates that the participant was concerned about introducing something new (help with making friends) into the life of the member with intellectual disability in the future.

For the purpose of service provision, measures of FQOL need to include questions about the past and the distant future in order to more fully understand present

FQOL and the way it has changed and is likely to change at different developmental stages. This information can also help current disability services provide more appropriate support, including relevant information about disability services for the future of the family. Such information might also enable disability services to schedule future specific support resources for families and to plan transition services that can prepare families to better cope with the developmental transitions when they occur. Being aware that such services will be available might also reduce the anxiety felt by parents about the future of their child with a disability and hence improve their present FQOL.

Conclusions & Recommendations for FQOL Measures

FQOL is an important area of research, because more people with disabilities are now living at home with their family rather than in alternative care settings. Results from the current study show support for a multidimensional framework to measure FQOL, including domains that encompass a wide range of objective and subjective aspects associated with family life such as support from disability-related services; leisure activities; involvement in the community; and material or physical well-being. This was to be expected given that both the International Survey and the Beach Center Survey were developed on the basis of the practical experiences of families having a member with a disability, and relevant statistical analyses by the developers have shown that the surveys are reliable. The current study contributes to cross cultural validation of the surveys, because both were found to be culturally relevant to issues concerning families that have a member with a disability in Australia. Both surveys also demonstrated good face validity and proved to be user-friendly insofar as there were no FQOL domains, or items in the surveys that seemed problematic or irrelevant to the FQOL of the participants. It can therefore be recommended that both surveys continue to be used as measures of FQOL. Within both surveys there were considerable similarities between the domains, and in each survey participants were asked to indicate their responses to Importance and Satisfaction levels on a 5-point Likert Scale. However, the International Survey also asked about Opportunities, Attainment, Initiative, and Stability, which, despite some issues with interpretation and understanding of the wording, provided additional useful information relevant to FQOL; even though it did make the International survey more repetitive than the Beach Center Survey. As a result, the International Survey does provide a more comprehensive assessment of FQOL domains, although its greater number of items means that it takes longer (average of 1 hr and 55 min compared with 55 min) than the Beach Center Survey to complete. The International Survey also elicited more qualitative comments because it presented all items in a domain/topic consecutively before moving on to the next domain/topic, with survey items organized into logical sections (as opposed to the Beach Center Survey design of items being presented in a random order).

Each survey may be more or less appropriate for research purposes or service provisions depending on the amount of detailed information required, the time available, the cost to administer, and/or the number of families to be assessed. Some research projects may only require particular information from the shorter Beach Center Survey, while some service assessments may find the longer, International Survey useful for individual families in crisis. The shorter Beach Center Survey may be more desirable for service providers undertaking outcome evaluations. However, the Beach Center Survey elicited less-detailed responses, and did not result in the substantial qualitative information required for other types of research that was provided by the International Survey. The International Survey developers have taken these different requirements into consideration by developing a short and long version of their survey. Since the short version was not used in the current study, it requires further research to evaluate its relative advantages and disadvantages. The extra qualitative data obtained from interviews with the Beach Center Survey in the current study cannot be compared with qualitative data from other studies using the Beach Center Survey, because they mostly used self-administration and have not specified whether follow-up interviews were conducted.

While all domains of FQOL were considered by participants to be important, Transportation was found to be a particularly important issue for many families. The Beach Center Survey covered this issue in detail and resulted in families explaining that having means (e.g., a family car, or taxi/bus service) for transporting the member with an intellectual disability around was critical to making life easier for the family. Another area of particular concern was being able to take care of the individual needs of every child in the family; for example, participants described the often negative effects on the siblings of the member with a disability, which in turn impacted the whole FQOL. For the six participants who had more than one family member with a disability, it was found to be necessary to provide them with the opportunity to talk about all family members with a disability (as allowed for by the International Survey) and not just the one who has "the most impact on the family" (as required in the Beach Center Survey). It was critical to understand the impact that more than one member with a disability can have on the family as a whole. Further to this, the Beach Center Survey item, "knowing others in the children's lives (i.e., friends, teachers)" from the "Parenting" domain did not appear to be as important as other items such as "teach the children to make good decisions" or "have time to take care of the individual needs of every child." Likewise, the International Survey domain "Influence of Values" was found to be of some importance to participants, but not of as high importance as other domains, such as "Health of the Family" or "Family Relationships." Revisions of these survey measures and future FQOL measures need to consider incorporating all of the abovementioned elements in order to provide a more comprehensive and useful assessment of FQOL.

During interviews with both surveys it was found useful, and in some cases necessary, to ask additional questions about family life in the past and in the anticipated future in order to adequately understand present FQOL issues. In many cases significant family events in the past were found to have an impact on present FQOL, and apprehension about anticipated FQOL issues in the distant future was also of present concern for many families. These concerns about the past and the future were raised in almost all domains of FQOL. For example, many Australian families were very concerned about the support from services that would be available in the future, because the amount and quality of support was perceived to vary according to the age of the member with a disability, with early childhood receiving the most family-based support. The results of the present study suggest that it is important to consider service provision, and information provided about such service provision, across the lifespan, because the impact of having a member with a disability can be different for different family members at different times.

Overall, the results of the present study suggest that both surveys are efficient measures of FQOL. However, both measures could be improved by some modifications, revisions, and refinement. For example, interview results suggested that it is critical to supplement quantitative data with qualitative information, and self-administered surveys should be followed up with face-to-face interviews where possible. Such interviews might involve asking questions about relevant past events and any concerns about the future. This is particularly important to clarify any apparent inconsistencies in the results. In a practical sense, it is not sufficient for service providers to acquire information that families are dissatisfied with respect to disability-related support; service providers need to know *why* main caregivers are expressing this dissatisfaction, and in order to obtain this information qualitative methods are required. Hence, it is suggested that face-to-face interviews using the surveys (rather than self-administration) should be preferred, in order to obtain more detailed, in-depth qualitative information. However, further research is needed with a larger sample of participants self-administering the surveys, in order to more accurately compare the user-friendliness, amount and quality of information obtained between the self-administered and interview formats.

Limitations to the Current Study and Further Research

The main aim of the current study was to compare the results of the two measures for the purpose of understanding the surveys' validity and applicability in an Australian context. This study did not consider the practical use of the surveys by service providers or policymakers. Internationally, both surveys have been found to be useful for service delivery and policymaking, but these applications are yet to be demonstrated in Australia, where there has been little research reported on the practical usefulness of FQOL measurement.

FQOL is a relatively new area of research in the disability field and further research is needed, particularly in the following areas:

- To assess not only the reliability and validity of FQOL measures but also their practical usefulness in different countries, including Australia.
- To assess the capacity of the measures to obtain relevant FQOL information from more varied family demographics and family circumstances (in the present study most families were lower middle class, two-parent families living in metropolitan areas).

- To compare both FQOL measures in larger groups using self-administered and interview formats in order to determine how the self-administered questions can be refined to obtain more of the critical qualitative information available from interviews.
- Conduct cross-cultural comparisons of the two measures controlling for different variables including the age(s) of member(s) with a disability and the types, levels, and combinations of disabilities. Such studies are needed to determine the extent to which family issues related to disability are similar across different countries and cultures.
- Evaluate the extent to which the practical use of FQOL measures by disability services advances the delivery of their services in terms of significant improvements in FQOL.

This study aimed to contribute to the evaluation of two existing FQOL measures and to investigate associated issues that might have implications for improved FQOL measures that could assist in appropriate provision of services to families having a member with a disability. Results suggested that the two measures of FQOL in the present study are both useful for the assessment of FQOL, but that both can and should be improved to facilitate the research, service provision, and policy development, that are required to improve the quality of life of individuals with an intellectual disability and their families.

References

ABS. (2001, 21 June 2007). Australian Bureau of Statistics 2001 Census QuickStats: Australia. Retrieved 6th May 2008, from http://www.censusdata.abs.gov.au/ABSNavigation/prenav/ViewData?action=402&documentproductno=0&documenttype=Main%20Features&order=1&tabname=Summary&areacode=0&issue=2001&producttype=QuickStats&javascript=true&textversion=false&navmapdisplayed=true&breadcrumb=PLD&&collection=Census&period=2001&producttype=QuickStats&method=Location%20on%20Census%20Night&

ABS. (2006, 1 August 2008). Australian Bureau of Statistics 2006 Census QuickStats: Australia. Retrieved 6th May, 2008, from http://www.censusdata.abs.gov.au/ABSNavigation/prenav/ViewData?action=402&documentproductno=0&documenttype=Main%20Features&order=1&tabname=Summary&areacode=0&issue=2006&producttype=QuickStats&javascript=true&textversion=false&navmapdisplayed=true&breadcrumb=LPD&&collection=Census&period=2006&producttype=QuickStats&method=Place%20of%20Usual%20Residence&

Aznar, A. S., & Castanon, D. G. (2005). Quality of life from the point of view of Latin American families: A participative research study. *Journal of Intellectual Disability Research, 49*(10), 784–788.

Bailey, D. B., McWilliam, R. A., Darkes, L. A., Hebbeler, K., Simeonsson, R. J., Spiker, D., et al. (1998). Family outcomes in early intervention: A framework for program evaluation and efficacy research. *Exceptional Children, 64*(3), 313–328.

Beach Center on Disability. (2003). *The Beach Center Family Quality of Life Scale* (Survey). Kansas: Beach Center, The University of Kansas, in partnership with families, service providers, and researchers.

Blacher, J. (2001). Transition to adulthood: Mental retardation, families, and culture. *American Journal on Mental Retardation, 106*(2), 173–188.

Brown, I., Anand, S., Fung, W. L. A., Isaacs, B. J., & Baum, N. T. (2003). Family quality of life: Canadian results from an international study. *Journal of developmental and physical disabilities, 15*(3), 207–230.

Brown, I., Brown, R., Cummins, R. A., Felce, D., Mattika, L., Keith, K., et al. (2000). *Quality of Life: Its conceptualization, measurement, and application* (A Consensus Document). Hastings, Nebraska: International Association for the Scientific Study of Intellectual Disabilities – Special Interest Research Group on Quality of Life (IASSID SIRG-QOL).

Brown, I., & Brown, R. I. (2004). Family quality of life as an area of study. In A. P. Turnbull, I. Brown, & H. R. Turnbull (Eds.), *Families and People with Mental Retardation and Quality of Life: International perspectives* (pp. 3–10). Washington: American Association on Mental Retardation (AAMR).

Brown, I., Brown, R. I., Baum, N. T., Isaacs, B. J., Myerscough, T., Neikrug, S., et al. (2006). *Family Quality of Life Survey: Main caregivers of people with intellectual disabilities*. Toronto, ON, Canada: Surrey Place Centre.

Brown, I., Isaacs, B. J., McCormack, B., Baum, N. T., & Renwick, R. (2004). Family quality of life in Canada. In A. P. Turnbull, I. Brown, & H. R. Turnbull (Eds.), *Families and People with Mental Retardation and Quality of Life: International perspectives* (pp. 183–220). Washington, DC: American Association on Mental Retardation (AAMR).

Brown, I., Neikrug, S., & Brown, R. I. (2000). Family Quality of Life Survey, *International Family Quality of Life Project: Australia, Canada, Israel.*

Brown, R. I. (Ed.). (1988). *Quality of Life for Handicapped People*. New York: Croom Helm.

Brown, R. I., & Brown, I. (2006). *Family Quality of Life Across Countries – Future Directions*. Paper presented at the E-IASSID Conference; Quality of Life Special Interest Research Group (QOL – SIRG), Maastricht, The Netherlands.

Brown, R. I., Davey, R., Shearer, J., & Kyrkou, M. (2004). Family quality of life in Australia. In A. P. Turnbull, I. Brown, & H. R. Turnbull (Eds.), *Families and People with Mental Retardation and Quality of Life: International Perspectives* (pp. 221–260). Washington, DC: American Association on Mental Retardation (AAMR).

Browne, G., & Bramston, P. (1996). Quality of life in the families of young people with intellectual disabilities. *Australian and New Zealand Journal of Mental Health Nursing*, *5*(3), 120–130.

Cummins, R. A. (1991). The comprehensive quality of life scale – intellectual disability: An initial report. *Australia and New Zealand Journal of Developmental Disabilities*, *17*(2), 259–264.

Cummins, R. A. (2003). Normative life satisfaction: Measurement issues and a homeostatic model. *Social Indicators Research*, *64*(2), 225–256.

Cummins, R. A. (2005). Moving from the quality of life concept to a theory. *Journal of Intellectual Disability Research*, *49*(10), 699–706.

Cummins, R. A. (2007, May 2007). Australian Centre on Quality of Life. Retrieved February 27, 2008, from http://www.deakin.edu.au/research/acqol/index.htm

Cummins, R. A., Eckersley, R., Pallant, J., Van Vugt, J., & Miasjon, R. (2003, November). Developing a national index of subjective wellbeing: the Australian unity wellbeing index. *Social Indicators Research*, *64*(2), 159–190.

Davis, K., & Gavidia-Payne, S. (2009). The impact of child, family, and professional support characteristics on the quality of life in families of young children with disabilities. *Journal of Intellectual and Developmental Disability*, *34*(2), 153–162.

Dennis, R. E., Williams, W., Giangreco, M. F., & Cloninger, C. J. (1993). Quality of life as context for planning and evaluation of services for people with disabilities. *Exceptional Children*, *59*(6), 499–512.

Devi, S. (2006). E-IASSID Conference; Quality of Life Special Interest Research Group (QOL – SIRG). Discussion about FQOL survey. Maastricht, The Netherlands.

Eacott, B. (2002). *Family quality of life for families who have a child, or children with an intellectual disability between the ages of twelve and sixteen*. Unpublished Masters of Special Education, Flinders University of South Australia, Adelaide.

Eisenhower, A. S., Baker, B. L., & Blacher, J. (2005). Preschool children with intellectual disability: Syndrome specificity, behaviour problems, and maternal well-being. *Journal of Intellectual Disability Research*, *49*(9), 657–671.

Esbensen, A. J., & Benson, B. A. (2006). A prospective analysis of life events, problem behaviours and depression in adults with intellectual disability. *Journal of Intellectual Disability Research, 50*(4), 248–258.

Glidden, L. M., & Jobe, B. M. (2007). Measuring parental daily rewards and worries in the transition to adulthood. *American Journal on Mental Retardation, 112*(4), 275–288.

Goode, D. (Ed.). (1994). *Quality of life for persons with disabilities: International perspectives and issues*. Cambridge, MA: Brookline Books.

Hodapp, R. M., Glidden, L. M., & Kaiser, A. P. (2005). Siblings of persons with disabilities: Toward a research agenda. *Mental Retardation, 43*(5), 334–338.

Hoffman, L., Marquis, J. G., Poston, D. J., Summers, J. A., & Turnbull, A. P. (2006). Assessing family outcomes: Psychometric evaluation of the beach center family quality of life scale. *Journal of marriage and family, 68*(4), 1069–1083.

Isaacs, B. J., Brown, I., Brown, R. I., Baum, N. T., Myerscough, T., Neikrug, S., et al. (2007). The International Family Quality of Life Project: Goals and description of a survey tool. *Journal of Policy and Practice in Intellectual Disabilities, 4*(3), 177–185.

Jokinen, N. S., & Brown, R. I. (2005). Family quality of life from the perspective of older parents. *Journal of Intellectual Disability Research, 49*(10), 789–793.

Kristine Peters Project Management Pty Ltd. (1998). *Review of the Family Support Services System Family Survey Results* (Review). Adelaide: Intellectual Disability Services Council (IDSC.

Llewellyn, G. (2004, 7 May). Family Support and Services Project. Retrieved February 26, 2008, from http://www3.fhs.usyd.edu.au/fssp/

Llewellyn, G., Dunn, P., Fante, M., Turnbull, L., & Grace, R. (1999). Family factors influencing out-of-home placement decisions. *Journal of Intellectual Disability Research, 43*(3), 219–233.

Llewellyn, G., Gething, L., Kendig, H., & Cant, R. (2003). *Invisible Carers: Facing an Uncertain Future* (Report of a study conducted with funding from the National Health and Medical Research Council, 2000–2002). Sydney: University of Sydney.

Llewellyn, G., Thompson, K., Whybrow, S., McConnell, D., Bratel, J., Coles, D., et al. (2003). *Supporting Families: Family Well-being and Children with Disabilities* (An ARC SPIRT collaborative research project). Sydney: University of Sydney in collaboration with the Spastic Centre of NSW.

Mackey, S., & Goddard, L. D. (2006). The experience of health and wellness in mothers of young children with intellectual disabilities. *Journal of Intellectual Disabilities, 10*(4), 305–315.

Mackey, S., & Goddard, L. D. (2007). *The Experience of Health and Wellness in Mothers of Children with Intellectual Disabilities and a Health Mentoring Intervention to improve their Health and the Health of their Families*. Paper presented at the Global Policy Summit on the Well-being of People with Intellectual Disabilities, Shanghai, China.

Mactavish, J. B., & Schleien, S. J. (2004). Re-injecting spontaneity and balance in family life: Parents' perspectives on recreation in families that include children with developmental disability. *Journal of Intellectual Disability Research, 48*(2), 123–141.

McVilly. (2007a). Beach Center on Disability Summary of International Family Quality of Life Research: Keith McVilly, *International Society for Quality of Life Studies (ISQOLS); QOL SIRG*. San Diego Conference.

McVilly. (2007b). FQOL Australia (subject of email communication). Australia: Rillotta, F.

Neikrug, S. M., Judes, J., Roth, D., & Krauss, B. (2004). Family quality of life in Israel. In A. P. Turnbull, I. Brown, & H. R. Turnbull (Eds.), *Families and People with Mental Retardation and Quality of Life: International Perspectives*. Washington, DC: American Association on Mental Retardation (AAMR).

Nuehring, M. L., & Sitlington, P. L. (2003). Transition as a vehicle: Moving from high school to an adult vocational service provider. *Journal of Disability Policy Studies, 14*(1), 23–35.

Owen, L., Gordon, M., Frederico, M., & Cooper, B. (2002). *"Listen To Us" – Supporting Families with Children with Disabilities: Identifying Service Responses that Impact on the Risk of Family Breakdown* (Executive Summary of The Family Resilience Project). Victoria: School of Social Work and Social Policy – La Trobe University.

Park, J., Hoffman, L., Marquis, J., Turnbull, A. P., Poston, D., Mannan, H., et al. (2003). Toward assessing family outcomes of service delivery: Validation of a family quality of life survey. *Journal of Intellectual Disability Research*, *47*(4/5), 367–384.

Poston, D. (2006). *Family Quality of Life: What We Have Learned Five Years Into a New Field of Study*. Paper presented at the E-IASSID Conference, Maastricht, The Netherlands.

Poston, D., Turnbull, A. P., Park, J., Mannan, H., Marquis, J., & Wang, M. (2003). Family quality of life: A qualitative inquiry. *Mental Retardation*, *41*(5), 313–328.

Rapanaro, C., Bartu, A., & Lee, A. H. (2008). Perceived benefits and negative impact of challenges encountered in caring for young adults with intellectual disabilities in the transition to adulthood. *Journal of Applied Research in Intellectual Disabilities*, *21*(1), 34–47.

Rapley, M. (2003). *Quality of Life Research: A critical introduction*. London: SAGE Publications.

Schalock, R. (2004a). The concept of quality of life: What we know and do not know. *Journal of Intellectual Disability Research*, *48*(3), 203–216.

Schalock, R. (2004b). Moving from individual to family quality of life as a research topic. In A. P. Turnbull, I. Brown, & H. R. Turnbull (Eds.), *Families and People with Mental Retardation and Quality of Life: International perspectives* (pp. 11–24). Washington, DC: American Association on Mental Retardation (AAMR).

Schalock, R. (2007, 6 December). *The development of concepts for new directions and challenges for quality of life*. Paper presented at the Quality of Life Special Interest Research Group Round Table, San Diego, USA.

Schneider, J., Wedgewood, N., Llewellyn, G., & McConnell, D. (2006). Families challenged by and accommodating to the adolescent years. *Journal of Intellectual Disability Research*, *50*(12), 926–936.

Seltzer, M. M., Greenberg, J. S., Krauss, M. W., Gordon, R. M., & Judge, K. (1997). Siblings of adults with mental retardation or mental illness: Effects on lifestyle and psychological well-being. *Family Relations*, *46*(4), 395–405.

Seltzer, M. M., & Krauss, M. W. (2001). Quality of life of adults with mental retardation/developmental disabilities who live with family. *Mental Retardation and Developmental Disabilities Research Reviews*, *7*(2), 105–114.

Shearer, J. (2000). *Aspects of the quality of life of children with a disability who are in inclusive educational settings*. Unpublished Master's Thesis, Flinders University of South Australia, Adelaide.

Strohm, K. (2002). *Siblings: Brothers and sisters of children with special needs*. Adelaide: Wakefield Press.

Summers, J. A., Marquis, J., Mannan, H., Turnbull, A. P., Fleming, K., Poston, D., et al. (2007). Relationship of perceived adequacy of services, family-professional partnerships, and family quality of life in early childhood service programmes. *International Journal of Disability, Development & Education*, *54*(3), 319–338.

Summers, J. A., Poston, D. J., Turnbull, A. P., Marquis, J., Hoffman, L., Mannan, H., et al. (2005). Conceptualizing and measuring family quality of life. *Journal of Intellectual Disability Research*, *49*(10), 777–783.

Turnbull, A. P., Brown, I., & Turnbull, H. R. (Eds.). (2004). *Families and People with Mental Retardation and Quality of Life: International perspectives*. Washington, DC: American Association on Mental Retardation (AAMR).

Verdugo, M. A., Córdoba, L., & Gómez, J. (2005). Spanish adaptation and validation of the Family Quality of Life Survey. *Journal of Intellectual Disability Research*, *49*(10), 794–798.

Wang, M., Summers, J. A., Little, T. D., Turnbull, A. P., Poston, D., & Mannan, H. (2006). Perspectives of fathers and mothers of children in early intervention programmes in assessing family quality of life. *Journal of Intellectual Disability Research*, *50*(12), 977–988.

Wang, M., Turnbull, A. P., Summers, J. A., Little, T. D., Poston, D., Mannan, H., et al. (2004). Severity of disability and income as predictors of parents' satisfaction with their family quality of life during early childhood years. *Research and Practice for Persons with Severe Disabilities*, *29*(2), 82–94.

Williams, B., Sawyer, S. C., & Wahlstrom, C. M. (2005). *Marriages, Families & Intimate Relationships: A Practical Introduction*. Boston, MA: Pearson.

Zuna, N., Beach Center on Disability, & Hu, X. (2007). *Beach Center Family Quality of Life Studies: What we know – and what we don't know* (Research Summary). Kansas: The University of Kansas.

Chapter 18
Quality of Life of the Families of People with Intellectual Disability in Spain

Climent Giné, Marta Gràcia, Rosa Vilaseca, and Anna Balcells

Introduction

The concept of family quality of life (FQoL) has emerged over the last few decades as a decisive construct both for improving families' capacity to cope with a child with disability and for evaluating the possible result of the services and support they receive. The importance researchers – especially at the international level – attach to the quality of life of families with a child with disability stands in contrast to the relative lack of studies in Spain looking at what families actually understand by quality of life and the impact on them of continually caring for and living with a person with disability, and in particular with intellectual disability (ID), throughout their life. Getting to know the critical components of a life of quality of Spanish families with a child with ID, with a view to producing an instrument for measuring QoL that will enable better planning, adjustment and provision of suitable support to these families, is a just and necessary goal.

The fact is that research on the QoL of families with people with ID in Spain began only recently, although some promising initiatives have already emerged in the last few years, especially in regard to research undertaken at the Institute of Integration into the Community (Instituto de Integración en la Comunidad – INICO) led by M. A. Verdugo at the University of Salamanca, and the work carried out by the "Disability and Quality of Life: Educational Aspects" research group led by C. Giné at the Blanquerna Faculty of Psychology, Education Sciences and Sport at Ramon Llull University in Barcelona.

The type of research proposed combines two traditions which, although they have gone their own ways for many years, have recently coincided on the need to pay attention to the QoL of families with a child with ID. We are referring, on the one hand, to research that in the past few decades has focused on the QoL of people with ID in different life contexts. In this connection it is necessary to mention the work, among others, of Brown, 1997; Cummins, 1996, 1997; Keith & Schalock,

C. Giné (✉)
Ramon Llull University, Barcelona, Spain
e-mail: climentgg@blanquerna.url.edu

R. Kober (ed.), *Enhancing the Quality of Life of People with Intellectual Disabilities*, Social Indicators Research Series 41, DOI 10.1007/978-90-481-9650-0_18,

2000; Schalock, 1996, 1997; Schalock et al., 2002; Schalock & Verdugo, 2002; and Schalock, Gardner, & Bradley, 2007.

On the other hand, there is the research on intervention into families as a development context aimed at assessing the impact of the presence of a child with a disability on their QoL and improving the parents' competencies. Nevertheless, research on the quality of life of families with a child with ID is extremely rare (Poston et al., 2003) compared with the tradition of research on the QoL of individuals with ID. Promoting the quality of life of such families must certainly be regarded as a necessary complement to the work done in relation to the QoL of individuals with disability, given the gradual recognition that FQoL is associated with the impact of disability on the family (Summers et al., 2005). Consequently, research in this field has focused both on the conceptualization of FQoL and on obtaining adequate instruments for gathering information on the current situation of this sector of the population with a view to promoting appropriate policies and services. In particular, several researches have been conducted over the past few years aimed at obtaining a more precise picture of what families understand by quality of life and studying the factors that may potentially have a positive impact on it. Indeed, the concept of QoL has not been systematically examined until very recently, although it is true to say that parents have been listened to for longer. However, it was not until the 1990s that two major projects dedicated to this were set in train. These studies were specifically designed to identify the basic components of family quality of life and develop instruments that could, on the one hand, provide information on the degree to which families perceive quality of life and, on the other, serve to identify more objectively the sources of support necessary to improve the quality of life of families with a children with ID and so enable them to demand the economic and personal resources required for this from the relevant government bodies and agencies. The studies in question are the one carried out at the University of Kansas and the one conducted by an international research group in Australia, Canada and Israel. (Brown, Anand, Fung, Isaacs, & Baum, 2003).

In summary, relevant work in this area includes that of Brown et al., 2003; Turnbull, Brown, & Turnbull, 2004; Turnbull, Turbiville, & Turnbull, 2000; Brown et al., 2006; Gallimore, Weisner, Bernheimer, Guthrie, & Nihira, 1993; Guralnick, 1999, 2001; Park et al. (2003); Wang et al., 2006; Jokinen and Brown, 2005; Peterander, 2000; Poston et al., 2003; Summers et al., 2005; and Verdugo, Córdoba and Gómez (2005).

A review of this work revealed the need to conduct a similar study in Spain to those undertaken at the University of Kansas Beach Center on Disability. We are well aware that the characteristics of American society are, in many ways, different from those of Spanish society, especially in the field of disabilities. That is why we considered that it was not sufficient to translate or adapt the scale developed in the United States (Summers et al., 2005), but that we would have to carry out the whole process from the beginning ourselves. This means that we are prepared to accept that the scale produced by our work may have similar features to that scale, but also others which are different, that reflect the differences between Spanish culture and American culture.

It should also be pointed out that the Beach Center Family Quality of Life Scale, on which we have based the design of our research, was constructed with the families of people with people with ID of up to 18 years old in mind. The challenge we have set ourselves is not only to produce a similar scale, which takes into account the context in which we live, but also to produce another scale that will be helpful to us in assessing the perception of QoL of the families of people with ID over 18 have. Although we will carry out the same steps in order to construct both scales, we are aware that in the case of the first scale (0–18) we have a clear model to guide us. In the second case (+18), however, we must be much more alert to new issues the families may identify, even if they go beyond those covered by the present American scale.

Therefore the goals we are pursuing in this research, to be covered in two stages, are as follows. The aims of the first stage are, first of all, to obtain a picture of what families with a child with ID and the people with ID themselves understand by QoL in relation to what may be regarded as the four basic stages in the development of people with disability: Preschool and primary education (0–11); secondary education (12–18); the transition to adult life and work (19–30); and adult life (>30).

Second, to explore which aspects the families regard as important for QoL and to what extent the services they receive help to promote it. Third, to identify the most important QoL dimensions and indicators. And finally, to compare our findings with those obtained in other countries, mainly the United States (Kansas University) and Canada (University of Toronto).

Based on the conclusions of the first stage and a comparison with the most relevant available research, the aims of the second stage are, first of all, to develop a scale for evaluating the QoL of families with an adult child with ID; second, to validate this adult scale in the Spanish population on the basis of a sample made up of families and persons with disability from various Autonomous Communities within Spain; and finally, to validate the Beach Center Family Quality of Life Scale (Summers et al., 2005) for the Spanish population.

The overall aim of all this is to put us in a better position to help in designing appropriate support services and programmes – as well as training programmes and refresher courses for the professionals involved – that will foster these families' QoL and, consequently the QoL of people with ID throughout the different stages of their lives.

In order to ensure that the sample is representative of the social composition of Spain, five Autonomous Communities have been selected: Madrid; Andalusia, the Basque Country, the Canary Islands and Catalonia; who account for more than 50% of the total population of Spain. As a result, researchers from the Autonomous University of Madrid, the University of Seville, the University of the Basque Country, the University of Las Palmas de Gran Canaria and Ramon Llull University in Barcelona are taking part in the study, which has been given a grant by the Spanish Ministry of Education and Science.

Method

Participants

The participants of this piece of research are 120 parents of people with ID, 40 siblings of people with ID and 45 people with ID. The parents, on the one hand, and the siblings, on the other, were allocated to various focus groups. The criteria for allocating the parents and siblings to the different focus groups were their child's or sibling's degree of disability (severe, slight, moderate), the age of the child or sibling with ID (0–18, over 18) and the family's place of residence (urban/rural area). Other variables that were taken into account, but did not constitute selection criteria, were culture of origin and socio-economic level.

The focus groups were arranged so that the participants in each one shared as many characteristics and were as homogeneous as possible with a view to guaranteeing that they would be predisposed and motivated to intervene. To ensure the reliability of the responses, measures were also taken so that, as far as possible, all the participants in a group came from different families, and, wherever possible, that none of them knew each other beforehand. In the end there were 12 parent focus groups (see Table 18.1) and 4 sibling focus groups (see Table 18.2) distributed among the different Autonomous Communities.

In summary, therefore, each Autonomous Community was to establish three or four parent focus groups and one sibling focus group.

In selecting the people with ID to be interviewed individually, age was one of the criteria taken into account, with an attempt made to ensure that the sample included people with different degrees of disability. In order to ensure that the people with ID had sufficient competence for their answers to the questions to be regarded as valid, it was decided to administer, by way of a pre-test, the *Protocolo para examinar la*

Table 18.1 Distribution of the parent focus groups among the different Autonomous Communities according to the age of the person with ID, the family's place of residence and the degree of disability of the person with ID

Focus group	Age of person with ID	Place of residence	Degree of disability	Autonomous Community
1	0–12	Urban	Severe	Canary Islands
2	0–12	Urban	Moderate	Madrid
3	0–12	Rural	Mild	Barcelona
4	12–18	Rural	Severe	Andalusia
5	12–18	Urban	Moderate	Barcelona
6	12–18	Urban	Mild	Canary Islands
7	18–30	Urban	Severe	Barcelona
8	18–30	Rural	Moderate	Madrid
9	18–30	Urban	Mild	Madrid
10	+30	Rural	Severe	Andalusia
11	+30	Urban	Moderate	Basque Country
12	+30	Urban	Mild	Basque Country

Table 18.2 Distribution of the sibling focus groups among the different Autonomous Communities according to the age of the person with ID, the family's place of residence and the degree of disability of the person with ID

Focus group	Age of person with ID	Place of residence	Degree of disability	Autonomous Community
1	0–18	Urban	Severe	Canary Islands
2	0–18	Rural	Mild	Barcelona
3	+18	Urban	Mild	Basque Country Madrid
4	+18	Rural	Severe	Andalusia

competencia discriminativa del entrevistado (Protocol for testing the discriminative competence of interviewees) drawn up on the basis of work by Cummins (Arostegui, 2002). Each Autonomous Community will carry out three interviews per age-group (12–18, 18–30, +30), resulting in 9 interviews per Autonomous Community and 45 interviews in all.

Design

The research we have set out to do is of the qualitative type and employs the procedures specific to participatory action research. Our aim is to gain knowledge of how families with people with ID perceive their family quality of life by enlisting their direct collaboration (Poston et al., 2003; Park et al., 2003).

Participatory action research is a systematic process of enquiry that is carried out in order to acquire a more thorough knowledge of the problems and possible solutions of a particular community by means of the direct involvement of the subjects comprising that community. The aim of participatory action is therefore not only to describe the problems of a particular community, but to generate, in conjunction with the agents involved, the necessary knowledge enabling a definition of the situation to be made and long-term lines of action to be undertaken leading to the transformation, change and improvement of the situation in question (Pérez, 1994).

The data-gathering techniques chosen for the research are interviews and focus groups. The interviews, carried out on an individual basis, facilitate direct interaction between the interviewer and the interviewee, which is important for getting to know the opinions of people with ID. The focus groups, on the other hand, provide a suitable context for encouraging people who are not used to being asked about their opinions to participate and share their views on important matters (Poston et al., 2003).

Once the methodological aspects of the project had been defined, a pilot study was designed to allow us to familiarize ourselves with the focus group technique. On the basis of this pilot study and a discussion of the results obtained, the adequacy of the methodology to the object of the study was evaluated and all the stages of the project were concretized, as described below.

Stage one of the research consisted in producing the necessary instruments for collecting the data. The instruments produced for this purpose were:

1. *A guide for conducting focus groups and a focus group observation grid*. The purpose of this guide is to ensure uniformity in the way all the focus groups in the different Autonomous Communities are conducted. This guide comprises two different parts and an appendix. The first part summarizes the features defining focus groups as a technique: the roles of the leaders, the structure of the sessions, the spatial arrangement of the participants, etc. The second part comprises the questions that are to guide the participants' interventions and which the leader must introduce during the sessions. These questions originate from those asked by the Beach Center on Disability research group in order to conceptualize family quality of life (Poston et al., 2003). The guide also contains observation grids with the previously agreed aspects to be identified by the group leaders.
2. *Guidelines for conducting the interviews with people with ID*. This second document was produced for a similar purpose to the first. It contains the questions to be put in the interviews with the people with ID to find out their views on family quality of life. Unlike those in the previous document, however, the questions in this one were drawn up by our research group. Nevertheless, it should be pointed out that in preparing them we based our questions on the *Cuestionario para Alumnos* (Pupils' Questionnaire), an instrument designed by the research group for the *Servicios y Calidad de Vida para las Personas con Discapacidad Intelectual* (Services and Quality of Life for People with Intellectual Disability) project funded by the Spanish Confederation of Organizations in Favor of People with Intellectual Disability (FEAPS) (Giné, 2004).

Stage two of the research focused on forming the focus groups bearing in mind the criteria listed above. The results are shown in Tables 18.1 and 18.2 above.

Stage three, which is under way at the moment, consists in conducting the focus group sessions with each of the groups and audio- and video-recording them (as decided by each Autonomous Community research group), using the ad hoc guidelines drawn up for this research.

Stage four will consist of the transcription by a team of suitably trained transcribers of the focus group discussions so that they can be analysed.

Stage five will consist of the analysis of the transcriptions using dedicated discourse-analysis software (ATLAS.ti). The main aim of this stage will be to find the general topics that are most often repeated so that we can work out the major dimensions that ought to form the skeleton of the scale and to proceed from there to gradually detect specific topics within each general topic in order to construct the items that will make up the scale.

Following this, in a subsequent stage, a pilot study will be held of the scales and the results used to design the definitive versions of the scales.

Data Gathering and Analysis

As previously mentioned, the main data-gathering technique to be used in this research will be the focus group, defined as a carefully planned series of discussions

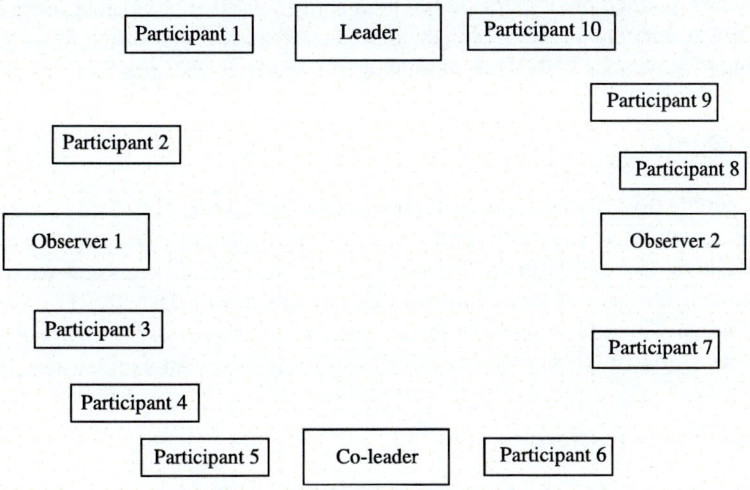

Diagram 18.1 Approximate seating arrangement of focus group participants

designed to obtain information on a defined area of interest (Krueger, 1988). The focus group sessions have been planned extremely systematically, not just in relation to the criteria for selecting the people forming each group, but also in relation to the type of issues that are going to be raised with them. Various matters, such as the following, have also been taken into account: having enough time to prepare the spaces where the sessions are going to be held; trying to get the participants to respect the layout of the chairs in the room, with the researcher leading the session (the leader) and the researcher helping her (the co-leader) sitting opposite each other, the two observers sitting perpendicular to the straight line between the leader and the co-leader, and the other people participating in the focus group distributed proportionally among the four segments formed by this arrangement (see Diagram 18.1).

The software we are going to use in analysing the data is ATLAS.ti, which is specifically designed for discourse and conversation analysis.

Pilot Study

Before starting the research proper, a pilot focus group was conducted which allowed us, as will be seen further on, to modify and improve our initial approach on the basis of the results of an analysis of this experiment.

The questions to be put to the groups were drawn up in accordance with our overall goal and the sample selected through contact with two services providing support to people with ID. In selecting the sample we took into consideration the following criteria: the age of the persons with ID and their degree of disability.

Two focus group sessions were scheduled with the same group of families with a week between the first and the second session. The sessions were video-recorded.

It should be pointed out that this initial pilot study consisted of a parent focus group only. It was not considered necessary to do a pilot study either of the focus groups of siblings of persons with ID or of individual interviews with persons with ID.

Participants

Seven people (five mothers and two fathers) took part in this pilot focus group. The participants were a reasonably homogeneous set of people who, with the exception of the mother and father of the same person with ID, did not know each other beforehand. The ages of their children with ID ranged from 16 to 42. Two families had children with autism and ID, three with a slight degree of ID and one with a moderate degree of ID. In one case the ID was associated with a motor disability.

Focus Group Sessions

The first session, which lasted 60 min, dealt with the more general aspects of QoL. The following matters in particular were discussed:

(a) When FQoL is mentioned, what is the first thing that comes to mind?
(b) On the basis of your own experience, say what things have gone really well in your family. What do you think helps things to go well?
(c) On the basis of your own experience, say what things have been especially hard or difficult in your family. What do you think contributes to making things hard or difficult?

Before the second session was held, the research group viewed the first session and commented on the aspects they regarded as most important.

This session allowed us, first of all, to get an overview of what families with a child with ID understand by FQoL and to explore which aspects families consider important for quality of life and to what extent they think the support services they receive help to promote it. Secondly, we sought to identify which dimensions were relevant and whether our findings were similar to those obtained in other similar studies.

In this first session, our families felt that for them to have a good quality of life, it was necessary:

1. For the family's primary needs (finances, work, housing, mobility and transport, etc.) to be covered.
2. For them to have services providing different types of support (emotional, educational, medical, employment, social, etc.) helping them to lead a "normal" life.
3. For family members to be able to spend time together as a family in a comfortable and relaxed way.
4. To have their own individual free time and leisure time.

5. For their children to be able to make progress in regard to their independence, improving their physical and mental health, and participating more in the social life of the community.
6. For children and parents to improve their relationship and their communication.
7. To receive support from the people around them.

This first session enabled us to identify some of the dimensions of FQoL that at first sight appear to be very similar to the categories developed by the Beach Center on Disability research group (Family Quality of Life Conversation Guide). Nevertheless, we considered it necessary to examine these matters a little further, which is why we decided to go ahead with the second session as originally planned.

The second session, which lasted 90 min, dealt with the more specific aspects of QoL. It took up again some of the aspects that had emerged in the first session, addressing also the degree of satisfaction in regard to them, and delved more deeply into the aspects the parents regarded as making a better FQoL possible. In this context, some of the questions that were put to the parents are listed below.

In regard to the influence the time they spend together has on their family quality of life, the following types of questions were asked: How do you think being able to spend time together as a family affects your family quality of life? Which aspects of your current situation concerning the time you spend together do you think need to change for you to achieve a better family quality of life? How do you think being able to sort out specially tricky or difficult situations together influences your family quality of life? How do you think being able to share good times with all the members of the family influences your family quality of life? Are you satisfied with how things have gone in regard to the time you spend together? Which aspects have enabled things to go well? Which aspects would you change or what would enable things to go better in regard to the time you spend together?

In regard to the influence having their material needs covered has on their family quality of life, the following types of questions were asked: How do you think having your material needs covered – for instance, being able to use public transport, getting medical attention if necessary, not having much higher expenses than other people with disability – influences your family quality of life? Which aspects would you change in this area or what would enable things to be better? What do you think about the benefits and/or support services you receive for your children with intellectual disability? How do you think these benefits and/or support services should be managed to enable you to have a better family quality of life?

The analysis of the second session, together with the findings from the first session, led us to a number of initial conclusions:

1. There appear to exist clear differences in regard to FQoL and in relation to the quality of the services received depending on the age of the person with ID, their degree of disability, and whether or not there are behaviour or mental health problems in addition to the disability.

2. There appear to exist differences to do with the rural/urban variable. Families living in an urban environment do not seem to have exactly the same needs as those living in a rural environment.
3. There appear to exist differences with regards to the knowledge parents have of the support and assistance services in general.
4. The families possess knowledge and good ideas that could be useful in improving the services currently available to help families with children with disability.
5. The families need places and time to meet each other to share needs and support.

Revision of Some of the Aspects in the Light of the Results of Our Pilot Study

Our pilot study has enabled us to reflect on the method used for gathering data, i.e. the focus group. The information provided by this data-gathering method is extremely rich and we regard it to be the most appropriate method given the aims we have set ourselves. What we have discovered is that leaving a week between the first and second sessions is too long. It is hard to maintain the same "scenery" and some of the issues dealt with in the first session seem a long way off, while others are gone over again without adding any more information.

So, although we consider it appropriate, with a view to the definitive data-gathering, to maintain the structure of two separate sessions, we think it is better to hold them both on the same day, with a break of about 30 min between them. This break will give the research team time to make an initial overall analysis of the first session and prepare the more specific questions for the second session.

Another conclusion the pilot study has enabled us to reach is that audio recordings of the focus group sessions need to be made with instruments that are technically sufficiently sophisticated to enable a good quality transcription to be made of what is said in them. In addition, we think that making a video-recording of the whole session with a different device may also be useful in analysing the transcriptions.

In regard to the composition of the sample, we think the gender variable should be taken into account and an attempt made, in so far as possible, to even up the balance between mothers and fathers, and between different social and cultural origins. Although in neither case do we think these should be selection criteria for the sample, we do feel that, as far as possible, such aspects should be borne in mind. We also think steps should be taken to avoid people who are related to each other participating in the same focus group.

Lastly, the pilot study has helped us in making the decision to include two mothers with children with ID in the research team, although this decision was not based only on the pilot focus group study and an analysis of its results. While considering the design of the guidelines for conducting the interviews with people with ID, we realized that the participation of parents of people with disability would be useful in developing the guidelines. Since they joined the team, we have seen how the presence of two mothers of people with intellectual disability aged 14 and 30 has brought a different and enriching view and perspective to the research group. This is doubtless yet another confirmation of the theoretical approach with which we have operated from the beginning, which stands for involving families in a collaborative partnership in the entire process of helping people with disability from the moment this is detected.

The Current Situation

Once the pilot study had been carried out and the results discussed, a number of adjustments were made in both the approach to, and the contents of, the focus groups, and the sample was selected as described in the foregoing sections. The focus group sessions are now under way and we hope to have completed them by the early part of 2009. We have already held a large number of focus groups in the different Autonomous Communities in which we are operating and are on schedule to finish them as planned. In particular, in the Autonomous Community of Catalonia, which is where the authors of this chapter are working, we have held three parent focus groups and one sibling group. Although we are not yet in a position to present definitive findings, our participation in these groups allows us to comment on certain aspects.

Without attempting to provide a systematic or exhaustive account, we think that most of the decisions we took after conducting the pilot focus group were appropriate, especially the one to hold both sessions on the same day with just a 30-min break between them. As already pointed out, in the pilot study there was a week between the first and the second session, which meant that in the second session ideas that had already come up in the first session had to be repeated and a great effort had to be made to pick up the thread of the discussion again. Another decision with which we are satisfied is not allowing both parents of a child with disability to take part in the same focus group, as it has become clear that parents feel freer to talk about their partners without causing an argument in the group if their partners are not present.

A second aspect we would like to highlight is that having parents of people over 18 – mostly around 30–35 – take part in the focus groups has highlighted the fact that the things that worry them and, therefore, the things they regard as affecting their quality of life, are appreciably different from those that concern parents of children under 18. Third, we would like to draw attention to the difficulties we have encountered in forming relatively homogeneous groups in regard to the degree of disability. We should also point out that very different dynamics were generated in the groups depending on the families' socio-cultural level. These are all aspects we will have to take into account at the data analysis stage.[1]

[1]This research was made possible by Spanish Ministry of Education and Science Grant SEJ2006-04773/PSIC.

Acknowledgments Those taking part in the research reported here were researchers from Ramon Llull University (C. Giné, Mª T. Pró, M. Dalmau, J. M. Mas, A. Balcells), the University of Barcelona (M. Gràcia, R. Vilaseca), as well as professionals working in various institutions dealing with people with intellectual disability (L. Zaurin, G. Fornés, N. Tresserras) and mothers of people with disability (N. Gotarda, G. Prats).

References

Arostegui, I. (2002). *Calidad de Vida y Retraso Mental*. Bilbao: Ediciones Mensajero, S.A.

Brown, I., Anand, S., Fung, W. L. A., Isaacs, B., & Baum, N. (2003). Family quality of life: Canadian results from an international study. *Journal of Developmental and Physical Disabilities, 15*(3), 207–230.

Brown, I., Brown, R. I., Baum, N. T., Isaacs, B. J., Myerscough, T., Neikrug, S., et al. (2006). *Family Quality of Life Survey (General Version)*. Toronto, ON, Canada: Surrey Place Centre.

Brown, R. I. (Ed.). (1997). *Quality of life for people with disabilities: Models, research and practice*. Cheltenham: Stanley Thornes Pub. Ltd.

Cummins, R. A. (1996). The domains of life satisfaction: An attempt to order chaos. *Social Indicators Research, 38*, 303–328.

Cummins, R. A. (1997). Self rated quality of life scales for people with an intellectual disability: A review. *Journal of Applied Research in Intellectual Disabilities, 10*, 199–216.

Gallimore, R., Weisner, T. S., Bernheimer, L. P., Guthrie, D., & Nihira, K. (1993). Family responses to young children with developmental delays: Accommodation activity in ecological and cultural context. *American Journal on Mental Retardation, 98*(2), 185–206.

Giné, C. (2004). Servicios y Calidad de Vida para Personas con Discapacidad Intelectual. *Siglo Cero, 35*(210), 18–28.

Guralnick, M. (1999). Family and child influence on the peer-related social competence of young children with developmental delays. *Mental Retardation and Developmental Disabilities Research Reviews, 5*, 21–29.

Guralnick, M. J. (2001). A developmental systems model for early intervention. *Infants and Young Children, 14*(2), 1–18.

Jokinen, N. S., & Brown, R. I. (2005). Family quality of life from the perspective of older parents. *Journal of Intellectual Disability Research, 49*(10), 789–793.

Keith, K. D., & Schalock, R. L. (Eds.). (2000). *Cross-cultural perspectives on quality of life*. Washington, DC: American Association on Mental Retardation.

Krueger, R. (1988). *Focus groups: A practical guide to applied research*. Newbury Park, CA: Sage.

Park, J., Hoffman, L., Marquis, J., Turnbull, A. J., Poston, D., Mannan, H., et al. (2003). Toward assessing family outcomes of service delivery: Validation of a family quality of life survey. *Journal of Intellectual Disability Research, 47*(4–5), 367–384.

Peterander, F. (2000). The best quality cooperation between parents and experts in early intervention. *Infants and Young Children, 12*(3), 32–45.

Poston, D., Turnbull, A., Park, J., Mannan, H., Marquis, J., & Wang, M. (2003). Family quality of life: A qualitative inquiry. *Mental Retardation, 41*(5), 313–328.

Pérez, G. (1994). *Investigación Cualitativa. Retos e Interrogantes*. Madrid: Editorial La Muralla.

Schalock, R. L. (Ed.). (1996). *Quality of life: Vol. I. Conceptualization and measurement*. Washington, DC: American Association on Mental Retardation.

Schalock, R. L. (Ed.). (1997). *Quality of life: Vol. II. Application to persons with disabilities*. Washington, DC: American Association on Mental Retardation.

Schalock, R. L., Brown, I., Brown, R., Cummins, R. A., Felce, D., Matikka, L., et al. (2002). Conceptualization, measurement and application of quality of life for persons with intellectual disabilities: Report of an international panel of experts. *Mental Retardation, 40*(6), 457–470.

Schalock, R. L., Gardner, J. F., & Bradley, V. J. (2007). *Quality of life for people with intellectual and other developmental disabilities*. Washington, DC: American Association on Intellectual and Developmental Disabilities.

Schalock, R. L., & Verdugo, M. A. (2002). *Handbook on quality of life for human services practitioners*. Washington, DC: American Association on Mental Retardation.

Summers, J. A., Poston, D., Turnbull, A. P., Marquis, J., Hoffman, L., Mannan, H., et al. (2005). Conceptualizing and measuring family quality of life. *Journal of Intellectual Disability Research, 49*(10), 777–783.

Turnbull, A., Brown, I., & Turnbull, R. (Eds.). (2004). *Families and people with mental retardation and quality of life: International perspectives*. Washington, DC: American Association on Mental Retardation.

Turnbull, A. P., Turbiville, V., & Turnbull, H. R. (2000). Evolution of family-professional partnership models: Collective empowerment as the model for the early 21st century. In J. P. Shonkoff & S. L. Meisels (Eds.), *The handbook of early childhood intervention* (pp. 630–650). New York: Cambridge University Press.

Verdugo, M. A., Córdoba, L., & Gómez, J. (2005). Spanish adaptation and validation of the family quality of life survey. *Journal of Intellectual Disability Research, 49*(10), 794–798.

Wang, M., Summers, J. A., Little, T., Turnbull, A. P., Poston, D., & Mannan, H. (2006). Perspectives of fathers and mothers of children in early intervention programmes in assessing family quality of life. *Journal of Intellectual Disability Research, 50*(12), 977–988.

Chapter 19
Quality of Life of Families with Children with Intellectual Disabilities in Slovenia

Majda Schmidt and Ralph Kober

Introduction

Qualityof life is determined by how an individual interprets their environment and the individuals and groups they interact with, and how this impacts on their well-being. It is based on an individual's own personal interpretation (Schalock et al., 2002). In the field of intellectual disability research, interest in researching family quality of life has been increasing in recent years (Turnball et al., 2004). The impact that a child with a disability may have on a family is not just felt by the parents, but also has an impact throughout the family system, including financially, vacations, social relations, and family satisfaction. As Brown et al. (2006) noted, family quality of life studies attempt to analyze how various domains of life are impacted when there is a child with a disability, and what the perceptions of family members are about family life in general. Such studies also explore the effects of services and community, as well as the influence of each individual member of the family, or the family as a whole. The study of family quality of life is no doubt complex, as we need to understand what supports are required for families to experience high levels of wellbeing (Brown & Brown, 2006, p.175).

The efforts and the activities of researchers from Canada, Australia, Israel, the USA, and other countries under the auspice of the International Family Quality of Life Project have contributed to the development of the concept family quality of life with the development of an instrument to measure family quality of life – FQoLS (Isaacs et al., 2007). It is expected that the information garnered from the FQoLS will be useful for a wide variety of purposes related to providing support to individuals and families.

Prior Slovene research on the quality of life of families who have a child with an intellectual disability has focused on: (1) the family life of the children; (2) the stress in families; (3) the position within the family of the children with intellectual disabilities; and (4) on the family dynamics (Mikuš-Kos, 1999; Novljan, 2004;

M. Schmidt (✉)
Faculty of Education, University of Maribor, Maribor, Slovenia
e-mail: majda.schmidt@uni-mb.si

R. Kober (ed.), *Enhancing the Quality of Life of People with Intellectual Disabilities*, Social Indicators Research Series 41, DOI 10.1007/978-90-481-9650-0_19,

Tomori, 1999). This chapter presents the first study in relation to family quality of life for families with children with intellectual disabilities in Slovenia. This chapter first discusses the care and support system for children with intellectual disabilities and their families in Slovenia followed by an empirical analysis of family quality of life.

Care and Support for Children with Intellectual Disabilities and Their Families

Under the auspice of deinstitutionalization and inclusion, Slovenia has, like many other European countries, passed or adopted the professional and legal grounds for the satisfaction of the needs and granting of rights to people with intellectual disabilities for education and training, learning, self confirmation through work in accordance with their abilities, active and meaningful pastime activities, personal integrity and intimacy, for the preservation of already acquired abilities, and for an appropriate quality of life. On the surface, given current Slovene legislation (Primary School Act, 1996, Placement Act, 2000), it would appear that there is relatively good care and support for children with intellectual disabilities. The view is further enhanced by the fact that you can observe a reasonable number of forms of care and support in practice. The reality, however, as we shall detail below, is somewhat different.

The majority of children with intellectual disabilities in Slovenia live with their families, that is, approximately 90% of children (Zaviršek, 2005). Parents can choose the option of including pre-school children with intellectual disabilities into mainstream kindergartens with additional professional support or into developmental units, or into care and educational institutions for children with moderate, severe and profound intellectual disabilities. During the pre-school years the Ministry of Health ensures Mental-hygiene Departments and Development Dispensaries (which enable and provide early identification and early holistic intervention) basic health care for children with intellectual disabilities and their families. Early holistic intervention includes pediatricians and developmental neurologists, psychologists, speech therapists, special rehabilitators/educators, social workers, and other therapists. However, non-governmental organizations in Slovenia like the Association Sožitje and Cerebral Palsy Association constantly emphasize in their reports that early identification and early intervention are neither equally available across Slovenia, nor are they sufficient in the extent of the interventions or treatments. Another major problem is in the qualifications (training, education) of professional personnel and the lack of certain professionals such as speech therapists, physiotherapists, and others. The services are typically more accessible to those families that live in major towns and cities (Kukova, Zaviršek, & Urh, 2005). A research study conducted by the Association Sožitje showed that 50% of parents did not have access to Development Dispensaries in the vicinity of their home and therefore had to drive their children to other places/towns. Parents also reported that they had to wait up to 6 months to be seen at a Development Dispensary. The report on availability of education and employment (2005) particularly emphasized the fact that the government should change the system of early intervention and improve the services for pre-school children, as well as developing and ensuring the quality of support programs for the parents of children with intellectual disabilities by including the appropriate information technology and emotional support (Kukova et al., 2005).

Similar to children without disabilities, it is compulsory for children with intellectual disabilities to receive schooling between the ages of 6 and 15. The Placement Act (2000) makes it possible for children with intellectual disabilities, particularly those with mild disabilities, to be included in adapted programs in certain schools on the basis of the diagnostic procedure performed by the placement commission. However, parents are not sufficiently included in the diagnostic procedures (Zaviršek, 2005), and they complain about the fact that procedures take too long. Furthermore, parents participatory role in the creation of the individualized programs – every child must have their own program – is very minor. A report by the Association Sožitje (2001) noted that the majority of parents of children with intellectual disabilities emphasized during interviews that they were not included in the education process. The report found that parents whose children attended schools with adapted programs partially participate in the education process through different forms, such as parent–teacher meetings, school open days, school councils, and also in some cases even directly in classes.

Children with intellectual disabilities, when compared with other groups of children with special needs, are not included together with their peers in regular schools or "schools for all," but typically undergo segregated schooling. Parents often complain of the fact that the state has not established a network of regular schools, which could accept children with moderate intellectual disabilities, and which could at the same time also make it possible for other children with moderate disabilities or with additional problems to transfer among programs. Consequently, social integration within the community is inhibited for children with intellectual disabilities, as well as for their families (Ombudsman Report, 2003).

Children with moderate, severe, and profound intellectual disabilities are included in programs within special schools or care and educational institutions where they can stay until they reach 21 or 26 years of age. There are ten such care and education institutions in Slovenia. Some institutions have opened day care centers; however, there still exists a lack of support, care, and treatment options for children with disabilities who live at home. It can be concluded from the education institutions report (2004) that the parents whose children are placed in those institutions wish to be more or better connected with the local community. The parents strongly emphasized the need for care at home, the possibility to rent orthopedic aids, for institutions to be closer to their homes; and to have more possibilities to participate in decision-making.

Parents whose children stay at home also claim that there is not enough support and home or community care to satisfy their needs and the needs of their children. Due to associated problems with mental health and other illnesses pediatric wards in general hospitals are included in the program of helping children with intellectual disabilities and their families. During hospitalization they provide counseling for the families as well as assistance with schools and social care institutions. The problems associated with hospital treatment are due to the lack of adequately trained professionals and overworked employees. During their schooling children and adolescents with intellectual disabilities and their parents receive some support from professionals in outpatient departments and counseling centers, which also provide treatment for other groups of children with special needs, as well as for children without disabilities.

In spite of the fact that the network of care and support for persons with intellectual disabilities is to some extent satisfactory, numerous authors and experts still express concern about the dominance of the medical model in diagnostics and intervention. It has been stated that such a medical model "ensures the development of individuality and integration into society for the young only at the formal level, but nevertheless in reality it only protects them and does not encourage the development of functional knowledge and skills" (Zaviršek, 2005, p. 234). In their work with children with intellectual disabilities and their families, many professionals focus too much on the child's inabilities and deficits, instead of on their skills or abilities and special needs. Although, it can be observed that parents' opinions have gradually become more listened, they are still not considered as equals in the process of decision-making on issues related to their children with disabilities. The parental role in relation to the process of diagnosis and intervention still remains a very minor one. It is also obvious that parents still do not have enough information and support. The partner-cooperative model with the emphasis on holistic approach for families with children with intellectual disabilities is still at the initial stages of development in Slovenia (Schmidt, 2007).

Providing social care for families with children with intellectual disabilities and financial assistance falls under the jurisdiction of Centers for Social Work. Families with children with intellectual disabilities are entitled to child support benefits and supplements for care. The latter are awarded to the families of children with moderate, severe, and profound intellectual disabilities until they reach 18 years of age. The amount of the care supplement differs according to whether the child lives with their parents, attends institutional day care, or lives permanently in a care and education institution. The parents whose children permanently stay with them at their home and take full care of them emphasize the fact that they do not have equal rights, since their children receive significantly fewer benefits and finances from the state than the children who are in institutional care (Educations Institutions Report, 2004). Parents of children with intellectual disabilities must often take sick leave because illnesses are far more frequent with these children than children without disabilities. Parental income is therefore lower and they often experience problems with their employers, with some parents even reporting the loss of their jobs. All these circumstances together with being overworked due to caring for a child with an intellectual disability, often lead to mental and physical parental exhaustion (Ombudsman Report, 2000).

In the field of health care the families of children with intellectual disabilities are legally entitled to comprehensive free public health care. The reality of the situation, however, is markedly different. Most parents have basic health care insurance, but must still pay themselves for their children to receive specialist services such as physiotherapy, which their children often require. Furthermore, parents also have to partially cover the cost of medications required by their children. Not surprisingly, half of parents report having financial difficulties in meeting these costs (Educations Institutions Report, 2004).

Among the non-governmental organizations, it is the Association Sožitje that provides most of the support for people (including children) with intellectual disabilities and their families. This association covers the whole of the Republic of Slovenia. They implement social programs such as: education and training to enable people with intellectual disabilities to lead independent and active lives; educating and counseling families with children with intellectual disabilities; providing assistance to maintain the health of people with intellectual disabilities and their families; providing adapted transportation for people with disabilities; organizing sporting and cultural activities; as well as providing special professional assistance like legal counseling. There is a special section within the Association Sožitje for children with Down syndrome and their parents. Another source of assistance is The Association for Cerebral Palsy Sonček, which is dedicated to assisting people with cerebral palsy and head. Civil initiatives within the past 2 years resulted in the establishment of The Association for Autism, which is dedicated to assisting autistic children or adolescents and their parents.

Family Quality Of Life

Having presented a brief picture of the situation for children with intellectual disabilities and their families in Slovenia, we will now present the results of an initial survey undertaken to establish the family quality of life of these families.

Research Method

Sample

The sample consists of 20 families with children with intellectual disabilities from north-eastern Slovenia; 10 of whom had children with intellectual disabilities who experience developmental issues and 10 of whom had children with intellectual disabilities and who experience behavioral issues. All the children attended special schools. The group comprising children with intellectual disabilities who experience developmental issues includes children who have motor functioning disabilities including cerebral palsy and speech and language disorders. Whereas, the group with children with intellectual disabilities who experience behavioral issues, consists of children who experience disruptive behavior, hyperactivity, and verbal aggression. All the children in both disability groups were professionally diagnosed by professional teams involving pediatric and/or psychiatric evaluation, psychological and special education assessment. The children were between 7 and 14 years of age.

Data Collection Procedure and Instrument

Data were collected between February and June 2007 using the Family Quality of Life Survey (Brown et al., 2006), which was adapted to Slovene conditions. The original survey consists of ten areas, however, the adapted version of the questionnaire consisted of only six areas (health, financial wellbeing, support from other people, support from disability-related services, community interaction, and overall family quality of life). The questionnaire utilized a four- or five-item scale and instructions explicitly that all the questions refer to the family as a whole. While we predominately concentrate on the quantitative results, we also make use of comments made to us by the parents of the children with intellectual disabilities during the interviews to gain a deeper understanding of our results.

Participation in this project was entirely voluntary and consent was obtained from the parents of children with intellectual disabilities. The Slovene version of the Family Quality of Life Survey was distributed to parents in person. After they had returned the completed questionnaires, we organized meetings with the parents and conducted interviews. The meetings served the dual purpose of checking the parents' comprehension of questions and also affording them the opportunity of elaborating on their responses should they so desire.

Results

Sample Demographics

Frequencies relating to our sample are presented in Tables 19.1 and 19.2. Table 19.1 presents characteristics of our sample related to the children with intellectual disabilities, while Table 19.2 presents characteristics related to the family. As can be seen from Table 19.1 our sample comprises of the same number of children with intellectual disabilities that experience developmental issues (10) and those that experience behavioral issues (10). All the children with intellectual disabilities in our sample required support at different levels – from temporary help in some cases to (55%) support in most or all aspects of life (45%) – and the children in the sample were able to communicate at least their basic needs and wants. Our sample comprises of predominately two-parent families (75%), with the mother typically being the primary carer (65%). Most participants perceive that having a child with an intellectual disability has resulted in them having a greater deal of responsibility, both toward the child with the intellectual disability (85%) and also the family as a whole (75%). These findings are similar to those reported in prior research (e.g., Hastings, 2003; Novljan, 1994; Roach, Orsmond, & Barratt, 1999).

Table 19.1 Characteristics related to the children with intellectual disabilities

		f	*f%*
Disability type	ID who experience developmental issues	10	50
	ID who experience behavioral issue	10	50
Level of disability-related support required	No support required	0	0
	Support required for only a few aspects of life	5	25
	Support required for some aspects of life	6	30
	Support required for most aspects of life	4	20
	Support required for almost all or all aspects of life	5	25
Level of communication	Able to communicate about a wide variety of topics	5	25
	Able to communicate within a limited range of topics	4	20
	Able to communicate needs, wants, and some ideas	8	40
	Able to communicate basic needs and wants	3	15
	Very little meaningful communication	0	0

f – abbreviation for frequency.
f% – abbreviation for frequency percentage.
ID – abbreviation for intellectual disability.

Table 19.2 Familial characteristics

		f	*f%*
Family type	One-parent	5	25
	Two-parent	15	75
Primary carer	Mother	13	65
	Father	0	0
	Equally shared	7	35
Degree of responsibility felt by primary carer toward family	Much less responsibility	0	0
	Less responsibility	0	0
	About the same amount of responsibility	5	25
	More responsibility	5	25
	Much more responsibility	10	50
Degree of responsibility felt by primary carer toward child with ID	Much less responsibility	0	0
	Less responsibility	0	0
	About the same amount of responsibility	3	15
	More responsibility	8	40
	Much more responsibility	9	45

f – abbreviation for frequency.
f% – abbreviation for frequency percentage.
ID – abbreviation for intellectual disability.

Family Quality of Life and Its Component Domains

Table 19.3 reports the means and standard deviations of the entire sample, as well as separately reporting the means and standard deviations for the two sub-samples (families with children with an intellectual disability who experience behavioral issues and families with children with an intellectual disability who experience developmental issues). As can be seen from the table, family quality of life is statistically significantly higher for families who have children with an intellectual disability who experience developmental issues compared with those families that have children with an intellectual disability who experience behavioral issues.[1] There are no statistically significant differences between the two samples for any of the domains of family quality of life. This is not surprising given the small sample sizes. However, looking at Table 19.3, it can be seen that for four of the five domains (the exception being health) families who have children with an intellectual disability who experience developmental issues report higher mean scores compared with those families that have children with an intellectual disability who experience behavioral issues.

Table 19.4 reports the percentage of scale maximum scores for family quality of life and its domains. Percentage of scale maximum involves the standardization

Table 19.3 Sample statistics and differences in family quality of life between the families with children with intellectual disabilities who experience developmental issues and the families of children with intellectual disabilities who experience behavioral issues

	Entire sample		ID – developmental		ID – behavioral		
Area	Mean	SD	Mean	SD	Mean	SD	Significance of t test
Health	26.15	2.739	25.70	3.093	26.60	2.413	.937
Financial wellbeing	36.75	5.721	38.30	5.832	35.20	5.453	.235
Support from other people	30.65	5.050	32.50	4.170	28.80	5.371	.102
Support from disability services	20.00	2.810	20.50	3.240	19.50	2.369	.441
Interaction with the community	28.50	3.502	29.50	3.567	27.50	3.308	.210
Total family quality of life	147.80	11.937	153.00	11.926	142.60	9.924	.048

ID – developmental – abbreviation for children with an intellectual disability who experience developmental issues

ID – behavioral – abbreviation for children with an intellectual disability who experience behavioral issues

[1]Kolmogorov-Smirnov tests were conducted to test whether the sample was non-normally distributed. Normality of the data could not be rejected at the 5% significance level, and as such all tests conducted are parametric.

Table 19.4 Percentage of scale maximum

Area	Entire sample	ID – developmental	ID – behavioral
Health (%)	46.47	46.39	48.89
Financial wellbeing (%)	45.67	48.65	42.69
Support from other people (%)	44.66	48.86	40.45
Support from disability services (%)	46.43	48.21	44.64
Interaction with the community (%)	54.17	56.94	51.39
Total family quality of life (%)	50.47	53.06	47.76

ID – developmental – abbreviation for children with an intellectual disability who experience developmental issues
ID – behavioral – abbreviation for children with an intellectual disability who experience behavioral issues

of a scale into a score that ranges from 0 to 100% (Cummins, 2000). This can be done using the following formula: [(score – theoretical minimum)/(theoretical maximum – theoretical minimum) × 100]. Converting the family quality of life scores to a percentage of scale maximum scores allows us to compare the relative scores of our Slovene sample with those of population norms form other quality of life studies. As noted in Chapter 3 by Cummins et al. (2010, this volume), the normal range for quality of life scores can be expected to lie within the range of 70–80% for western populations and 60–80% for a broader international sample (Cummins, 1995, 1998), with scores below this indicating a defeat of homeostasis.[2] That is, the environment experienced by that population "has become so aversive that, on average, it exceeds the average person's adaptational capacity" (Cummins, 2000, p. 137). Chapter 3 by Cummins et al. (2010, this volume) proposes that this is the cause of depression.

As can be seen from Table 19.4 for our Slovene sample of families with children with intellectual disabilities (and the two sub-samples), they are below 60% sale maximum for total family quality of life as well as for each domain, indicating that the families are finding their environment that aversive that they are not able to function effectively; one may even wish to consider the family-unit being in a depressed state. The two areas that receive consistently low scores are support from other people and support from disability services. Comments made by participants attest to the lack of support received by these families. One of the mothers summarized her experiences and her reflections in connection with the support from services: "We could not benefit from those services. Our part of Slovenia is poorly organized regarding support in the area of health, physiotherapy hydrotherapy, and the rehabilitation services do not really work. I wish for active cooperation and participation in education which would be of help to me and my child." Another mother of a girl attending a special school with an adapted program mentioned: "The services whose support we benefit from do not provide enough help. If you are motivated yourself

[2]For an explanation of homeostasis and homeostatic theory of subjective wellbeing see Cummins (1995, 1998, 2003).

to help your child, you will find a way and get the assistance you are entitled to." In regards to the future, all participants saw their situation of a lack of appropriate support as remaining the same or deteriorating.

While the above result are not entirely surprising given the description of support systems detailed in the first part of the chapter, it is nevertheless still a matter of concern to note that homeostasis has been defeated to such an extent and across all domains of family quality of life. It is clear that there is the need for an increase in professional attention and support across all areas of family quality of life, so that Slovene families with children with intellectual disabilities can lead lives of quality.

Table 19.5 examines the correlation coefficients for each domain in relation to total family quality of life for the entire sample as well as for the two sub-samples (families who have children with intellectual disabilities who experience developmental issues and families who have children with intellectual disabilities who experience behavioral issues). As can be seen from Table 19.5, the correlation between financial wellbeing is statistically significant for the entire sample as well as for both sub-samples. This result highlighting the importance of financial matters in family quality of life is consistent with the arguments of Cummins (2000) that income can act as an external buffer that can protect a person from negative input from the surrounding environment. For example, if a person falls sick and they are financially well-off they can use their income to purchase the best medical treatment and thus minimize the negative effect of the sickness on their quality of life. However, if the person is poor, such premium medical treatment is not available to them and as such they are unable to buffer themselves against the negative effects of the sickness on their quality of life. As such, Cummins (2000) contends that income does not have a primary effect on quality of life, but a secondary effect, in that greater income levels enhance the availability of external resources which can be used by the person to buffer themselves from negative events.

Table 19.5 Correlations between individual domains and total of family quality of life

Domain	Entire sample FQOL ($n = 20$)	ID – developmental FQOL ($n = 10$)	ID – behavioral FQOL ($n = 10$)
Health	0.359	0.516	0.069
Financial wellbeing	0.690*	0.750*	0.550**
Support from other people	0.146	0.308	−0.279
Support from disability services	−0.165	−0.333	0.0000
Interactions with the community	0.190	0.014	0.302

ID – developmental – abbreviation for children with an intellectual disability who experience developmental issues

ID – behavioral – abbreviation for children with an intellectual disability who experience behavioral issues

* Significant at or beyond the 5% level (two tail)

** Significant at or beyond the 10% level (two tail)

Given the financial pressures experienced by Slovene families who have children with intellectual disabilities it is not surprising that the greatest correlation between any domain and overall family quality relates to financial wellbeing. Comments made by interviewees support the finding of a high correlation between financial wellbeing and family quality of life. Comments were often made in relation to the fact that children with intellectual disabilities required extra supports, which were costly and therefore families should be eligible for benefits from the state. However, interviewees noted that families were not receiving any financial support from services, although in almost all cases they required additional financial support for special care, medication, aids for the child, etc. Comments relating to a lack of opportunities in regards the ability to earn additional income were also made. Unfortunately, most interviewees express concern in regards to their financial future and foresaw the situation remaining the same or getting worse. From the interviews and our results, it is apparent that this lack of financial support is impacting on the family quality of life experienced by Slovene families with children with intellectual disabilities.

Discussion of Results and Conclusions

This chapter had two primary purposes; first to present a description of the current situation in Slovenia for families with children with intellectual disabilities, and second to present statistics relating to the family quality of life of these Slovene families. We used an adapted version of the Family Quality of Life Survey (Brown et al., 2006) and surveyed 20 families; 10 who had children with intellectual disabilities who experience developmental issues, and 10 children with intellectual disabilities who experience behavioral issues. The results we believe that are of particular interest are (1) the low family quality of life for Slovene families with a child with an intellectual disability relative to international averages; (2) a statistically significantly higher family quality of life in the families with children with intellectual disabilities who experience developmental issues compared with families with children with intellectual disabilities who experience behavioral issues; and (3) financial wellbeing, being statistically significantly correlated to total family quality of life.

The interviews enabled us to gain a greater level of understanding about the personal lives of the families with children with disabilities. Many families told us that they had never had an opportunity to discuss their situation in a similar way. The data and the interviews highlighted an urgent need to identify appropriate ways of providing support, which would improve the quality of life of families with children with intellectual disabilities. With a particular need to develop services employing trained professionals that provide support for the family as a whole and not only for the child with an intellectual disability. This need especially applies to the regional areas where most of the families included in this research came from.

Comments made during the interviews emphasized the necessity of respecting and taking into account the needs of the entire family and not just those of the child with an intellectual disability. Participants commented on not knowing where to look for support, and that if found, there was a lack of professional commitment in support services, who do not take family problems into consideration. Support provided to families by professionals needs to be based on partnership and on the principles of empowerment (Lucyshyn, Horner, Dunlap, Albin, & Ben, 2002). We also believe that our results highlight the need for families with children with intellectual disabilities to have ready access to family support workers (as is the situation in many other countries) who would provide the connections between the families and different forms of formal and informal support (Singer, Goldberg-Hamblin, Peckham-Hardin, Barry, & Santarelli, 2002).

Comments made during interviews also highlighted a lack support from family members, neighbors, and friends, and also indicate a lower level of understanding, solidarity, and willingness to help. It is therefore advisable to include the wider community in assisting families with children with intellectual disabilities, by establishing the mechanisms for self-assistance, which would bring together members of the families, other organizations, and volunteers. The community can contribute to a great deal in ensuring equal opportunities for people with intellectual disabilities and the improvement of family life (Mikuš-Kos, 1999).

The financial hardship faced by families was often commented on by participants during interviews. The majority of families did not receive any financial allowances, although the children with intellectual disabilities had increased needs in regards to medication, therapies, equipment, aids, etc. As emphasized by Kukova et al. (2005), for families that support their children with intellectual disabilities at home, this minimal or no financial support means that those families with low incomes are unable to satisfy their needs.

Comments were also made by participants in regards to their dissatisfaction with the education system for children with intellectual disabilities; as the system does not offer any alternative forms of education in regular primary schools and thereby hinders the social and emotional development of their children. This is the same as was found by Kukova et al. (2005) in their report.

Our study does have several limitations. The primary ones being the small sample size and the fact that all participants are drawn from one geographical region. Furthermore, the Family Quality of Life Survey included only six areas and not the full ten of the original instrument; excluded areas were family relationships, influence of values, careers and leisure, and recreation. Future research should also consider these areas so as to obtain an insight into all areas of family quality of life. Another drawback, which is not uncommon in the area of family quality of life research, is that only mothers participated in the interviews. This means the views expressed were those of the mothers and not necessarily the entire family. Future research should investigate methods of incorporating the views of all members of the family, especially both parents.

From what we have presented in this chapter it is clear that there is a substantial amount of work to be done in providing the required support for Slovene families with children with intellectual disabilities so that they these families can lead lives of quality. We believe the time has come that Slovene researchers and practitioners make a concerted effort to investigate the quality of life of families with children with intellectual disabilities in a systematic manner over all periods of life. As well as gaining a better understanding of the current family quality of life of these families, it is essential that the information gained be used to identify areas of need so as to improve the care and support received by Slovene families with children with intellectual disabilities, so that these families can indeed lead a life of quality.

References

Association Sožitje Report. (2001). Available via www.zveza-sozitje.si/uploads/nacionalno_porocilo.doc accessed 18 Nov 2007

Brown, I., & Brown, R. I. (2006). *Quality of life and disability. An approach for community practitioners*. London and Philadelphia, PA: Jessica Kingsley Publishers.

Brown, I., Brown, R. I., Baum, N. T., Isaacs, B. J., Myerscough, T., Neikrug, S., et al. (2006). *Vprašalnik o raziskovanju kvalitete življenja družine: Glavni skrbniki oseb z motnjami v intelektualnem razvoju* (M. Schmidt, trans.). Toronto, ON: Surrey Place Centre.

Brown, R. I., MacAdam-Crisp, J., Wang, M., & Iarocci, G. (2006). Family quality of life when there is a child with a developmental disability. *Journal of Policy and Practice in Intellectual Disabilities*, *3*(4), 238–245.

Cummins, R. A. (1995). On the trail of the gold standard for life satisfaction. *Social Indicators Research*, *35*, 179–200.

Cummins, R. A. (1998). The second approximation to an international standard of life satisfaction. *Social Indicators Research*, *43*, 307–334.

Cummins, R. A. (2000). Personal income and subjective well-being: A review. *Journal of Happiness Studies*, *1*, 133–158.

Cummins, R. A. (2003). Normative life satisfaction: Measurement issues and homesotatic model. *Social Indicators Research*, *64*, 225–256.

Education Institutions Report, Republic of Slovenia Ministry of Labour, Family and Social Affairs. (2004). Available via www.mddsz.gov.si/fileadmin/mddsz.gov.si/pageuploads/dokumenti_pdf/zavodi_usposabljanja_vizija_koncno.pdf accessed 18 Nov 2007

Hastings, R. P. (2002). Parental stress and behaviour problems of children with developmental disability. *Journal of Intellectual and Developmental Disability*, *27*, 149–160.

Isaacs, B. J., Brown, I., Brown, R. I., Baum, N., Myerscough, T., Neikrug, S., et al. (2007). The International Family Quality of Life Project: Goals and description of a survey tool. *Journal of Policy and Practice in Intellectual Disabilities*, *4*(3), 177–185.

Kukova, S., Zaviršek, D., & Urh, Š. (2005). *Rights of people with intellectual disabilities. Access to education and employment : Slovenia : monitoring report = Pravice oseb z intelektualnimi ovirami. Dostopnost izobraževanja in zaposlovanja : Slovenija : poročilo*. Budapest, New York: Open Society Institute. Available via www.eumap.org/topics/inteldis/reports/national/slovenia/id_si2.pdf accessed 10 Nov 2007

Lucyshyn, J. M., Horner, R. H., Dunlap, G., Albin, R. W., & Ben, K. R. (2002). Positive behavior support with families. In Lucyshyn, J. M., Dunlap, G., Albin, R. (Eds.), *Families and Positive Behavior Support* (pp. 3–43). Baltimore, London, Toronto, ON, Sydney: Paul H. Brookes Publishing Co.

Mikuš-Kos, A. (1999). Kakovost življenja kronično bolnih in invalidnih otrok. In A. Mikuš-Kos (Ed.), *Različnim otrokom enake možnosti* (pp. 147–174). Ljubljana: Zveza prijateljev mladine Slovenije.

Novljan, E. (1994). Položaj družine z otrokom z motnjo v duševnem razvoju. *Naš zbornik*, *27*(1), 1–5.

Novljan, E. (2004). *Sodelovanje s starši otrok s posebnimi potrebami pri zgodnji obravnavi*. Zveza Sožitje: Ljubljana.

Ombudsman Report. (2003). Available via www.varuh-rs.si accessed 19 Nov 2007

Ombudsman Report. (2000). Available via www.varuh-rs.si accessed 19 Nov 2007

Placement Act. (2000). Uradni list Republike Slovenije 54/00.

Primary School Act. (1996). Uradni list Republike Slovenije 12/96.

Roach, M. A., Orsmond, G. I., & Barratt, M. S. (1999). Mothers and fathers of children with Down syndrome. Parental stress and involvement in childcare. *American Journal on Mental Retardation, 104*, 422–436.

Schalock, R. L., Brown, I., Brown, R. I., Cummins, R. A., Felce, D., & Mattikka, L. (2002). Conceptualization, measurement, and application of quality of life for persons with intellectual disabilities: results of an international panel of experts. *Mental Retardation, 40*, 457–470.

Schmidt, M. (2007). Podpora družinam z otroki z motnjami v duševnem razvoju. In B. Aberšek, M. Kordigel Aberšek, & M. Schmidt (Eds.), *Starši: Najuspešnejši člen pri podpori in usposabljanju ljudi s posebnimi potrebami* (pp. 11–17). Maribor: Pedagoška fakulteta, Fakulteta za naravoslovje in matematiko.

Singer, G. H. S., Goldberg-Hamblin, S. E., Peckham-Hardin, K. D., Barry, L., & Santarelli, G. E. (2002). Toward a Synthesis of family support practices and positive behavior support. In Lucyshyn, J. M., Dunlap, G., Albin, R. (Eds.), *Families and positive behavior support* (pp. 155–183). Baltimore, London, Toronto, Sydney: Paul H. Brookes Publishing Co.

Tomori, M. (1999). Družina in duševno zdravje otrok. In E. Kraševec-Ravnik (Ed.), *Varovanje duševnega zdravja otrok in mladostnikov* (pp. 150–155). Ljubljana: Kolaborativni center Svetovne zdravstvene organizacije za duševno zdravje otrok pri Svetovalnem centru za otroke, mladostnike in starše: Inštitut za varovanje zdravja Republike Slovenije.

Turnbull, A., Brown, I., & Turnbull, H. R. (2004). *Families and people with mental retardation and quality of life: International perspectives*. Washington, DC: American Association on Mental Retardation.

Zaviršek, D. (2005). Položaj otrok z ovirami: od formalne enakosti do resnične vključenosti. In A. Črnak-Meglič (Ed.), *Otroci in mladina v prehodni družbi: analiza položaja v Sloveniji* (pp. 221–238). Ljubljana: Ministrstvo za šolstvo in šport, Urad Republike Slovenije za mladino.

Chapter 20
Family Quality of Life in Several Countries: Results and Discussion of Satisfaction in Families Where There Is a Child with a Disability

Roy I. Brown, Keumja Hong, Joanne Shearer, Mian Wang, and Shin-yi Wang

Introduction

This chapter is about quality of life in families where there is a child, regardless of age, with an intellectual or developmental disability. The results are from Australia, Canada, South Korea, and Taiwan and particularly involve the perceptions of the primary carers (mostly mothers) as respondents. The material has been collected from Australia and Canada, although additional findings from Taiwan and South Korea are also included. The procedure involved asking families to complete, through the primary caregiver, the *Family Quality of Life Survey*, first edition (Brown, Brown et al., 2006) across nine domains, with particular reference to family satisfaction.

The challenge for the field is that many children with disabilities are now living in the regular community. Many people support this move, because it did away with the types of institutional settings, often of vast size, which caused concern in many countries. Previously, thousands of children and adults had little opportunity to return to the community and live an integrated and inclusive life. Although this development has been critically important in the lives of a large number of people, a serious challenge arises for many families (see Turnbull, Brown, & Turnbull, 2004). How do they cope when there is a child who is severely disabled, or a child with multiple diagnosis or extreme emotional behavioral problems within the family (see Brown, MacAdam-Crisp et al., 2006)? What happens to the family, what issues arise, and how can we ensure that the vast burden of responsibility of care and support is alleviated when making our society truly inclusive, while providing the types of support services that are required? The overall aim of society, through government policy and community services, is to enable the child with a disability to function as effectively as possible, and also to enable parents and other siblings to function effectively, and wherever possible, live lives of quality (Brown & Brown,

R.I. Brown (✉)
University of Calgary, Calgary, AB, Canada; Flinders University, Adelaide, SA, Australia
e-mail: roybrown@telus.net

R. Kober (ed.), *Enhancing the Quality of Life of People with Intellectual Disabilities*, Social Indicators Research Series 41, DOI 10.1007/978-90-481-9650-0_20,

2003). Family is the environment, which enables the individual members to develop and grow effectively.

The present chapter is primarily concerned with how disability affects those in the family who are not disabled and how we can develop ways of mitigating negative effects so each member, including the person(s) with intellectual disability, can function optimally. The issue is not just a child with a disability in a family but the interaction of disability with the family members as a whole.

Family Definitions

Families are seen in many societies as consisting of one or two parents and their children. Because of changes in social norms, a wide range of family constructs must now be taken into account, which were not seen as so relevant in the past. Families may be small or very large and wage earners may be none or several. The range and the complexity of families vary considerably and each structure brings rewards and challenges. This also applies to families where there are children with intellectual or developmental disabilities. We now recognize that there are various definitions of family, and in the research we have carried out we accept the parent's, generally the mother's, definition of how the family is constructed (see Brown & Brown, 2003, 2004).

Family Quality of Life Survey

The *Family Quality of Life Survey* is made up of domains of family functioning (see Isaacs et al., 2007). All impact the family in some way or other, but often in different ways. The survey was completed by individual family members who responded to the questions in the survey either on their own, through a face-to-face interview, or by telephone. At the respondent's request, this sometimes included a lengthy, on occasion up to 2 h, session where the respondent wished to elaborate at length on the answers. The detailed interviews provided amplification of qualitative information provided in this chapter.

The survey begins with information about the family and the duties each member performs. It then leads into nine domains of family life. The domains in the *Family Quality of Life Survey* are

1. Health of the family
2. Financial Well-Being
3. Family Relationships
4. Support from Other People
5. Support from Disability Related Services
6. Spiritual and Cultural Beliefs
7. Career and Preparing for Careers
8. Leisure and Enjoyment of Life
9. Community and Civic Involvement

Many of the domain questions in the survey are based on Likert scales. In this chapter, we are particularly interested in the satisfaction with family quality of life in each domain. The Likert measure on this dimension (FQOL Satisfaction) uses a 5-point scale ranging from very dissatisfied to very satisfied.

The survey question, for example, from the Health domain took the following form:

All things considered, how satisfied are you with the physical health of your family as it is today?

Very satisfied
Satisfied
Neither satisfied or dissatisfied
Dissatisfied
Very dissatisfied

The satisfaction questions from other domains take a parallel form. The results are presented in a series of figures covering satisfaction in each domain across samples in several countries. The study samples are from Australia (South Australia), Canada (British Columbia), South Korea, and Taiwan. The studies represent a continuum of exploration by the authors. We present the results in this form so that readers can see the sequence of our studies over the period of data collection and note how discussion and conclusions developed, including the variables that have come into play. We now believe these results should be considered very carefully in future studies and that outcome recommendations should be further explored and applied in policy and practice.

One of the most important aspects of Family Quality of Life is whether a family believes they have a life of quality across the nine major domains of family life. In the following figures the data reflect the highest 2 scores – that is "satisfied" and "very satisfied" combined. In the rest of this chapter, we refer to this combination as representing satisfaction. We argue that because if services are provided and family needs are met, then it is necessary that the family respondent record satisfied or very satisfied. Agency services and policymakers would presumably expect that their support and intervention contributions would lead to satisfaction. This is certainly the expectation of family members. Our aim is to measure domain satisfaction and through the qualitative addition of commentary associated with each domain isolate where needs occur, their frequency, and then how they affect family quality of life. From this we suggest ways in which families can be strengthened and increase the viability of each member including that of the individual with a disability.

Family Satisfaction Data from Four Countries

We have been fortunate to be able to collect data from four places, and this information is presented below. The data from Australia and Canada are presented in the order in which they were collected, along with discussion. These results are then followed with data from South Korea and Taiwan.

Australian Results

The sample families were obtained through agencies working with children with intellectual disabilities in South Australia and involved both city and rural communities. The sample, of 55 families, consisted of parents who agreed to be involved in the study. It can be regarded as a convenience sample. The children were aged between 2 and 41 years, so there is a wide age span that included children who are now adults.[1] The sample represents a mixed group of people. The individuals with intellectual disabilities included some with Down syndrome and a few with autism. In our initial research, these diagnostic groups were not separated, which is fairly consistent with other studies carried out in the family quality of life area (e.g., Brown, Anand, Fung, Isaacs, & Baum, 2003).

Figure 20.1 shows the pattern of responding across domains. The vast majority of families were satisfied in the domain of Family Health, and in the majority

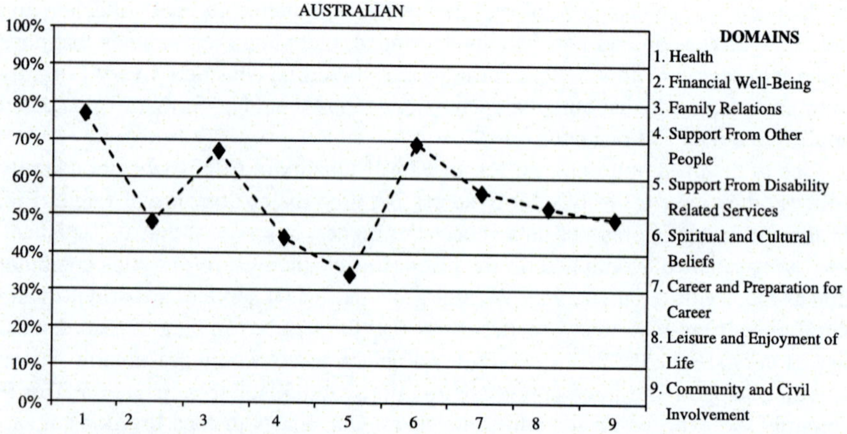

Fig. 20.1 Data percentage ofrespondents satisfied or very satisfied with family quality of life for each domain (Notes: Total Australia (n = 55); Respondent: Mean Age = 49 years; Age Range = 32–77. Child: Mean Age = 15 years; Age Range = 2–41. The *graph line* shown in this figure has been used for reasons of clarity (differences between domains). The domains are in the order used in the Family Quality of Life Survey instrument and the sequence of domains has no social or behavioral significance.

[1] "Children" is the term used to cover persons of all ages who are the individuals who have been raised by adult members of the family. Unless otherwise stated these children represented a wide age range.

of instances, Family Relations were seen as satisfactory, as they were in families' Spiritual and Cultural Beliefs. Career and Preparation for Careers were just above the 50% mark in terms of satisfaction, as was Leisure and Enjoyment of Life. Families were less satisfied about the Financial Well-Being domain that fell just below the 50% level. There are other domains such as Support from Other People, as well as support from disability-related services, whether private or public, which fell below the 50% satisfaction mark. Disability-related services showed the lowest domain satisfaction level which was within the 30% range.

The domains can be divided into what might be termed:

(1) Internal family quality life, which relates to how families see themselves functioning in terms of health, family relations, and their spiritual and cultural beliefs, which were all at least at the 60% level of satisfaction, and the highest domain percentages recorded. These domains are intrinsically about internal aspects of family life, which to a large degree relate to family values and internal relationships.
(2) External family quality of life, which relates to aspects of outside events, impacts the family somewhat differently. This includes domains, such as Financial Well-Being (i.e., essentially what the family earned from outside employment including disability allowances), support from other people in the community, and disability-related services, which were the lowest three domains in terms of satisfaction.

The differences between internal and external quality of life may be important, particularly if reflected in other studies. We are not suggesting that these two aspects are independent, for externally related domains are likely to have negative or positive impacts on family functioning. Very often internal and external domains or areas interact, e.g., a mother who is sensitive about her child's behavior may be reluctant to see neighbors, but responses from people in the community may make her more sensitive about the child's behavior which can influence family life. The internal domains are more associated with the behavior and development of families, in terms of their internal structure – their members' health, the relationships between family members and the rewards and satisfaction associated with these, and what can be termed the family's emotional, spiritual, and cultural factors.

Ageing and Family Satisfaction

There is now some evidence that older families show higher levels of satisfaction across domains than younger families. Chapter 16 by Jokinen and Brown in this book gives information on high levels of satisfaction in many older families consistent with the data below.

Using the Australian data, it is possible to compare satisfaction levels in aging families (parents 55 years and older) with younger ones. Figure 20.2 shows higher satisfaction scores on seven of the nine domains compared with the younger parent families in the sample. The two exceptions are Support from Other People and

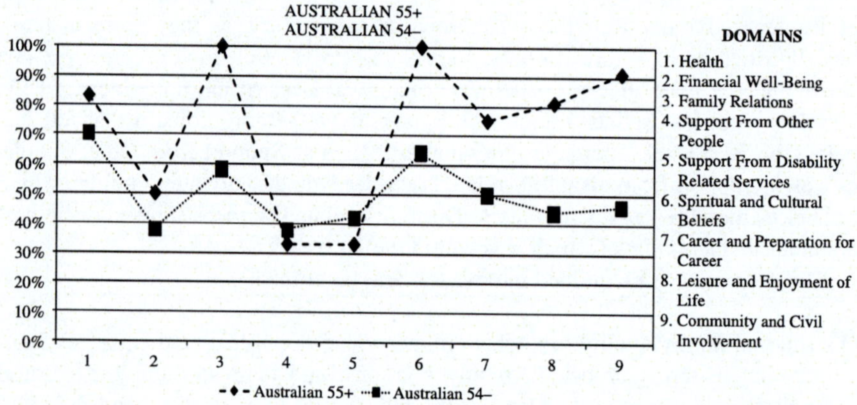

Fig. 20.2 Data percentage of respondents satisfied or very satisfied with Family Quality of Life for each domain (Notes: Australian 55+ ($n = 12$); Parent: mean age = 63 years; Age Range = 56–77; Child: Mean Age = 26; Age Range = 14–41. Australian 54– ($n = 27$); Parent: Mean Age = 43 years; Age Range = 32–54; Child: Mean Age = 12; Age Range = 5–34. The *graph lines* shown in this figure have been used for reasons of clarity (differences between domains). The domains are in the order used in the Family Quality of Life Survey instrument and the sequence of domains has no social or behavioral significance.

Support from Disability Services, both of which are the only ones in the ageing group to fall well below the 40% levels, and the mean score is lower than in the younger group of parents.

The question that arises is whether the satisfaction levels are a result of different social norms associated with the two age groups, for as data noted in the Jokinen and Brown chapter (Chapter 16) indicates, higher happiness levels are shown among a random sample of older people from the United States' general population. Alternatively, the difference associated with changes in the relationship between older parents and their child with disabilities may be associated with improved or more satisfying relationships, e.g., "my spouse has died and my son with a disability gives me company", and "she (the person with a disability) now makes the beds and carries the shopping." It seems possible that both aspects may be occurring, and in addition, older people with disabilities may in our sample be less disabled than individuals in the younger cohort.

Canadian Results

This section presents results from Canadian research in British Columbia. The families were from a large city and surrounding areas including a major island area of the Province. The sample mainly consisted of younger families and their children. There were 51 families in this group with children aged between 2 and 11 years. The satisfaction results are shown in Fig. 20.3.

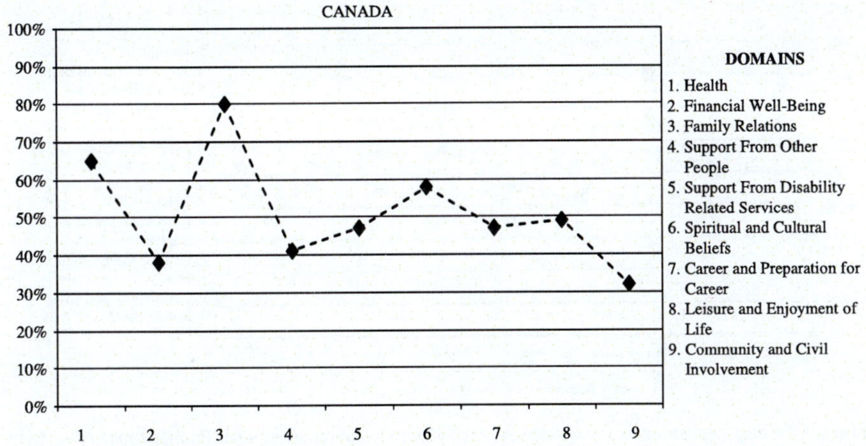

Fig. 20.3 Data percentage of respondents satisfied or very satisfied with Family Quality of Life for each domain (Notes: Canada ($n = 51$); Parent: Mean Age = 40 years; Age Range = 27–60. Child: Mean Age =7.6 years; Age Range = 2–13. The *graph lines* shown in this figure have only been used for reasons of clarity (differences between domains). The domains are in the order used in the Family Quality of Life Survey instrument and the sequence of domains has no social or behavioral significance.

Like the Australian data, Family Relationships, Family Health, and, then, Family Spiritual and Cultural satisfaction were the most highly rated domains. Family Leisure and Enjoyment of Life, Careers and Preparing for Careers plus Financial Well-Being, Support from Other People, and Disability-Related Services were all rated below the 50% level in terms of satisfaction. In the areas of Career Development and Preparation for Careers, as well as Leisure and Enjoyment of Life, the ratings were just below 50% satisfaction, while Community and Civic Involvement was substantially low and Financial Well-Being returned the second lowest satisfaction rating.

Australian and Canadian Comparisons

It is interesting to show the Australian and Canadian data in one figure (see Fig. 20.4.)

These satisfaction results show very similar patterns for both the Australian and the Canadian groups. The relative lows and highs are similar. Health of the Family, Family Relationships, and Spiritual and Cultural Values show the highest domain percentages in both groups, the first two lie in the 60–80% range. Spiritual and Cultural Beliefs are above the 60% level for the Australian data, and the Canadian result is only just below. The remaining domains for Canada lie below the 50% level. Both Financial Well-Being and Support from Other People, that is those in the surrounding neighborhood and extended family (i.e., family members not living

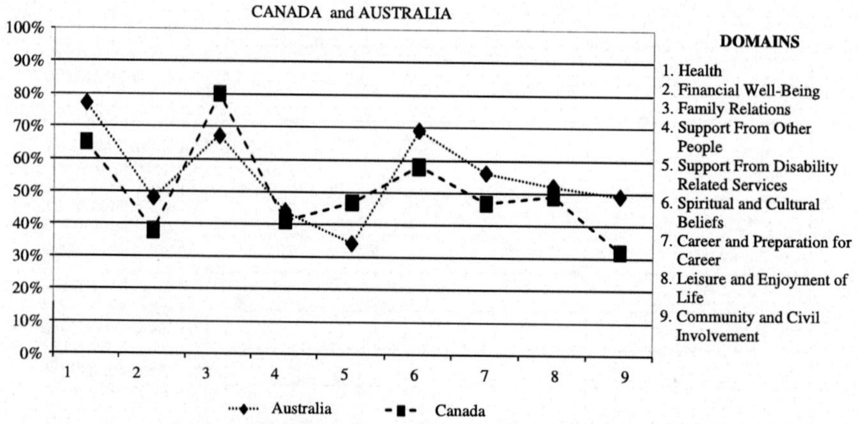

Fig. 20.4 Data percentage of respondents satisfied or very satisfied with Family Quality of Life for each domain (Notes: Australia ($n = 55$); Respondent: Mean Age = 49 years; Age Range = 32–77; Child: Mean Age = 15 years; Age Range = 2–41. Canada ($n = 51$); Respondent: Mean Age = 40 years; Age Range = 27–60; Child: Mean Age = 7.6 years; Age Range = 2–13. The *graph lines* shown in this figure have only been used for reasons of clarity (differences between domains). The domains are in the order used in the Family Quality of Life Survey instrument and the sequence of domains has no social or behavioral significance.

with the nuclear family), are below the 50% level and are among the lowest domain scores in both countries. Support from Disability-Related Services in terms of family is the lowest satisfaction domain in the Australian group, below 40%, while the Canadian sample lies in the 40% range. The questions arising relate to impact on the family by such services, not just the person with a disability i.e., "All things considered, how satisfied are you with disability related services your family receives?" Service to and support for the family, rather than just the individual with a disability, is discussed later.

The results from both of these samples seem reasonably consistent, and the suggestion made earlier that domains can be divided in terms of internal and external areas seems reasonable. However the types of support or intervention required, where families are low on the first set of domains, maybe very different from that required in the case of poor responses in the second set of domains. One obvious difference is that more families are satisfied on the internal set of domains while less than half are satisfied in the external set of domains. The data suggest that a portion of families face considerable internal family dissatisfaction when there are major challenges in families, namely, Family Health, Personal Family, and Relations plus the lack of satisfaction or absence of support or spiritual and cultural beliefs. In fact, where there are strong spiritual and cultural beliefs, family viability appears to remain strong.

The types of supports required are somewhat different. Support services for such families need to consider how these families can be helped further. The results suggest a gap in service policy and support services. Generally, families are not seen by services as the major focus for such impact, and it is suggested these are areas where greater support is required. It therefore appears that we can separate out at least two types of families: (1) those who have positive and satisfactory internal family dimensions, but lacked adequate support for aspects of external family life and (2) those families who have low levels of satisfaction in both internal and external aspects of family life.

Although there is obviously variability within and between groups, it does suggest that in families with high satisfaction in what we have termed internal family domains, but with low external satisfaction, personal support needs to be provided along with direct funding, which is an economic proposition for particular families (see later). In terms of other aspects of external support, for example, the domain of Community Support including neighbors is often an area of low satisfaction, indicating a need for society to provide information and example. A number of quotes from both the Canadian and Australian records support this view, e.g., "I thought I was the only Mum who was ignored by neighbors." Other examples relate to employment, including financial earnings and career and career preparation. Careers and Preparation for Careers within the family, which includes schooling as well as tertiary education and/or employment satisfaction for children and parents, lies around the 45–56% level in samples from both countries, for example, " I had to give up my employment which involved travel for a lower paid, but local job, so I could support my wife." "I am a single mother who has had to give up my university studies as my child (with intellectual disability) takes up most of my time." The implication is that this concern is shared by around half of the families. The question is, can we identify who these are? These types of concern are also true of Leisure and Enjoyment of life, while Community and Civic Involvement is low in the Canadian data compared to Australian.

The families who have challenges in both the internal and external domains are apparently much more vulnerable and need additional and often emotional or direct personal support as illustrated by many qualitative quotations. Such families frequently show low ratings on Leisure and Enjoyment of Life. Such areas as family leisure and enjoyment of life are generally not a factor associated with priorities for policy and support services. The results here indicate major concerns with areas of outstanding need, because they relate to the ability to function effectively. Associated with this are issues of mental health, a key consideration in families where there is low satisfaction on these internal measures an aspect discussed in some detail by Esbensen, Seltzer and Greenberg (2006). They also illustrate an important principle in quality of life, namely, holism, which indicates that support in one area of functioning can affect other areas or domains in a positive fashion (see Schalock et al., 2002).

It may be asked whether these domains are related to some causal pattern? Do they reflect the holistic and interconnected nature of well-being and quality of life? One method of examining this possibility is to compare families where there are children showing different diagnostic categories. It is possible to look at and compare the Canadian data in terms of diagnostic criteria, since two disability groups were separately selected, Down syndrome and Autism.

Down Syndrome and Autism compared

Figure 20.5 shows a breakdown of the Canadian data into two groups: Autism and Down syndrome. The sample represents a fairly young group of families, where the children have similar mean and reasonably similar ranges in terms of age. The families were of comparable size, parental age, and economic background (see Brown, MacAdam-Crisp et al., 2006). The data now tell a new story. Although some domains in both groups show similar satisfaction percentages there are two major domains where the families with a child with Autism are much lower than in the Down syndrome group of families. These are the family members' Careers and Preparation for Careers, and their Leisure and Enjoyment of Life. Both of these domains show below 50% satisfaction within the Autism group, unlike the Down group which lies near the 60% satisfaction level, a difference which is significant. It is tempting to see these differences resulting from Autism but, as Brown et al. (2006) point out, disruptive behavior and its effects on the family is possibly the aspect which causes distress and therefore low family satisfaction. If this is the case it seems likely that other groups, such as families who have children with Fetal

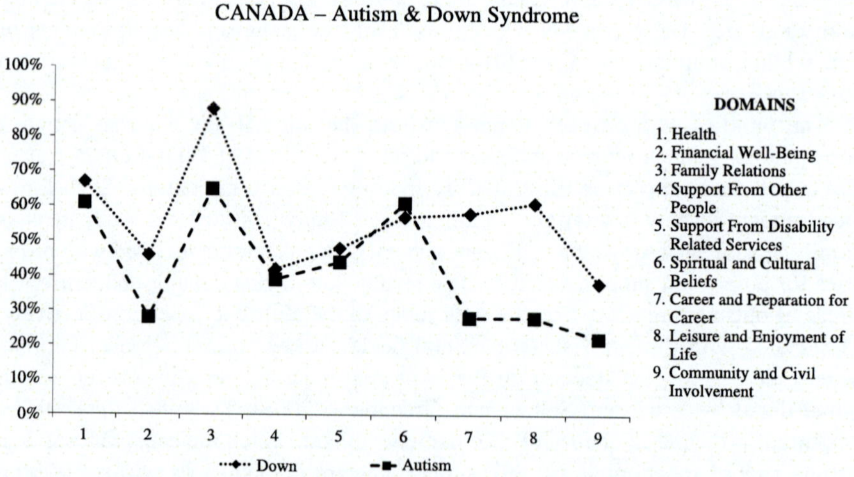

Fig. 20.5 Data percentage of respondents satisfied or very satisfied with family quality of life for each domain (Notes: Autism ($n = 18$); Mean Age: 7.78 years; Age Range: 6–13. Down ($n = 33$); Mean Age: 7.55 years; Age Range: 2–12. The *graph lines* shown in this figure have only been used for reasons of clarity (differences between domains). The domains are in the order used in the Family Quality of Life Survey instrument and the sequence of domains has no social or behavioral significance.

Alcohol Spectrum Disorder and Prader Willi syndrome, may show similar results in terms of satisfaction. This needs to be explored in further research.

Disability groups contrasted with families where there is no child with a disability

The Canadian research was also designed to provide us with an opportunity to compare the two disability groups with families with a similar number of children of similar age where there is no child with a disability. There is an absence, of course, of scores for the domain, Support from Disability Services, in the last mentioned group (see Fig. 20.6). Overall there is a significant difference between the domains of the contrast group and the other two groups in favor of the former. This is particularly marked in terms of the level of satisfaction in the contrast group, which reports higher satisfaction levels in all eight domains where the comparisons could be made.

The first three domains (Health, Financial Well-Being, Family Relationships) show a similar pattern for each group but at different levels, with the Down syndrome group lying in an intermediate position above Autism but below the contrast group. It is of interest that the percentage for Family Relations is nearly as high in the Down syndrome group as in the contrast group but the Autism group is around 25% lower. The question is why should this be? Possibly, the answer lies in the nature of emotional and disruptive behavior as discussed in the previous section.

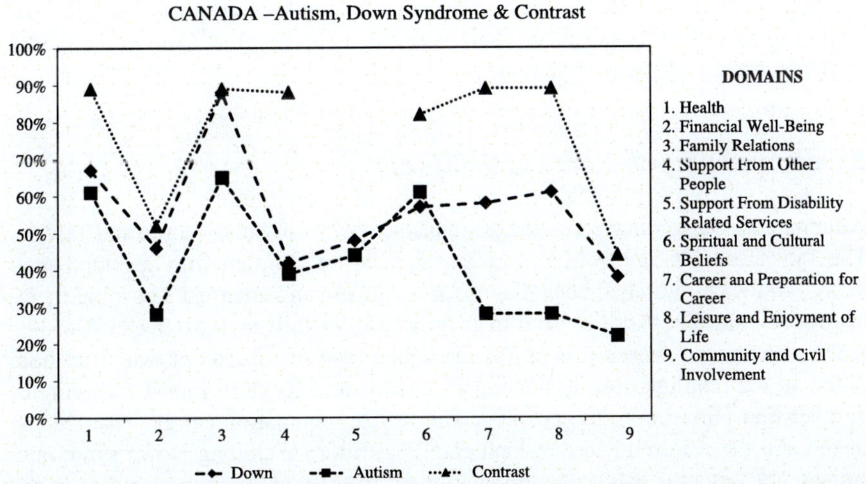

Fig. 20.6 Data percentage of respondents satisfied of very satisfied with family quality of life for each domain (Notes: Autism (n = 18); Mean Age: 7.78 years; Age Range: 6–13. Down (n = 33); Mean Age: 7.55 years; Age Range: 2–12. Contrast (n = 18) Mean Age: 6.81 years; Age Range: 4–12. The *graph lines* shown in this figure have only been used for reasons of clarity (differences between domains). The domains are in the order used in the Family Quality of Life Survey instrument and the sequence of domains has no social or behavioral significance.

In addition, the contrast group shows a higher satisfaction level in Support from Other People which is around 50% greater when compared with the other two groups, a difference which will be commented upon later. The contrast group also has higher levels of satisfaction in the Spiritual and Cultural Beliefs domain, and the highest level of satisfaction in Careers and Preparation for Careers and Leisure and Enjoyment of Life. Community and Civic Involvement in the contrast group is higher in terms of mean score than the other two groups, but very close to that of families with a child who has Down syndrome. The results appear to show that families who do not have a child with a disability enjoy a higher perceived quality of life overall compared with the two other groups, with the Down group showing an intermediate position, lying above the Autism group. Even so, it should be noted that there are families in each group who perceived satisfaction in overall quality of life.

The survey employed in this research allows us to identify families with a relatively low satisfaction compared with others, and to identify particular domains where major challenges appear to occur. The ability to provide a fairly basic measure of domain variation and group similarity and dissimilarity represents a step toward providing information, which allows decisions to be made, their outcomes to be evaluated (See Verdugo & Schalock, 2009), and research to be focused on more specific questions and hypotheses. The results are also relevant to the clinical use of the survey (see Wang & Brown, 2009, for further elaboration). Indeed, when there are lower levels of life satisfaction in the Down syndrome group, the presence of emotional disturbance and challenging behavior appeared to be present and not necessarily in the child with Down syndrome. In one family identified through a Down Syndrome Association, we could not understand the very low overall satisfaction levels until we recognized there was also a child with Autism in the family who had marked disruptive behavior.

Results from South Korea and Taiwan

Later on data were collected on the same instrument from South Korea and Taiwan. The Taiwanese data are from a sample of families of children with developmental delay. All the children had been diagnosed as autistic and attended a hospital therapeutic program. The families lived in an urban area in Taiwan, most in a city located at the western and central part of Taiwan with a total population of over 1 million. A few of the families lived in the county nearby, and spent 30 min–1 h driving or in other transportation to the hospital. The Korean population can be described as mixed. All the children had developmental disabilities including Down syndrome, autism, and cerebral palsy. The population is diagnostically similar to that of the Australian sample.

The satisfaction results for both South Korea and Taiwan are seen in Fig. 20.7 and in several domains show lower levels of satisfaction than the Australian and Canadian data. This is particularly true of the Taiwanese results. The South Korean data are also considerably lower than Australian and Canadian data in terms of

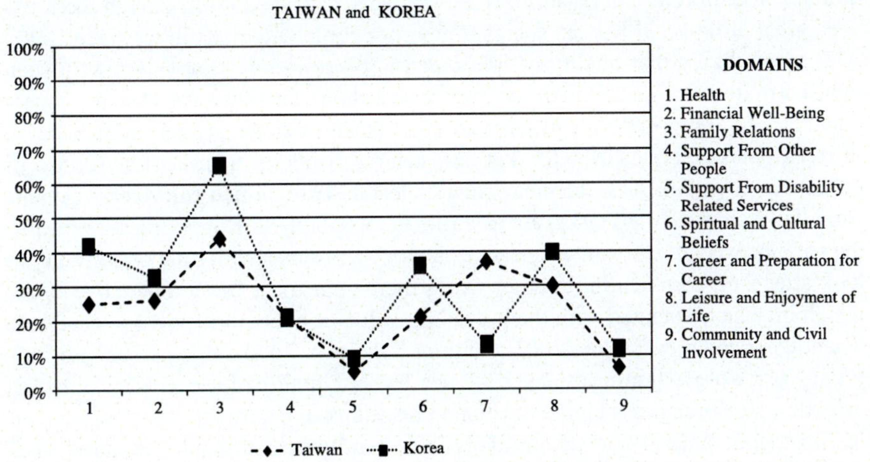

Fig. 20.7 Data percentage of respondents satisfied or very satisfied with Family Quality of Life for each domain (Notes: Taiwan ($n = 83$) Parent: Mean age = 37.9 years; Age range = 26–58; Child: Mean age = 5.4 Age Range = Child 1–14. Korea ($n = 81$); Parent: Mean age = 37.7 years; Age Range = 21–51; Child Mean Age = 8.4; Age Range = 4–18. The *graph lines* shown in this figure have only been used for reasons of clarity (differences between domains). The domains are in the order used in the Family Quality of Life Survey instrument and the sequence of domains has no social or behavioral significance.

Family Health, Support from Other People, Careers and Preparation for Careers, Leisure and Enjoyment of Life, and Community and Civic Involvement. The South Korean data show only one domain, Family Relationships, where the majority of people are satisfied with their quality of life. It is also the highest domain for satisfaction for the Taiwanese data, although that is within the 40% range. The Taiwanese data, unlike other data reported so far, shows a very low rating in support from Disability-Related Services, though not significantly different from the South Korean percentage. The other lowest areas are Support from Other People and Spiritual and Cultural beliefs. It is of concern that issues of Family Health and Financial Well-Being are reported at low satisfaction levels in the Taiwanese data.

Research in South Korea recognizes issues of children with developmental disabilities necessarily involve the whole family. However, interventions have only focused on children with disabilities, and circumstances involving the family have been overlooked (Chung, Lee, & Chung, 2003). It is also important to take into account Korean perspectives about children and disabilities if one is to understand the quality of life of Korean families. The idea that children's disabilities result from sins committed by their parents in a previous life is a traditional and pervasive among Koreans (Yang, 1998). Therefore all problems or suffering which result from children's disabilities are expected to be solved by their parents. It is probably because of this belief that social rights of children with disabilities and their families have developed in a passive way. As a result, social policy and social services for the families of children with disabilities are still very restricted, even though there has been great progress in Korean social policy for people with disabilities since 2000.

It seems likely that quality of life which is perceived as relatively low in such families may be associated with society's views about disability, and then the consequent lack of appropriate social services. Parents who provide primary care, because of lack of these services even for day care, can rarely pursue a professional career or obtain employment. Also, services such as respite care, which can release parents from daily physical care tasks, are as a rule not available in Korea. Because of this, the parents execute labor-intense care tasks for themselves with little opportunity to look after their own health. In other words there appears to be an interactive cycle, which may be associated with the prevailing value or belief system associated with disability (Brown & Brown, 2003; Keith & Schalock, 2000). It is perhaps not surprising that Korean families showed a lower level of quality of life in terms of health even though Korea has a highly developed institutional health insurance system.

In general, Asian societies are likely to be family or community-centered, so it was expected that Korean families would be relatively more satisfied with supports from other people. However, interestingly, the result showed that this expectation was not supported. Korean parents, due to their beliefs about children and disability, are inclined to conceal that they are raising children with disabilities and therefore isolate themselves from neighbors (see Lee, 2002).

One of the critical difficulties families with a disabled child experience is a financial problem. Families raising a disabled child incur extra expenses but have less time and opportunity than members of other families to pursue a career and find a job (Kim, 1997). Indeed this is not unique to South Korea and is a challenge faced by a large portion of the families reported from other countries in this chapter, along with concern that the parent, generally the mother, has more responsibilities for caring than they would like, an aspect which probably influences satisfaction levels in most if not all domains of family quality of life.

Since 2006 the South Korean government has provided financial support to families raising children with disability, which was approximately $50 per child per month in 2008. This amount of support was insufficient to significantly reduce the financial burden on the family, and most of the families reported financial difficulties. In addition financial difficulty probably plays a significant role in limiting social service use, and this is supported by the finding that the level of support from disability-related services domain was lower than other areas. However, once again it is likely that this is an interactive issue where each domain impacts or is impacted by the other.

Taiwanese satisfaction results appear, overall, to be lower than data recorded in Australia and Canada, though reasonably similar to those from South Korea. However, it should be noted that the children were all diagnosed with Autism, the group which also showed much lower satisfaction levels across domains in the Canadian Group. This is of particular interest because some work by Chou and Schalock (2009), using quality of life data from Taiwan, notes that average quality of life scores for "social belong/community integration" among all Taiwanese residents from three residential models were lower than the residents in the studies conducted by Schalock and Keith (1993) in the United States and Otrebski (2000) in Poland. Chou and Schalock's conclusion is that policy changes are desirable so that quality of life can be taken into account in service delivery. Their data applied to persons with intellectual disabilities, but they also suggest that expectations for quality of life were easily satisfied for many individuals.

Research in Canada Brown, Bayer & Brown (1992) suggests that introducing a quality of life approach raises expectation and helps individuals focus on raising their own quality of life – one of the reasons that an intervention model needs to be replaced by a support model encouraging personal choice and decision making, which is then supported through services and community action. The present chapter suggests that the same may well apply to the families of children with intellectual disabilities. This also seems consistent with the Taiwanese family quality of life research. Further exploration is necessary, as is the case with the South Korean group. For example, the lowest score in support from Disability-Related Services may be associated with insufficient welfare support for the participants. Further, the major act providing welfare support to people with disability in Taiwan, Welfare Act for People with Disability was established in 1990 with a focus on the provision of medical, educational, and vocational supports to the persons older than 6 years with disabilities. Children younger than 6-year old and the families of people with disability were not seen as a central focus of the welfare system. Most of the participants in the Taiwanese study were the families of young children with Autism that tend to benefit least from the current welfare system. Furthermore, the low scores in Support from Disability Services, Support from Other People and Spiritual Culture dimensions may be explained by the negative views toward disabilities in society and this, too, appears consistent with the South Korean data where having a child with Autism can be viewed as a punishment from God or through wrongdoing of the family members. Families may isolate themselves and avoid seeking supports from the government and others in the community, including religious organizations, in order to avoid being seen as of "bad family." However, the connection between the core family members can become stronger, because sharing the responsibilities for taking care of the child with disability within the family is taken for granted and honored in Taiwanese culture. In terms of the Taiwanese low scores in Family Health and Financial Well-Being, it is not clear if having a child with disability increases the anxiety toward Family Health and Financial Well-Being. Most families in Taiwan emphasize the importance of physical health and saving money. A sense of crisis toward physical health and saving money can arise when a family has a child with disability. Insufficient support and the nature of support from the government, the cost spent on the child with a disability by the family, and the income loss caused by caring for the child may prevent the family from saving money both for the future needs of the child with a disability and for other members of the family in the future, and thereby increasing their dissatisfaction.

Overall it would appear that the two sets of data from South Korea and Taiwan show much lower satisfaction response rates compared with either the overall Canadian or Australian results. The South Korean sample is a mixed sample and, like the Taiwanese data, underscores the importance and relatively high level of satisfaction with family relations. However, the Taiwanese data, which is based on families where there is a child with Autism, have some similarities with the Autism sample from Canada. In both cases where there is a child with Autism, Leisure and Enjoyment of Life falls below the 40% level. This must be regarded with concern and should result in changes to policy and support.

Discussion

It is important to remind the reader that the questions in this survey are directed toward issues about the family, not just the person with a disability. The responses represent perceptions of the respondent. Researchers (e.g., Andrews, 1974) have recognized for a long time that perceptions are a major driving force of human behavior, that is, what is perceived and believed affects how the individual or, in this case family members behave. This includes how a family is affected by its belief and value system, the nature of disability services, whether they are private or public; health and the satisfaction of health in the family, and so on. This means any and all members of the family may have experiences that cause the person filling in the survey to rate the family higher or lower on the 5-point satisfaction scale. In the Canadian and Australian data where qualitative information was recorded in addition to ratings, it was clear, for example, that though the respondent recognized that direct support had often been given to the person with a disability, no mention was made of services supporting the family needs resulting from disability. This is one possible explanation for the relatively low ratings on the support from Disability-Related Services domain in all four countries. In this context, there are often pressing challenges, for the disability of one member of the family negatively influences the behavior or resources of the family as a whole, for example, when a mother has to give up her job to look after her child.

It is also important to stress that the survey is an attempt to measure individual aspects of life through the domains, as well as document interaction between domains. It is likely that the level of satisfaction in one particular domain influences and is influenced by other domain values and experiences. Factors, such as behavioral disruption, can become the focus of concern in some families. In other words, this survey approach provides an opportunity to look at all aspects of life and their integration.

The holistic hypothesis needs further investigation. It seems plausible and underscores the possibility that intervention and support in one key area is likely, because of the holistic nature of human behavior, to improve other aspects of family functioning and therefore overall family satisfaction. Key areas differ to some extent from family to family, or over time in the same family, arguing for an individual approach to support. We have also noted that there appeared to be families where internal aspects of family life were positive and the challenges largely arose from outside the family, e.g., community reaction, lack of support, and lack of appropriate respite when required. These challenges necessitate careful and considered observation, reflection, and flexibility on the part of policy and service personnel.

Additionally, combining intervention and/or support in more than one domain, e.g., Family Health and support for the family in terms of enjoyment of life (Leisure and Recreation or Career Preparation) is likely to have greater and possibly wide-ranging effects on a family's overall satisfaction and quality of life. This would need much close collaboration between different service groups and would require much greater coordination of policy between different departments and agencies. If such arguments are correct such an approach: (a) requires an accent on service and support across agencies; and (b) should have long-term economic savings, since such coordinated intervention might be expected to have holistic benefits, such as an increase in family overall health and economic viability. However, as stressed by Brown and Brown (2009), such intervention and coordination should critically involve the family perception of needs and choices. It is important to consider how domains may link together. The lowest domains, in terms of satisfaction, are Financial Well-Being, Support from Other People, and Support from Disability Services so the interplay between these domains warrants further examination. In addition to these domains, in some families, particularly those where there is behavioral disturbance as in the Autism group, low levels of satisfaction are returned for Careers and Preparation for Careers and in overall Enjoyment of Life. Also, Family Relationships appear lower in the families where there is Autism compared with both the Down and the contrast group. The challenge may not be Autism per se, but disruptive behavior which influences the family as a whole. This suggests challenging behavior by the individual, which can sometimes be severe, such as screaming and rocking behavior and aggressive outburst toward others, is a highly relevant factor, and this is consistent with a study carried out by Brown in Scotland and to be reported in the near future. It is important to put the notion of disruptive behavior into context. In some of these families isolation due to separation of the parents often appears to exacerbate the situation. There are exceptions to this where breakdown between the parents resulted in an improved quality of life according to a few qualitative comments, e.g., "life became better when he left."

Sometimes some of these behaviors occur in the Down syndrome group. However, there seems much less dissatisfaction around a number of the domains where Down syndrome families are concerned. Where there is challenging and disruptive behavior there appears to be greater negative family impact on quality of life for all of the members of the family. It seems likely that this is why such families do not see the disability and support services responding to their needs. What then are these concerns across domains in such families? They include:

- Lack of short-term respite care when required and necessary for acceptable family life
- Longer term respite where a child has major behavior disturbance
- Lack of necessary information and how to get existing information about services and supports
- Challenging behavior which is continuously disruptive to all family members
- Lack of relief for parents who may have had no vacations over many years
- Parents unable to have time for themselves or together with their spouse or partner

- The inability of children or adults to study at home in a suitable atmosphere
- Instances where employment has to change or to terminate in order that one or both parents can provide better support for their child in the home.
- Financial impact on each member of the family.
- The above and particular challenges associated with single-parent status

Siblings may be impacted in terms of studying, and having friends to their home. Further, it may be difficult to invite guests or have neighbors over because of major behavioral disturbance. Quite frequently there is a lack of desired support from neighbors and community. This occurs in both the Down syndrome and Autism groups and also other developmental disabilities, although the lack of support appears much higher where multiple disability occurs, and includes lack of appropriate support from community agencies such as religious organizations. The result is that families, and therefore people with the disabilities, are then effectively cut off from necessary support and community interaction. This is a major form of exclusion and raises important questions when many agencies and individuals go to some length to advocate inclusive policies, though to address this community knowledge and experience in handling such needs are relevant. Although such occurrences are not universal, they appear frequently in the records of our data. There is a need to carefully examine the practical impacts of exclusion and what this entails (see Brown and Brown, 2003).

In some instances a parent has indicated that they feel ignored by neighbors, but occasionally concede that this may sometimes come from their own concerns about what neighbors might think. There is a lack of consistency of service, and among those parents who are older, concerns for adequate services after they themselves cannot cope, or will have died. On top of this, lack of knowledge about services, and the inability to get needs met remain major issues from primary carers whether they are parents or siblings (see also Chapter 16 by Jokinen and Brown, this volume for further details).

It is important in further studies in the disability field to ensure there is a comparison age group without disabilities (compare Brown, MacAdam-Crisp et al., 2006). The results underscore the importance of comparative data from the general community. This may be relevant, not only in terms of differences between countries, but also in terms of comparisons across cultures, and may be used as a yardstick or, as in the cases described here, to pinpoint some of the issues which are of major concern and particularly impact families across the lifespan where a child with a disability is involved. In all the studies described, the support from disability-related services are regarded as among the lowest in terms of satisfaction, whether that is from the Australian data including older families, Canadian data involving young families with Down or the Autism groups, with the greatest concerns being stated in those families where there is a child with challenging behavior. The interpretation of this is important. Disability-related services do provide considerable support for the child with a disability, yet many families remain highly vulnerable and require additional assistance that would enable the whole family to function more effectively economically, socially, and emotionally. The areas of concern for family members include challenges in education and employment. Both these challenges lower family economic status particularly when behavioral and emotional disturbance are involved. Behavioral and emotional disturbance reduce the family's ability to work and study, and has some wider and damaging effects on siblings who live in such families. It is suggested that both on economic and health grounds, it would be prudent for disability-related services and policymakers to provide more direct family support than currently is the case, and that support needs to be specific and targeted to families where there are particularly low satisfaction ratings. Such support is likely to positively influence family relations and resilience, through reduction in relentless stress, which often results in individuals experiencing fatigue, should positively influence overall family quality of life. Such measures underscore the changing focus of studies which are moving from a deficit model to the promotion of well-being and quality of life (Ylvén, Bjôrck-Åkesson, & Granlund, 2006).

A guiding principle in this context comes from quality of life research which underscores the importance of choice by family members (For details see Brown & Brown, 2009), which enables families to feel in charge of their life situation and helps to stabilize family units. Importantly, from a government policy point of view, this should, in the long run, result in reduced economic need and also promote quality of health for the family as a whole.

The above means a fundamental change in how we set policy, administer disability services, and then carry out practices at the managerial and frontline levels. It also requires changes to the way we educate personnel. An understanding of the interaction of the holistic nature of lifestyle among families with children with disabilities, and the major causes of family disruption, are therefore critically important.

The Family Quality of Life Survey seems sensitive to, and can pick up cultural and local community differences. However, such aspects need much further examination. This should not cause a delay in providing family supports, for the evidence across our samples indicates many similar results and these are largely consistent with that, for example, of Zuna, Turnbull, and Summers (2009) and is also reflected in the papers by Werner, Edwards, and Baum (2009), findings supported by the work of Wilgosh and Scorgie (2006)

A Word of Caution

There are a number of families who are satisfied across the domains of family quality of life, although in most instances in this chapter, those who record satisfaction may still have important needs at a family level. Cummins' (2001b) research on individuals with intellectual disabilities and their satisfaction levels suggests that a number may indicate that aspects of the child's life are satisfactory, when in fact there are major needs and concerns. This may also apply to family situations. Such families may have less apparent needs or may be reluctant to expose people outside their family circle to their predicament. However, it seems possible that family respondents may reflect family issues more accurately than when an individual is refereeing to their own satisfaction (see Brown, Schalock, & Brown, 2009). Further it seems likely that the populations in the present studies represent families who have the time and interest to participate in the FQOL survey. This suggests that families with greater challenges may not be appropriately represented. However, it seems possible that more disabled samples were obtained in the Taiwanese and South Korean studies, but further exploration will be necessary to determine whether this is in fact correct. For example, the Taiwanese findings came from a specific agency and are believed to be representative of that agency's families having a child with autism. Because they benefited little from general education or had been rejected by general childcare service most were brought to the hospital by the families for further treatment. Furthermore, the families in the sample are more likely to represent the families with limited resources who could not get sufficient supports or needed public funding to pay for the intervention for their child. The intervention program at the hospital was funded by the national health insurance of the government. It is also noted that families varied considerably, and it is likely that families also vary over time. It is critically important that family behavior is monitored on a regular basis. For example, the ability to access family quality of life, even on the short version of the survey (Brown et al., 2006, website), on at least a yearly or biannual basis may be important. Furthermore, there should be a means of noting when family circumstances are believed to change, and particular attention needs to be given to indicators provided by parents or other primary carers. Change in a family's life in one domain is likely to affect other domains.

Acknowledgements We would like to acknowledge the support and assistance of:

Brian Eacott and Hilary Hayes for their involvement in collecting the Australian data while at Flinders University.

Jacqueline Crisp, University of Victoria, Canada, for help with the original Canadian study.

Hyeji Choi, Seoul Women's University, South Korea.

Cheng-Yea Ma, Psychiatrist, Tsaotun Psychiatric Center, Department of Health, Tsao tun, Nan-Tou, Taiwan.

Also thanks to Patricia M. Brown for editorial suggestions and Cathy Craft, Canada, for graphical preparation.

We also appreciated the support of Office for Disability and Client Services of the South Australian Department for Families and Communities for their assistance in the Australian data collection and The Ministry of Children and Family Development through the Human Early Learning Partnership (HELP) for the Canadian material. The views stated are those of the authors and do not necessarily represent the views of government or HELP.

References

Andrews, F. M. (1974). Social indicators of perceived life quality. *Social Indicators Research, 1*, 279–299.

Brown, I., Anand., S., Fung, W., Isaacs, B., & Baum, N. (2003). Family quality of life: Canadian results from an international study. *Journal of Developmental and Physical Disabilities, 15*, 207–230.

Brown, I., & Brown, R. (2004). Concept for beginning study in family quality of life. In A. Turnbull, I. Brown, & R. Turnbull (Eds.), *Families and people with mental retardation and quality of life: International perspectives* (pp. 25–47). Washington, DC: American Association on Mental Retardation.

Brown, I., & Brown, R. I. (2003). *Quality of Life and Disability: An Approach for Community Practitioners*. London, UK: Jessica Kingsley.

Brown, I., & Brown, R. I. (2009). Choice as an aspect of quality of life for people with intellectual disabilities. *Journal of Policy and Practice in Intellectual Disabilities, 6*, 10–17.

Brown, I., Brown, R. I., Baum, N. T., Isaacs, B. J., Meyerscough, T., Neikrug, S., et al. (2006). *Family Quality of Life Survey: Main Caregivers of People with Intellectual or Developmental Disabilities*. Toronto: Surrey Place Centre.

Brown, R. I., Bayer, M. B., & Brown, P. M. (1992). *Empowerment and developmental handicaps: Choices and quality of life*. Toronto: Captus.

Brown, R. I., MacAdam-Crisp, J., Wang, M., & Iarocci, G. (2006). Family quality of life where there is a child with a developmental disability? *Journal of Policy and Practice in Intellectual Disabilities, 3*(4), 238–245.

Brown, R. I., Schalock, R. L., & Brown, I. (2009). Quality of life: Its application to persons with intellectual disabilities and their families – introduction and overview. *Journal of Policy and Practice in Intellectual Disabilities, 6*(1), 2–6.

Chou, Y.-C., & Schalock, R. (2009). Survey outcomes and cross-national comparisons of quality of life with respect to people with intellectual disabilities in Taiwan. *Journal of Policy and Practice in Intellectual Disabilities. Intellectual and Developmental Disability, 6*(1), 6–9.

Chung, Y., Lee, S., & Chung, B. (2003). *Children with developmental disability and family welfare*. Seoul: Hyunhaksa.

Cummins, R. A. (2001b). The subjective wellbeing of people caring for a family member with a severe disability at home: A review. *Journal of Intellectual and Developmental Disability, 26*(1), 88–100.

Esbensen, A. J., Seltzer, M. M., & Greenberg, J. S. (2006). Depressive symptoms of adults with mild to moderate intellectual disability and their relation to maternal well-being. *Journal of Policy and Practice in Intellectual Disabilities, 3*(4), 229–237.

Isaacs, B. J., Brown, I., Brown, R. I., Baum, N., Myerscough, T., Neikrug, S., et al. (2007). The international family quality of life project: Goals and description of a survey tool. *Journal of Policy and Practice in Intellectual Disabilities, 4*(3), 177–185.

Keith, K. D., & Schalock, R. L. (Eds.). (2000). *Cross-cultural perspectives on quality of life*. Washington, DC: American Association on Mental Retardation.

Kim, N. (1997). *Social work Intervention model for mothers of children with auditory impairment*. Busan: Busan University.

Lee, H. (2002). Parenting social network for the children with developmental disabilities. *Korean Journal of Special Education, 37*(3), 57–74.

Otrebski, W. (2000). Quality of life of people with mental retardation living in two different environments. In K. D. Keith & R. L. Schalock (Eds.), *Cross-cultural perspectives on quality of life* (pp. 83–92). Washington, DC: American.

Schalock, R. L., Brown, I., Brown, R., Cummins, R. A., Felce, D., Matikka, L., et al. (2002). Conceptualization, measurement, and application of quality of life for persons with intellectual disabilities: Report of an international panel of experts. *Mental Retardation, 40*, 457–470.

Schalock, R. L., & Keith, K. D. (1993). *Quality of Life Questionnaire*. Worthington, OH: IDS Publishing.

Turnbull, A., Brown, I., & Turnbull, R. (Eds.). (2004). *Families and people with mental retardation and quality of life: International perspectives*. Washington, DC: American Association on Mental Retardation.

Verdugo, M. A., & Schalock, R. L. (2009). Quality of life: From concept to future applications in the field of intellectual disabilities. *Journal of Policy and Practice in Intellectual Disabilities, 6*, 62–64.

Wang, M., & Brown, R. (2009). Family quality of life: A framework for policy and social service provisions to support families of children with disabilities. *Journal of Family Social Work, 12*, 144–167.

Wilgosh, L., & Scorgie, K. (2006). Theoretical model for conceptualizing cross-cultural applications and intervention strategies for parents of children with disabilities. *Journal of Policy and Practice in Intellectual Disabilities, 3*(4), 211–218.

Werner, S., Edwards, M., & Baum, N. T. (2009). Family quality of life before and after out-of-home placement of a family member with an intellectual disability. *Journal of Policy and Practice in Intellectual Disabilities, 6*, 32–39.

Yang, O. (1998). Social stigma on people with mental disorder. *The Korean Journal of Social Welfare, 35*, 231–260.

Ylvén, R., Bjôrck-Åkesson, E., & Granlund, M. (2006). Literature review of positive functioning in families with children with a disability. *Journal of Policy and Practice in Intellectual Disabilities, 3*(4), 253–270.

Zuna, N. I., Turnbull, A., & Summers, J. A. (2009). Family quality of life: Moving fro measurement to application. *Journal of Policy and Practice in Intellectual Disabilities, 6*, 24–31.

Part VI
Enhancing QOL

Chapter 21
Developing Numeracy to Enhance Quality of Life

Rhonda M. Faragher

Introduction

Have you needed to learn something new recently? Most of us have. Learning can be difficult and may take considerable effort, so why bother? Most adults will make the commitment to learning if they see there is value. When we learn we may do so to improve our quality of life. We might learn how to operate the new photocopier in the office so that we are able to perform required tasks. We might learn how to calculate the fabric we need to make curtains to save paying someone else to measure up the windows for us. Potential improvements to our quality of life can motivate us to learn many things, including those we do not particularly enjoy at the time – perhaps aspects of mathematics. This will be explored in this chapter.

The use of mathematics in our daily activities (numeracy) can contribute to our quality of life. Numeracy is about being able and willing to use mathematics in the contexts of our lives (AAMT, 1997). It seems self-evident that numeracy would be important and certainly it is a major goal of schooling in many jurisdictions (see, for example, MCEETYA, 1999). Surprisingly, the importance of numeracy for adults with intellectual disabilities is not always as clearly appreciated. The manager of a large provider of services for adults with disabilities told me her clients had no need for numeracy development. Certainly, it is possible to reduce the numeracy demands of life but that comes at the cost of empowerment and independence. In this chapter, I contend that numeracy is important for all, especially those with an intellectual disability. Further, it is possible for everyone to develop their personal numeracy throughout their life. For people with intellectual impairments, numeracy development needs to be deliberately encouraged.

R.M. Faragher (✉)
Australian Catholic University (Canberra), P.O. Box 256, Dickson, ACT 2602, Australia
e-mail: Rhonda.Faragher@acu.edu.au

R. Kober (ed.), *Enhancing the Quality of Life of People with Intellectual Disabilities*, Social Indicators Research Series 41, DOI 10.1007/978-90-481-9650-0_21,

Numeracy and Quality of Life

The quality of life of a person with an intellectual impairment can be enhanced by numeracy development (Faragher & Brown, 2005). Quality of life has a number of facets including the importance of perception, choice and a lifespan approach (Schalock et al., 2002). Each of these interacts with aspects of numeracy in complex ways so that numeracy and quality of life influence each other. For example, how people view themselves and the perceptions of others can be affected by the ability or inability to do the mathematics they need. If you have difficulty tendering cash for purchases, every shopping transaction is a potential source of stress and embarrassment. Similarly, choices influence quality of life and are fundamental to numeracy. Being able to do mathematics opens opportunities for choice to engage in more life contexts. New contexts, in turn, offer opportunities to learn and use new mathematics. Throughout our lives, our contexts change and our numeracy needs change as well. A lifespan approach, necessary for quality of life is also important for numeracy. Life-long numeracy development is essential for all of us.

For most adults, we learnt the foundations of the mathematics we need in school and have adapted these techniques for personal use (Willis, 1990). Throughout our lives we also learn mathematics as we need to, often in work contexts (Riall & Burghes, 2000). For adults with intellectual disabilities, opportunities to learn mathematics may have been limited throughout life, due to limited schooling, lack of adult employment, and unavailable workplace training (Faragher, 2006). Limited opportunities to learn mathematics vicariously can be debilitating for adults with intellectual disabilities.

In this chapter, the role of numeracy is considered through the lens of the quality of life model where it is argued that since numeracy matters, its development needs to be planned and not left to chance. This chapter explores the need for systematic development of numeracy throughout life. A Numeracy Development Plan is proposed as one approach to do this. A Numeracy Development Plan is a way to purposefully develop numeracy when incidental opportunities may be limited.

- *It is not* about learning school mathematics again
- *It is not* about doing exercises
- It *is* focused on what an individual needs and wants to learn
- It *is* about choice in how to learn and what to learn

Numeracy Development Plan (NDP)

Numeracy development for individuals with intellectual disabilities is too important to be left to chance. Unfortunately, if numeracy development is not planned, the chance of success depends on having support people around the person with an intellectual impairment who value numeracy development and recognize the teaching component in their support role. Of course, carers have a complex role and adding numeracy development may be seen as one task too many. However, the positive effects on quality of life are such that the effort is essential. Numeracy development can improve the independence of a person – someone who has learned how to set their alarm clock no longer needs to be woken for work; the person who can interpret bath scales can monitor their own weight.

A systematic approach to numeracy development can be achieved using a numeracy development plan. This plan can be considered as a specific form of person-centred planning (see, for example, Adams, Beadle-Brown, & Mansell, 2006). In the Robertson et al. study (2007), it was found that the effectiveness of person-centred plans was linked to the commitment of those involved with the implementation. Acknowledging the connection between numeracy development and quality of life may help those involved to be committed to the effort of implementation.

The Planning Process

There are six main steps in the Numeracy Development Planning process. These are outlined in the following sections. To help explain the process, I have provided an example of the preparation of a Numeracy Development Plan for Tanya Boulton, a young woman with an intellectual impairment. She, and her mother, Helen, worked with me to develop the plan.

Tanya lives in supported accommodation with three other clients and rostered carers. Through disability support agencies, she is employed in three separate contexts undertaking office cleaning and folding brochures. She enjoys walking and swimming with her carer. When visiting her parents' home, she works on 1,000 piece jigsaw puzzles and enjoys playing with her nieces and nephew.

Step 1: Undertake a Context Audit

The first step in the numeracy development plan is to identify the contexts of the life of the person. It may help to list activities on a weekly planner. An example is shown in Fig. 21.1, completed for Tanya. I wrote while Tanya and her mother told me Tanya's daily activities. The text of the handwritten document is as follows:

Sunday: Church; Lunch at Mum and Dad's – jigsaws, watch cricket, play with nieces and nephew, call from sister; Home at 5

Monday: 8:30 collected by ute [utility vehicle]; Work – cleaning crew 3+ support worker, mop, brooms, toilets, offices, lunchroom; come home about 3:30 – watch TV; Carer comes at 5; 9 to bed after tablets. Webster packs for medicine.

Tuesday: Work cleaning – different support worker and clients

Wednesday: 9 Paperworks – support worker collects, make booklets, notepads. 3+2 part-time workers; afternoon recreation with Alison [carer] – art at Narrabunda, movies, Tillies [café], shopping – take money; Wendy [carer] comes at 5 pm

Thursday: About 9:30 Lead Office in Civic – fold City News, put in envelopes with address stickers, one other; Respite care afternoon – swimming, + one other; Home to rinse swimmers.

Step 1 What do you do?

This step involves identifying all the contexts of a person's life – what they do day-to-day. Also, it is a place to list what a person would like to do in the future – perhaps they want to prepare for a new job.

What is your week like?

SUNDAY	MONDAY	TUESDAY	WEDNESDAY	THURSDAY	FRIDAY	SATURDAY
Church Lunch at Mum + Dad's – jigsaws – watch TV (cricket) – play with nieces + nephew – call from Sister Home at 5pm	8:30 collected by ute Work cleaning crew – 3+ support worker tasks – sweeping – mopping – toilets, offices, Lunchroom ~3:30 Home - Watch T.V. - carer comes at 5 pm 9:00 – medication (Webster packs) - Bed	Work Cleaning - different spt worker and clients	9:00 collected by support worker Work "Paperworks" – make booklets + notepads – 3+ 2 support workers Afternoon Recreation with Alison (money) – Art at Narr. – Movies – cafe – Shopping 5:00 Wendy comes	9:30 'LEAD' office in city - Fold 'City News' – put in envelope with address labels – one other staff client Respite care afternoon – Swimming – with one other Home – rinse swimmers	Walk with respite carer Games – Skip Bo – Yahtze – Rummy Q (number game) 'Music for Everyone' – singing – dancing – playing percussion – Karaoke	Day out with Rick. e.g: museum – Floriade – War Mem. Lunch out Haircuts etc at Belcon. Cleaning room

Fig. 21.1 Tanya's weekly activities

Friday: Walk with respite care; Game of Skip Bo, Yahtze, Rummy Q – number game; Music for Everyone – singing, dancing, playing drums, percussion, karaoke.

Saturday: Rick [carer] takes out, e.g. museum, War Memorial, Floriade; Lunch out; Haircuts, etc. at Belconnen; Cleaning your room.

Next, we added other contexts – some from the past, some for the future. The sheet in Fig. 21.2 shows the result. Helen needed to explain the notion of ideas in the head of the cartoon person to Tanya. The two 'thought clouds' say, 'Literacy and Numeracy at Reid CIT' and 'Horticulture and Office Skills at CIT'. CIT is a provider of adult vocational education programmes.

Step 2: Establish What Will Be Taught

Once the contexts have been identified, the numeracy requirements of those contexts must be established. This can be quite complex – some are obvious, such as telling the time or counting coins, but mathematics is a broad discipline and aspects such as interpreting graphs and estimating volumes are easily overlooked. In trials of the NDP, it was found in some cases to be easier to consider one context at a time and thoroughly detail the aspects of mathematics. It is certainly easier to spot the mathematics in a context when one is used to looking for it and it may help to seek the assistance of a mathematics teacher at this stage.

As the identification of mathematics unfolds, it is important to entertain the possibility of new contexts. A friend wished to work in a dress shop, although at

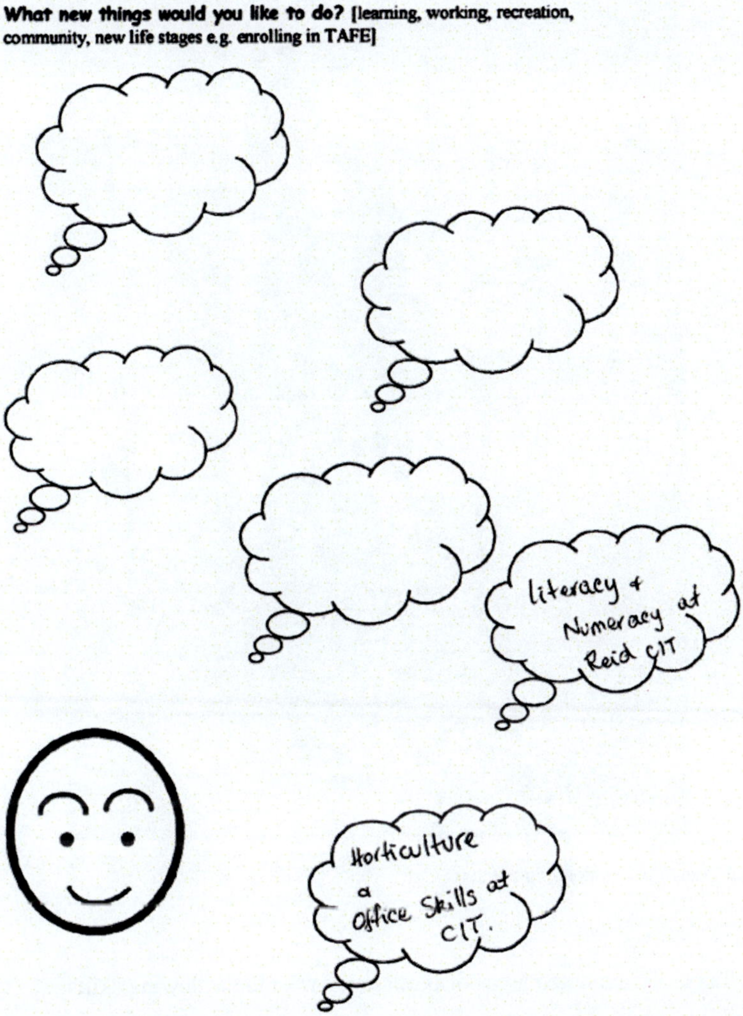

Fig. 21.2 Tanya listed other activities

the time she was employed in a rag factory. Before she could move to the new employment, she needed to develop her ability to identify and interpret clothing sizes on labels to the stage where she could order the sizes on a rack. Identification of mathematics needed for new contexts should be included in a list of skills. Tanya is also about to be a co-leader of a church fellowship group. This context will present new opportunities for her numeracy development (Fig. 21.3).

Once a list of mathematics has been established (for one or all contexts) determine which of these demands need to be explicitly taught. No doubt there will be some skills the person is already using proficiently.

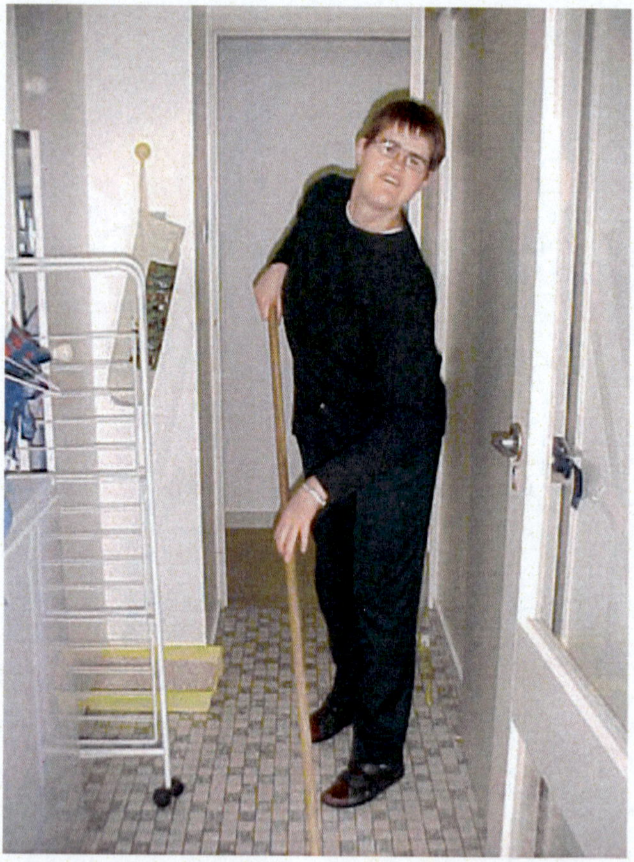

Fig. 21.3 Tanya in her cleaning context

For Tanya, Helen noted areas of proficiency with the following skills:

- Each week, Tanya is given money in small denominations by her parents and takes this back to her group home. There the carer helps her write what the money is for on envelopes (for example, $3 for the church collection, $5 for swimming pool entry) and then checks the correct money has been placed in each envelope. Figure 21.4 shows Tanya organizing her money.
- Tanya is able to read digital and analogue time. Her mother noted that she had learnt this early in life and with surprising ease.
- The arrival of a new carer meant development of Tanya's skills in measurement. Previously, her weight had been measured for her. Recently, with encouragement from her carer, she has learned to read her own weight. This involves pressing a button to 'zero' the scales prior to stepping on them and then reading the digital display of a two-digit number. Her weight is recorded by the carer.

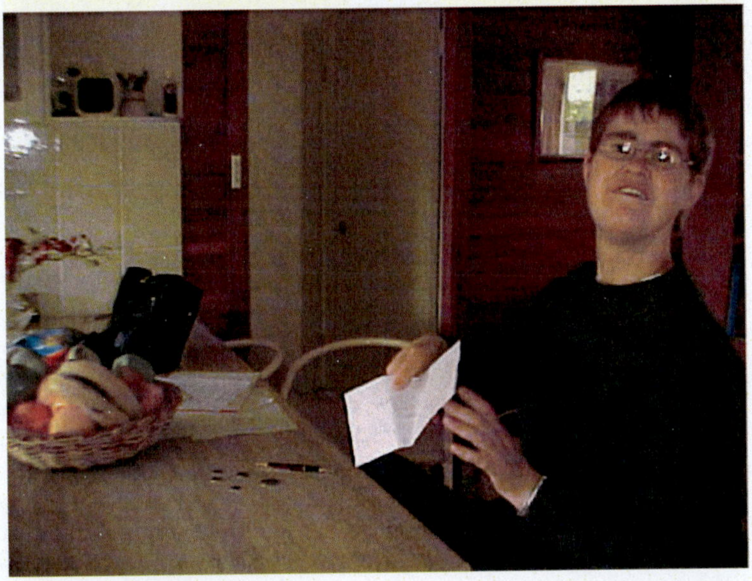

Fig. 21.4 Tanya organizing her money

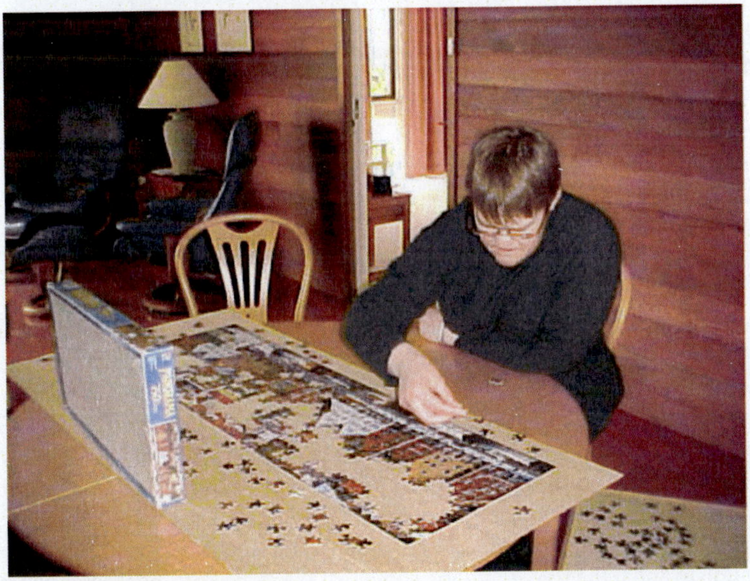

Fig. 21.5 Tanya working on her jigsaw

- Observation of Tanya placing jigsaw pieces demonstrated an awareness of pattern shape and colour matching (see Fig. 21.5).

While Tanya is able to count coins, her mother indicated that she is yet to develop conceptual understanding of the value of money.

At the end of Step 2, this is Tanya's list:

- Further development of the conceptual understanding of money
- Recording her weight once measured. This could be extended to graphing the weight to learn about the visual representation of data.
- The new position of group coordinator will make use of Tanya's ability to read the time. Planning programmes will involve generating and reading tables.

Step 3: Prioritize the List

No matter how much mathematics we already know, there will always be more to learn! The list of skills to be learned may be long. Success requires choice. The list needs to be prioritized and pruned. Ask the person to prioritize the list, allowing choice – as a core idea of quality of life, the principle of choice is important in allowing the person involved to have direct control over what they wish to learn. The right to make decisions and choices is a feature of adult learning.

For Tanya, conceptual understanding of money is a long-term goal and under the regular support of her carers and parents. More imperative at this stage of Tanya's life is the development of the numeracy needs of her new position as a fellowship coordinator.

Step 4: Establish Who Will Do the Teaching and Where It Will Occur

The list has been prepared, the order determined and now, decisions about how the learning will occur are needed. First, who will be responsible for teaching? Not all parents or relatives are available or able to teach new skills. In addition, inexperienced, untrained paid carers may not be confident teachers. To help make the decision, decide where the learning will occur. Learning in the context where the skills are needed is likely to be most effective. However, some contexts are too public to allow teaching. For example, learning how to tender amounts for purchases could be embarrassing if undertaken in a shopping centre, at least in the initial stages. Private teaching in a home setting before moving to the actual context may be needed.

Having established where the teaching will occur, the person to be responsible for the teaching is likely to be the adult present in the context with the learner. This may be a paid carer. The teaching role of carers needs to be identified. For many carers, however, teaching is not clearly identified in role descriptions, resulting in teaching occurring only in situations where individual carers have a particular interest or disposition to adopt the role. It will be noted that the arrival of a new carer in Tanya's house led to development of numeracy.

Step 5: Establish How the Teaching Will Occur

It is natural for people who may doubt their own mathematical ability to feel anxious about being asked to teach mathematics to others. However, anxiety can be reduced if it is remembered that the learning is needed for a context. If the adult assisting in the context is able to do the mathematics required, for example, measure the required quantity of liquid for a recipe, they will be able to demonstrate the skill to the person needing to learn. Modelling is a most effective method for teaching mathematics in contexts.

Modelling needs to be followed by opportunities for practice and consolidation. Skills learned but not consolidated will be forgotten. Opportunities to make use of skills learned are vital. Communication if carers change is essential to avoid underestimating the accomplishments of an individual. For example, if a person has learned to set their alarm for work in the morning, the skill may be lost if a new carer automatically takes over the task.

Tanya's family were initially a little uncertain about the process of numeracy development, with hesitation noting that Tanya had left school some time ago and had little formal teaching of mathematics since then. This is a legitimate concern that has been voiced by many parents. However, the purpose of the NDP is to learn in the contexts where the skills are needed, often using modelling and practice, rather than written procedures and exercises more common in school.

Step 6: Review the Plan

Numeracy development is life-long. To make plans that are effective, a regular process of review is needed.

There are six main steps in the Numeracy Development Planning Process and these are summarized in Fig. 21.6 below.

Summary of the Numeracy Development Planning Process

Step 1 – Undertake a context audit
Identify the contexts of a person's life.
Identify new contexts the person would like to explore.

Step 2 – Establish what will be taught
List all the mathematics involved in each context.
Distinguish between mathematics the person can perform competently and aspects that need development.

Step 3 – Prioritize the list
In consultation with the person, determine which aspects will be taught first.

Step 4 – Establish who will do the teaching and where it will occur
Teach in contexts where the mathematics is needed, if appropriate.
The adult present in the context with the person is likely to be in the best position to do the teaching.

Step 5 – Establish how the teaching will occur
Modeling with opportunities for practice and consolidation.

Step 6 – Review the plan
Determine appropriate review times.

Fig. 21.6 Summary of the planning process

The Value of a Plan

A mother of a young person with an intellectual disability once challenged me about the value of a Numeracy Development Plan. She argued that adults with ID have plans and everyone else has a life! This view is worth consideration and serves as a useful brake on enthusiasm long enough to critically reflect on the value of a plan. In the case study, Tanya was able to count out her money to allocate it to her spending needs. However, it was not until a change of carer, who supported her to do so that she was able to demonstrate and develop her ability. In the past, the task of allocating money had been undertaken by the carer alone. On-going numeracy development is important and should not depend on the chance allocation of carers.

For adults with limited access to, or success with, school mathematics, those supporting them can feel that numeracy development is no longer possible. The value of a numeracy development plan is in its individual approach and reliance on contexts. Learning is therefore tailored to the individual's needs and taught where the skills are required.

Conclusion

Numeracy, the use of mathematics in the contexts of a person's life, is important for all. Numeracy matters! It has direct impact on a person's quality of life. For people with intellectual impairments, numeracy development may not happen vicariously. For many, it can be the 'luck of the draw', depending on prior access to mathematics education and the allocation of a carer who is willing and able to teach aspects of numeracy and also recognizes the need to do so. Numeracy development is too important to be left to chance. A Numeracy Development Plan is one way to focus attention on this important area, and thereby enhance a person's quality of life.

Acknowledgments I wish to acknowledge with gratitude the assistance given by my friends, Tanya and Helen Boulton in the preparation of this chapter. I am also grateful for Prof. Roy Brown's assistance with the conceptual development of this work.

References

AAMT. (1997). *Numeracy = everyone's business. The report of the numeracy education strategy development conference*. Canberra: Commonwealth of Australia.

Adams, L., Beadle-Brown, J., & Mansell, J. (2006). Individual planning: An exploration of the link between quality of plan and quality of life. *British Journal of Learning Disabilities, 34*, 68–76.

Faragher, R. M. (2006). *Numeracy in the context of adulthood and Down syndrome*. Unpublished Doctoral Thesis, Flinders University of South Australia, Adelaide.

Faragher, R. M., & Brown, R. I. (2005). Numeracy for adults with Down syndrome: It's a matter of quality of life. *Journal of Intellectual Disability Research, 49*(10), 761–765.

MCEETYA. (1999). *The Adelaide declaration on national goals for schooling in the twenty-first century*. 10th Ministerial Council on Education, Employment, Training and Youth Affairs (MCEETYA), Adelaide, Australia.

Riall, R., & Burghes, D. (2000). Mathematical needs of young employees. *Teaching Mathematics and its Applications*, *19*(3), 104–113.

Robertson, J., Emerson, E., Hatton, C., Elliott, J., McIntosh, B., Swift, P., et al. (2007). Person-centred planning: Factors associated with successful outcomes for people with intellectual disabilities. *Journal of Intellectual Disability Research*, *51*(3), 232–243.

Schalock, R., Brown, I., Brown, R. I., Cummins, R. A., Felce, D., Matikka, L., et al. (2002). Conceptualization, measurement, and application of quality of life for persons with intellectual disabilities: Report of an international panel of experts. *Mental Retardation*, *40*(6), 457–470.

Willis, S. (1990). *Being numerate: What counts?* Hawthorn, VIC: Australian Council for Educational Research (ACER).

Chapter 22
Increasing Quality of Life Through Social Capital: Life Without the Workshop

Cathy Ficker Terrill and James Gardner

Introduction

The success of large-scale organizational change is facilitated by action grounded in theory and sound measurement of key variables. The Ray Graham Association for People with Disabilities (RGA) closed its workshops and offered people with intellectual disabilities a variety of alternative opportunities within community settings. The RGA developed a new Community Learning Centers model. RGA based the change on the documented impact of social capital on people and measured the success of the change with the *Personal Outcome Measures*. The purpose of this chapter is to (1) discuss the contribution of social capital theory and research to organizational change; (2) describe the effectiveness of the closure of the sheltered workshop in personal outcomes and quality of life measures.

Social Capital: Concept and Research

For the purposes of this chapter, social capital is defined as, "the networks and norms of trust and reciprocity that govern people's interactions with each other" (Putnam, 2000). Researchers concur that social capital influences our quality of life (Adler & Kwon, 2002; Lesser, 2000; Lin, 2001; Putnam & Feldstein, 2003; Putnam, 2000; Rothberg, 2001; Stone & Hughes, 2002; Stone, 2001). Social capital impacts the viability of civic institutions, community life, and the economic and social measures of wellness in neighborhoods. The quality of life and social equity for individuals with disabilities is an issue of profound interest to groups and organizations around the world.

Schneider (2006) used social capital to explore welfare reform. Finke (2003), Iannaccone (2003) Malloch (2003), and Woodberry (2003) have approached spiritual capital as a subset of social capital. The Saguaro Seminar (2000a, 2000b, 2002)

C.F. Terrill (✉)
President and CEO, Ray Graham Association for People with Disabilities, Downers Grove, Illinois, USA
e-mail: cathyfickerterrill@yahoo.com

R. Kober (ed.), *Enhancing the Quality of Life of People with Intellectual Disabilities*, Social Indicators Research Series 41, DOI 10.1007/978-90-481-9650-0_22,

at Harvard University has explored the definitions and theory of social capital and disseminated Social Capital Community Benchmark Survey instruments. The World Bank measures social capital and the potential impact of social capital as a condition for capital investment (Krishna & Shrader, 1999; World Bank, 1998).

Social Capital theory, measurement, and interpretation vary across research settings and academic orientation (Edwards & Foley, 2001). They noted (p. 5) "striking differences across disciplines both in how the term is understood and how it is employed." In addition, researchers do not agree on the current or historical status of social capital within communities. Social capital, like any community or economic indicator, has fluctuated across time. Putnam (2000) describes decreasing trends over the last 40 years in the number of people who participate in social and philanthropic clubs and activities, organized religion, and other aspects of community life. He concludes that social capital in the United States has dropped precipitously. McPherson, Smith-Lovin, and Brashears (2006, p. 372) have recently provided additional information that supports Putnam's argument that Americans have decreased their social ties. They argue that "The types of bridging ties that connect us to community and neighborhood have withered . . .."

In contrast, Wellman (1999) has noted the transformation in our definitions of community and social networks. The widespread use of the Internet has accelerated the shift from local geographical communities to broader and more diverse social networks. People now seek out a variety of people, resources, and supports in emerging networks. These networks can be electronic and worldwide. The networks can also consist of people who cross neighborhood and community boundaries to share common interests. The Pew Internet and American Life Project (Boase, Horrigan, Wellman, & Rainie, 2006) concluded that communities are not disappearing; rather they are transforming:

> The traditional human orientation to neighborhood – and village-based groups is moving toward communities that are oriented around geographically dispersed social networks. People communicate and maneuver in these networks rather than being bound up in one solidary community. (2006, p. i)

Social Capital: Model for Change

The RGA used social capital theory as a model for change. We recognized the many complexities in social capital definition, measurement methodology, and interpretation, but we isolated the basic principles of social capital. We began with Putnam's definition of social capital as the networks and the norms of trust and reciprocity that govern people's interactions with each other. We also view social capital as a resource for individuals, groups, and indeed the community:

> the basic idea of social capital is that a person's family, friends, and associates constitute an important asset, one that can be called on in a crisis, enjoyed for its own sake, and/or leveraged for material gain . . . What is true for individuals, moreover, also holds for groups. (Woodcock & Narayan, 2000, p. 236)

Putnam states, "the idea at the core of the theory of social capital is extremely simple: Social networks matter. Networks have value." (2002, p. 6). In an analysis of the work of significant contributors to social capital theory and research (Bourdieu, 1986; Coleman, 1988, 1990; Putnam, 2000), Winter (2000) finds common agreement that social capital is a network resource for collective action.

The RGA adopted a change strategy that rested on the premise that our lives are enhanced by social ties with other people – our families, friends, neighbors, community groups, and co-workers. Increases in these social contacts have been associated with improved mental and physical health, lower rates of social problems and greater access to economic security. People who belong to organized social groups live longer than those who do not belong to such groups. Children with increased social capital do better in school (Putnam, 2000).

These social ties also produce reciprocity – we ask for favors or for help, knowing that we will return the favor in the future. Social ties and reciprocity build trust. We believe that we can make commitments to each other that will be honored and not require extensive bargaining or negotiating.

Increasing social capital benefits us all. With greater social capital we will live healthier and happier lives, increase out community affiliations, and be able to exercise choice and self-determination. Social capital offers a common meeting point for people receiving services and supports, families, employers, employees, and community organizations, both public and private.

Social capital redefines the organization's role and purpose. Organizations and systems focus their services and supports on increasing people's social capital. Organizations and systems support people's social capital within the context of the community to facilitate their alliances with others and create access to generic resources.

Developing trusting relationships and social ties is also important for families. Assisting families to develop social capital within communities increases their connections to other more generic resources.

Social capital provides an additional opportunity for leadership. Organizations, by building social capital for all employees, increase the richness of their ties to each other, their families, and the community. Organizations evaluate their effectiveness by the impact they have on the social capital of their employees, as well as that of the people they support.

The common unifying task for the organization is to build social capital for the community of interests it serves – people with intellectual disabilities, families, volunteers, and employees. The purpose of the organization goes beyond the provision of services and supports. The role of the organization is to connect people within their communities, to serve as a bridge to community for people with intellectual disabilities, their families, volunteers, and employees.

Personal Outcome Introduction and Summary

CQL (The Council on Quality and Leadership) introduced a person-centered outcome assessment instrument – the *Outcome Based Performance Measures* in 1993. CQL developed the measures from focus groups with people with intellectual disabilities in the United States and Canada. The *Outcome Based Performance*

Measures were revised in 1997 and renamed the *Personal Outcome Measures*. CQL has maintained a national Personal Outcome Measure database since 1993 that now includes interviews with over 6,000 people who have participated in CQL accreditation reviews since 1993. CQL has reported on the reliability and validity of the instrument, its application across a wide range of services and supports and to people with very diverse disabilities, and the results of its analysis of 3,630 interviews conducted during the period 1993–2002 (Gardner & Carran, 2005; Gardner, Carran, & Nudler, 2001; Gardner, Nudler, & Chapman, 1997).

CQL has maintained an international data base on over 6,500 Personal Outcome Interviews conducted under uniform protocols with CQL-certified reviewers. During the past 15 years CQL has revised the Personal Outcome Measures based on factor analysis research of our data base. The most recent factor analysis resulted in the following Personal Outcome Measures:

My Self
People are connected to natural support networks
People have intimate relationships
People are safe
People have the best possible health
People exercise rights
People are treated fairly
People are free from abuse and neglect
People experience continuity and security
People decide when to share personal information

My World
People choose where and with whom they live
People choose where they work
People use their environments
People live in integrated environments
People interact with other members of the community
People perform different social roles
People choose services

My Dreams
People choose personal goals
People realize personal goals
People participate in the life of the community
People have friends
People are respected

CQL has also discussed the difficulty and complexity of obtaining reliable and valid information from some people with significant disabilities, and the people who support them, of communicating with people who use nontraditional communication methods, and making decisions about "choice" by people who have had very limited opportunity to experience different options in their lives (Gardner & Carran, 2005; Gardner et al., 1997; 2001; CQL, 2000, 2005).

The application of the *Personal Outcome Measures* results in the identification of specific supports and resources that have facilitated, or would facilitate, the outcome as defined by the individual. Instead of managing uniform program activities, organizations must now individualize supports to facilitate the outcomes as defined by the individual. Moreover, the individualized supports cannot be identified until after the person had defined the individualized meaning of the outcome.

This individualization of process reverses the traditional quality management methodology. If all people receiving services and supports defined all outcomes in the same manner, and if all of those same people learned and interacted with other people in the same way, then process might be standardized as in the production of toasters or computers. However, because different people define their outcomes in a unique manner, the processes that facilitate the outcomes will vary. This link between personally defined outcomes and individualized supports leads to two conclusions about the limitations of the workshop environment. (a) Organizations cannot provide supports without first identifying the outcome for which the supports are designed. (b) Continued measurement of the organizational process alone after identifying the outcome creates the possibility of measuring process that is no longer relevant because the person has redefined the outcome.

The nature of the contractual work and repetitive process of the workshop make it nearly impossible to continuously realign supports around personal outcomes. The individualization of supports and organizational process is negated by the routine and repetition required by workshop economics, staffing, and program goals.

Planning and Elimination of the Sheltered Workshop for People with Intellectual Disabilities

Adults with intellectual disabilities have historically been isolated and institutionalized in the United States since the early 1600s. But, since 1980, changes in social norms and public policy within the United States have enabled more adults with intellectual disabilities to become contributing members of society.

Sheltered workshops have been a part of the institutionalization of people with intellectual disabilities. For more than 50 years, sheltered workshops were the primary employment option for adults with intellectual disabilities. Work centers were created that separated and isolated these individuals from typical work force places of employment.

Due to changes in social norms and public policy, self advocates and their supporters are seeking alternatives to large, sheltered workshops. This has enabled many of these same individuals to now work along side their non-disabled peers. However, adults with intellectual disabilities have little experience building social capital, which enhances the quality of one's life.

One of the greatest challenges faced by reformers and disability advocates is the development of alternatives to sheltered workshops. RGA's Community Learning Center is one model which has proven effective as an alternative to large, segregated sheltered workshops. RGA designed this alternative approach after soliciting individual's expectations for social capital and community affiliation and the design of supports around their expectations.

Our hypothesis was that an individual's score on the Personal Outcome Measures, in the areas of social capital and community affiliation would increase as the individual moved from a large sheltered workshop to a small decentralized environment, where the focus was placed on developing social capital within the community.

Social capital enables people to coordinate action to achieve desired goals (World Bank, 1998). People need certain things to be present in order to develop social capital. All people need space and time to connect; time to demonstrate trust; a means to effectively communicate; and an opportunity for genuine participation, not mere presence (Putnam, 2000). In a sheltered workshop there is not much private space, little community participation or affiliation, and limited opportunity to connect to non-disabled peers.

Leaders within the organization decided to pursue a new vision for employment for people with intellectual disabilities. Many of the stakeholders receiving support services from the organization had expressed a desire to work, wanted an opportunity to connect in their communities, and wanted days that were filled with meaningful opportunities. Multiple focus groups were conducted with all levels of stakeholder and employee participation. Input from the focus groups resulted in creating new options that facilitated the return of people with intellectual disabilities to their communities doing paid work, volunteer work, and networking. The program focus totally changed from the outcome of piece work to a focus on community connecting and building social capital. All stakeholders were encouraged to join one of the many implementation teams and be part of the organizational change. Some staff who were wedded to the workshop model left and found employment elsewhere, but most staff recognized the need for change and joined a team to help with implementation. This major organizational change was budget neutral. Property costs remained about the same, transportation costs significantly decreased, some staff costs increased, while other staff positions, not needed in the new model were eliminated for a cost savings.

RGA is a non-profit organization with a unionized direct care staff. The union did not serve as a barrier with the implementation of this organizational change. The union presence did require new forms of communication and exchange with its leadership. Management had to remind union stewards that this change was based upon best practice, the input of the primary stakeholders, and was driven by the need to support people to have meaningful outcomes in their lives. Although the union reviewed the new job description, they worked with us as partners in the process.

This pilot examined ways to expand social capital and enhance the quality of life for adults with intellectual disabilities. The RGA exploration was centered on two questions:

- How can we use social capital to channel diversity and creativity?
- How can we offer people the opportunity and advantages that accrue to people through their membership in groups?

RGA management and staff answered these questions through a reframing process. Instead of the CEO being the "RGA member" of the local Chamber of Commerce, individuals with disabilities who were starting micro-industries represented the association at Chamber meetings. Volunteers were brought in, not to help people with intellectual disabilities, but rather to assist men and women with disabilities to launch micro-businesses. Medicaid funding continued at the new locations with the focus on community participation. Local businesses carved out employment opportunities. Church groups, elder service organizations, animal shelters, and park districts embraced us and welcomed us.

The RGA also significantly changed staff positions. Management eliminated a Production Coordinator and General Manager of the Workshop, and in turn created a Community Learning Center Administrator, Work Services Team Leader, Community Liaison, and Marketing Specialist. The new positions all included an external community focus as well as an overall expectation for staff to support individuals to create their own meaningful day. The new program was not designed around existing employees and current positions, but rather the program designed positions to meet expectations of the new model.

Results as Measured by Personal Outcome Scores

The RGA designed the Community Learning Center model. Community Learning Centers provide adults with intellectual disabilities choices in how they spend their day. Each adult participates in those activities which are of interest to them as an individual and which meet their personal goals. The six Community Learning Centers serve 225 adults with intellectual disabilities. The adults range in age from 21 to 85. Each of the six Community Learning Centers provides a unique set of services and activities. No two Centers are exactly alike. Each is designed to have a goodness-of-fit with the community in which it operates and they are dynamic, changing as new opportunities arise. To date, the Community Learning Centers have focused on four areas: (a) developing micro enterprises and small businesses, (b) volunteerism, (c) community participation, and (d) employment opportunities.

The Association measures the quality of its programs through Personal Outcome Measures developed by The Council on Quality and Leadership. Personal Outcome Measures are defined as "what people expect from the services and supports they receive." On a quarterly basis, the RGA interviews a sample of individuals served using the Council's 25 Personal Outcome Measures.

By comparing aggregate Personal Outcome Measures from 2003, the last year of our large workshop, with outcome measures from 2006, when the Community Learning Centers had been operating for two and a half years, the scores in measures related to adult day services improved. This indicates that individuals have experienced an improved quality of life reflected in higher aggregate scores in outcomes related to adult day services.

Table 22.1 shows a sampling of the 21 Personal Outcome Measures to measure quality indicators in the form of outcomes. The six outcome areas listed in

Table 22.1 Outcomes present in people's lives

Outcome measure	Aggregated scores 2003 (%)	2006 (%)	Percent change Increase/decrease (%)
• People choose service	47	87	+40
• People realize personal goals	63	100	+37
• People are connected to natural supports	52	81	+29
• People perform different social roles	21	50	+29
• People have friends	58	81	+23
• People use their environments	78	100	+22

Table 22.1 show a remarkable increase in outcomes present in the lives of individuals with intellectual disabilities from 2003 until 3 years later in 2006. In particular with the emphasis on building social capital, the individuals in the sample indicated a 29% increase in performing different social roles; 29% increase in being connected to natural supports in their communities; and a 23% increase in having friends.

The only thing that changed in the lives of the individuals in the study was the closing of the sheltered workshop and the opening of a new model of supports for people called Community Learning Centers. These centers were smaller facilities located as store fronts in local communities. The emphasis moved from entirely training on piece work to training and supports in being volunteers, starting micro industries, community participation, and real employment options.

- Micro Enterprises: Individuals served in Community Learning Centers have developed eight new, small businesses, which they operate. The micro enterprises provide creative, income generating, self-employment opportunities. They include *Bow-Wow Dog Products*, *Save-The-Planet Aluminum Recycling*, *Hip-Hop Craft Shop*, and *Monarch Inc*, an on-line book resale business.
- Volunteerism: Individuals served have established 17 volunteer relationships with organizations in their communities such as *The Community House*, *Graue Mill*, *Public Library*, *Sunrise Senior Center*, *Fullersburg Woods Nature Education Center*, to name a few. This demonstrates that people with intellectual disabilities are contributing members of their community who share their talents and skills with others. The DuPage County Senior Services division recognized volunteers supported by RGA at a county wide event for community volunteerism.
- Community Participation: To avoid isolation and segregation, which is often the case in sheltered workshops; individuals in the Community Learning Centers regularly participate in community events and activities. Community activities are diverse and include; cultural activities, adult education, sports, and fairs and festivals. Data is maintained on the number of events in which each individual participates.
- Employment: Community Employment Services are available through the Community Learning Centers. In 2005, 102 individuals found and maintained employment. Full-time, part-time, and seasonal employment offers many choices

to meet the interests and talents of each individual. The hourly wage for individuals, $8.11 an hour, is significantly above the minimum wage in Illinois.

New friendships have developed between individuals in the Community Learning Centers and other community citizens. For instance, the senior citizens, who receive Meals on Wheels delivered by individuals with disabilities, genuinely look forward to greeting the individual delivering their meal. They know the person by name and engage them in conversation about their life, interests, family, and current events. Friendships such as these were not made possible when individuals attended the sheltered workshop because they were isolated from the community at large.

As Table 22.2 illustrates, the Community Learning Centers demonstrate innovative organizational change, moving from a large, centralized system, which had been in place for 42 years, to a smaller, decentralized system. This innovation has significantly improved the quality of life of individuals with disabilities served by RGA.

The implementation of the community learning center model has resulted in numerous stories for participating individuals. Michelle had been looking for a job for 2 years. She had several opportunities along the way, but right before Thanksgiving 2005, she finally connected with the right job match at Kmart. She was originally hired to greet and check out customers as they leave the store. However, parts of this position presented some challenges for Michelle. Her supervisor then decided that her skills would be better utilized on the loading dock and throughout the store greeting customers. She has since blossomed into a great Kmart associate. She currently works 3–4 days a week. In addition to finding the right job match, Michelle has increased her social skills, resulting in being more outgoing, friendly, and confident about herself.

Janet has been supported by Ray Graham since 1973. She loves to work and is usually very quiet and shy. Since being hired as the Lead Inventory Specialist at the Snack Bar at Main Street, Janet has opened up tremendously. She is much more talkative and outgoing with co workers and staff. She has participated in going into the community, in particular to Sam's Club to get more supplies. Janet is a very conscientious and reliable worker, and she has many new friends.

In September 2005 Hurricane Katrina devastated the Gulf region of the United States. When talking about the hurricane in the current events group, everyone wanted to do something to help. With staff support, everyone put donations together, which were shipped through a connection with the Chicago Bulls and White Sox training camp. We called September our Katrina Kare month. These success stories coupled with the outcome data, convinced staff that the Association was making progress in supporting people to build social capital in their lives and to connect within their communities.

RGA has initiated a monthly quality campaign to connect the *Personal Outcome Measures* implementation to social capital attainment. Every month a team selects one outcome as the focus. A cross-organizational team plans the quality campaign. Everyone in the organization is involved. There are quality games, contest, activities, prizes, and a grand finale with a program, skit, or major contest. The focus of the activities is all related to that one outcome, but the focus of the learning is fun.

Table 22.2 Comparison on two different models of support

Sheltered workshop	Community learning center
Location	
• One city	• Six villages and cities throughout the county
Size	
• One 40,000 sq ft building	• Six buildings, averaging 4,500 sq ft each
Facility cost	
• Building leader and operating costs $403,000 per year	• Leases for six buildings and operating costs $405,000 per year
Individuals served	
• 165	• Average 35 per location
Paid work	
• One major, manufacturing "assembly" contract for $400,000 with an external company. When contract was not renewed individuals experienced excessive downtime with no pay	• Entrepreneurial model with eight small businesses and micro enterprises operated by individuals served. Products sold on web. • In 2005, 102 individuals found paid employment in the community. • In 2006, 110 individuals found paid employment in the community.
Volunteer opportunities	
• None	• Individuals volunteer weekly at 17 community locations
Community connections	
• None	• Individuals participate in an average of 190 activities in their communities per quarter.
Transportation	
• 5 large 36-passenger buses • $75,000 cost per bus • Separate bus drivers requiring CDL license • Buses traveled throughout county • 90 min, average door-to-door ride time for individuals • Large buses problematic for community access due to size	• 21 smaller 6 to 15-passenger vans • Average costs per van $35,000 • Staff who work in program serve as van drivers, no CDL needed • Vans travel in cities/villages served by each location • 40 min, average door-to-door ride time for individuals • Smaller vans allow for more community access
Staffing	
• One staff per 20 individuals served (1:20 ratio)	• One staff per seven individuals served (1:7 ratio) • New job title and job description: "life skills instructor" requiring experience to supervise programs

Guidelines and Recommendations for Other Organizations

The RGA used the theory and practice of social capital to guide this major organizational change. The Association transformed itself from an organization that provided traditional social services to adults with intellectual disabilities, to an organization that is focused on the mission of, "full participation of all people with intellectual disabilities in a quality of life by providing leadership that supports the accomplishment of individuals, strengthens families and inspires community involvement." We do this by staying focused on the mission of supporting individuals to build a better life through the development of social capital.

The Association mobilized organizational energy to close the sheltered workshop.

The Association identified champions to help with organizational change. The Personal Outcome Measures provided the fundamental map for the future. Throughout the process it was critical to be honest with everyone, clearly communicate the basic road map, and allow people to discuss real issues. A comprehensive action plan was developed with multiple stakeholder input. It was circulated widely, both internally and externally. The action plan was defined using outcomes. There were timetables and there was a quarterly review of progress, barriers, and the need to revise or expand implementation strategies.

The organization was transparent in planning and implementing activities related to the organizational redesign to alleviate fears and stress, while focusing on security. The RGA leadership focused on consistent and constant communication throughout the process, to assure that everyone had the information they believe they needed. The new organizational design was developed not to redirect resources around more or less new work, but rather to reframe staff engagement in an innovative work environment. RGA did not ask staff to perform more work; rather it asked staff to undertake different work.

The RGA leadership identified opportunities for networking and building social capital. Many of the staff were not connected to their community, and so a volunteer coordinator was hired who not only coordinated internal volunteers, but more importantly, identified volunteer opportunities external to the organization. People with intellectual disabilities became active needed volunteers. Staff devised means to ask individuals to define their own outcome measures for personal success. Individual preferences for being active in the community were collected in a variety of nontraditional ways. Staff will often do what is measured, and so, we regularly measured community affiliation, community participation, and the development of social roles.

Progress was monitored at the individual level, the program level, and also at the policy level. At each step staff worked with individuals to creatively find ways to assist people to successfully accomplish their outcomes. Management teams started meetings celebrating individual outcomes. Outcomes related to friendships, mutual respect, and interdependence became key indicators of success. People now have friends they can confide in and share their confidences. Individuals are now known as neighbors, co-workers, church members, Chamber of Commerce members, and volunteers, rather than simply, a person with a disability. Friends, neighbors, and family are linking people to employment, home ownership, and new modes of transportation. There are new opportunities for genuine participation, rather than a mere presence in the community. As an indicator of success, only 2 individuals with disabilities out of 455 people chose to leave the program after the organization shift from the sheltered workshop to community learning centers.

The Association measured organizational change through the impact on each person's quality of life. Once adults with intellectual disabilities were given opportunities to develop new social relationships, they discovered times and places to connect with others. People not only registered to vote, but they started attending political rallies. Some people asked staff to support them to pre-program their augmentative communication devises to ask candidates tough disability questions. In January 2006, Barrack Obama invited one of the women to join his advisory group on disability issues. People are not only attending the religious service of their choice, but some have joined the choir and been invited to become deacons of their place of worship.

Conclusion

The transition from the sheltered workshop to the Community Learning center resulted in increases in people's personal quality of life as measured by the *Personal Outcome Measures*. The transition also enabled people with intellectual disabilities to build social capital. As a result, individuals with disabilities are using social capital to make change. They are partnering with branches of government to restructure funding and control of resources. Some are networking with elder advocates, local mayors, and business leaders in their community. Individuals are strengthening ties that bind them into new communities, communities of influence. As they build trust and understanding, they are also building friends, networks, and power for the future.

References

Adler, P. S., & Kwon, S. W. (2002). Social capital: Prospects for a new concept. *Academy of Management Review, 27*, 17–40.

Boase, J., Horrigan, J. B., Wellman, B., & Rainie, L. (2006). *The strength of Internet ties*. Washington, DC: PEW Internet and American Life Project.

Bourdieu, P. (1985). The forms of capital. In J. G. Richardson (Ed.), *Handbook of theory and research for the sociology of education* (pp. 241–258). New York: Greenwood Press.

Coleman, J. (1988). Social capital and the creation of human capital. *American Journal of Sociology, 94*, 95–120.

Coleman, J. (1990). *Foundations of social theory*. Cambridge, MA: Harvard University Press.

Council on Quality and Leadership. (2000). *Personal outcomes measures: 2000 edition*. Towson, MD: Author.

Council on Quality and Leadership. (2005). *Quality measures 2005*. Towson, MD: Author.

Edwards, B., & Foley, M. W. (2001). Civil society and social capital: A primer. In B. Edwards, M. W. Foley, & M. Diani (Eds.), *Beyond Tocqueville: Civil society and social capital debate in comparative perspective* (pp. 1–14). Hanover, NH: University Press of New England.

Finke, R. (2003). *Spiritual capital: Definitions, applications, and new frontiers*. Paper delivered at the Spiritual Capital Planning Meeting, October 10–11, 2003, Cambridge, MA.

Gardner, J. F., & Carran, D. (2005). Attainment of Personal Outcome Measures by people with development disabilities. *Mental Retardation, 43*, 157–174.

Gardner, J. F., Carran, D. T., & Nudler, S. (2001). Measuring quality of life and quality of services through personal outcome measures: Implications for public policy. *International Review of Research in Mental Retardation, 24*, 75–100.

Gardner, J. F., Nudler, S., & Chapman, M. (1997). Personal outcome measures of quality. *Mental Retardation, 35*, 295–305.

Iannaccone, L. R. (2003). *Spiritual capital: An introduction and literature review*. Paper delivered at the Spiritual Capital Planning Meeting, October, 10–11, 2003, Cambridge, MA.

Krishna, A., & Shrader, E. (1999). *Social capital assessment tool.* Paper Prepared for the Conference on Social Capital and Poverty Reduction. The World Bank, June 1999, Washington, DC.

Lesser, E. L. (Ed.). (2000). *Knowledge and social capital.* Woburn, MA: Butterworth-Heinemann.

Lin, N. (2001). *Social capital: A theory of social structure and action.* New York: Cambridge University Press.

Malloch, T. R. (2003). *Social, human and spiritual capital in economic development.* Paper delivered at the Spiritual Capital Planning Meeting, October 10–11, 2003, Cambridge, MA.

McPherson, M., Smith-Lovin, L., & Brashears, M. (2006). Social isolation in America: Changes in core discussion networks over two decades. *American Sociological Review, 71*, 353–375.

Putnam, R. D. (2000). *Bowling alone: Collapse and revival of American community.* New York: Simon & Schuster.

Putnam, R. D. (Ed.). (2002). *Democracies in flux: The evolution of social capital in contemporary society.* New York: Oxford University Press.

Putnam, R. D., & Feldstein, L. M. (2003). *Better together: Restoring the American community.* New York: Simon & Schuster.

Rothberg, R. I. (Ed.). (2001). *Patterns of social capital: Stability and change in historical perspective.* New York: Cambridge University Press.

Saguaro Seminar. (2000a). *Better together: The report of the Saguaro Seminar: Civic engagement in America.* Cambridge, MA: Author.

Saguaro Seminar. (2000b). *Social capital community benchmark survey*, final version, August 4, 2000. Cambridge, MA: Author.

Schneider, J. A. (2006). *Social capital and welfare reform: Organizations, congregations, and communities.* New York: Columbia University Press.

Seminar, S. (2002). *Social capital community benchmark survey,* short form, September 2002 draft, release 1.1. Cambridge, MA: Author.

Stone, W. (2001). *Measuring social capital: Toward a theoretically informed measurement framework for researching social capital in family and community life (Research paper #24).* Melbourne: Australian Institute of Family Studies.

Stone, W., & Hughes, J. (2002). *Measuring social capital: Toward a standardized approach.* Paper presented at the 2002 Australasian Evaluation Society International Conference. Melbourne: Australia, Australian Institute for Family Studies.

Wellman, B. (Ed.). (1999). *Networks in the global village: Life in contemporary communities.* Boulder, CO: Westview Press.

Winter, I. (2000). Major themes and debates in the social capital literature: The Australian connection. In I. Winter (Ed.), *Social capital and public policy in Australia* (pp. 57–81). Melbourne: Australian Institute for Family Studies.

Woodcock, M., & Narayan, D. (2000). Social capital: Implications for development theory, research, and policy. *The World Bank Observer, 15*, 225–249.

Woodberry, R. D. (2003). *Researching spiritual capital: Promises and pitfalls.* Paper delivered at the Spiritual Capital Planning Meeting, October 10–11, 2003, Cambridge, MA.

World Bank. (1998). *The initiative of defining, monitoring, and measuring social capital: Overview and program description* (Social Capital Initiative Working Paper No. 1). Washington, DC: World Bank.

Gardner, J. F., Nudler, S., & Chapman, M. (1997). Personal outcome measures of quality. *Mental Retardation, 35*, 295–305.

Iannaccone, L. R. (2003). *Spiritual capital: An introduction and literature review*. Paper delivered at the Spiritual Capital Planning Meeting, October, 10–11, 2003, Cambridge, MA.

Krishna, A., & Shrader, E. (1999). *Social capital assessment tool*. Paper Prepared for the Conference on Social Capital and Poverty Reduction. The World Bank, June 1999, Washington, DC.

Lesser, E. L. (Ed.). (2000). *Knowledge and social capital*. Woburn, MA: Butterworth-Heinemann.

Lin, N. (2001). *Social capital: A theory of social structure and action*. New York: Cambridge University Press.

Malloch, T. R. (2003). *Social, human and spiritual capital in economic development*. Paper delivered at the Spiritual Capital Planning Meeting, October 10–11, 2003, Cambridge, MA.

McPherson, M., Smith-Lovin, L., & Brashears, M. (2006). Social isolation in America: Changes in core discussion networks over two decades. *American Sociological Review, 71*, 353–375.

Putnam, R. D. (2000). *Bowling alone: Collapse and revival of American community*. New York: Simon & Schuster.

Putnam, R. D. (Ed.). (2002). *Democracies in flux: The evolution of social capital in contemporary society*. New York: Oxford University Press.

Putnam, R. D., & Feldstein, L. M. (2003). *Better together: Restoring the American community*. New York: Simon & Schuster.

Rothberg, R. I. (Ed.). (2001). *Patterns of social capital: Stability and change in historical perspective*. New York: Cambridge University Press.

Saguaro Seminar. (2000a). *Better together: The report of the Saguaro Seminar: Civic engagement in America*. Cambridge, MA: Author.

Saguaro Seminar. (2000b). *Social capital community benchmark survey*, final version, August 4, 2000. Cambridge, MA: Author.

Schneider, J. A. (2006). *Social capital and welfare reform: Organizations, congregations, and communities*. New York: Columbia University Press.

Seminar, S. (2002). *Social capital community benchmark survey*, short form, September 2002 draft, release 1.1. Cambridge, MA: Author.

Stone, W. (2001). *Measuring social capital: Toward a theoretically informed measurement framework for researching social capital in family and community life (Research paper #24)*. Melbourne: Australian Institute of Family Studies.

Stone, W., & Hughes, J. (2002). *Measuring social capital: Toward a standardized approach*. Paper presented at the 2002 Australasian Evaluation Society International Conference. Melbourne: Australia, Australian Institute for Family Studies.

Wellman, B. (Ed.). (1999). *Networks in the global village: Life in contemporary communities*. Boulder, CO: Westview Press.

Winter, I. (2000). Major themes and debates in the social capital literature: The Australian connection. In I. Winter (Ed.), *Social capital and public policy in Australia* (pp. 57–81). Melbourne: Australian Institute for Family Studies.

Woodcock, M., & Narayan, D. (2000). Social capital: Implications for development theory, research, and policy. *The World Bank Observer, 15*, 225–249.

Woodberry, R. D. (2003). *Researching spiritual capital: Promises and pitfalls*. Paper delivered at the Spiritual Capital Planning Meeting, October 10–11, 2003, Cambridge, MA.

World Bank. (1998). *The initiative of defining, monitoring, and measuring social capital: Overview and program description* (Social Capital Initiative Working Paper No. 1). Washington, DC: World Bank.

Gardner, J. F., Nudler, S., & Chapman, M. (1997). Personal outcome measures of quality. *Mental Retardation, 35*, 295–305.

Iannaccone, L. R. (2003). *Spiritual capital: An introduction and literature review*. Paper delivered at the Spiritual Capital Planning Meeting, October, 10–11, 2003, Cambridge, MA.

Krishna, A., & Shrader, E. (1999). *Social capital assessment tool*. Paper Prepared for the Conference on Social Capital and Poverty Reduction. The World Bank, June 1999, Washington, DC.

Lesser, E. L. (Ed.). (2000). *Knowledge and social capital*. Woburn, MA: Butterworth-Heinemann.

Lin, N. (2001). *Social capital: A theory of social structure and action*. New York: Cambridge University Press.

Malloch, T. R. (2003). *Social, human and spiritual capital in economic development*. Paper delivered at the Spiritual Capital Planning Meeting, October 10–11, 2003, Cambridge, MA.

McPherson, M., Smith-Lovin, L., & Brashears, M. (2006). Social isolation in America: Changes in core discussion networks over two decades. *American Sociological Review, 71*, 353–375.

Putnam, R. D. (2000). *Bowling alone: Collapse and revival of American community*. New York: Simon & Schuster.

Putnam, R. D. (Ed.). (2002). *Democracies in flux: The evolution of social capital in contemporary society*. New York: Oxford University Press.

Putnam, R. D., & Feldstein, L. M. (2003). *Better together: Restoring the American community*. New York: Simon & Schuster.

Rothberg, R. I. (Ed.). (2001). *Patterns of social capital: Stability and change in historical perspective*. New York: Cambridge University Press.

Saguaro Seminar. (2000a). *Better together: The report of the Saguaro Seminar: Civic engagement in America*. Cambridge, MA: Author.

Saguaro Seminar. (2000b). *Social capital community benchmark survey*, final version, August 4, 2000. Cambridge, MA: Author.

Schneider, J. A. (2006). *Social capital and welfare reform: Organizations, congregations, and communities*. New York: Columbia University Press.

Seminar, S. (2002). *Social capital community benchmark survey*, short form, September 2002 draft, release 1.1. Cambridge, MA: Author.

Stone, W. (2001). *Measuring social capital: Toward a theoretically informed measurement framework for researching social capital in family and community life (Research paper #24)*. Melbourne: Australian Institute of Family Studies.

Stone, W., & Hughes, J. (2002). *Measuring social capital: Toward a standardized approach*. Paper presented at the 2002 Australasian Evaluation Society International Conference. Melbourne: Australia, Australian Institute for Family Studies.

Wellman, B. (Ed.). (1999). *Networks in the global village: Life in contemporary communities*. Boulder, CO: Westview Press.

Winter, I. (2000). Major themes and debates in the social capital literature: The Australian connection. In I. Winter (Ed.), *Social capital and public policy in Australia* (pp. 57–81). Melbourne: Australian Institute for Family Studies.

Woodcock, M., & Narayan, D. (2000). Social capital: Implications for development theory, research, and policy. *The World Bank Observer, 15*, 225–249.

Woodberry, R. D. (2003). *Researching spiritual capital: Promises and pitfalls*. Paper delivered at the Spiritual Capital Planning Meeting, October 10–11, 2003, Cambridge, MA.

World Bank. (1998). *The initiative of defining, monitoring, and measuring social capital: Overview and program description* (Social Capital Initiative Working Paper No. 1). Washington, DC: World Bank.

Index

R. Kober (ed.), *Enhancing the Quality of Life of People with Intellectual Disabilities*, Social Indicators Research Series 41, DOI 10.1007/978-90-481-9650-0,